Drug-Induced
Hepatic Injury

Drug-Induced Disorders Vol. 1

Series Editor: M.N.G. Dukes

Drug-Induced Hepatic Injury

A comprehensive survey of the literature on adverse drug reactions up to January 1985

B.H.Ch. Stricker

Netherlands Center for Monitoring of Adverse Reactions to Drugs, Leidschendam, and Department of Gastroenterology and Hepatology, University Medical Center, Leiden, The Netherlands

P. Spoelstra

Department of Gastroenterology and Hepatology, University Medical Center, Leiden, and Department of Internal Medicine, Medical Center, Leeuwarden, The Netherlands

ELSEVIER

ISBN 0 444 90342 9

Published by:
Elsevier Science Publishers B.V.
P.O. Box 1126
1000 BC Amsterdam

Sole distributors for the USA and Canada:
Elsevier Science Publishing Co. Inc.
52 Vanderbilt Avenue
New York, NY 10017

Printed in the Netherlands by Casparie, Amsterdam

ACKNOWLEDGEMENTS

The authors wish to thank the following persons for their advice or assistance in preparing the manuscript:

M.J.A. van Berge Henegouwen; G.P. van Berge Henegouwen, M.D.; C.P.H. van Dijke, M.D.; A.R. Janssens, M.D.; R.H.B. Meyboom, M.D.; L. Offerhaus, M.D.; D.J. Ruiter, M.D., Professor of Medicine; P.A.G.M. de Smet, Pharm. D.; and H.J. Zimmerman, M.D., Professor of Medicine.

We are indebted to the Koninklijke Nederlandse Maatschappij ter bevordering der Pharmacie, The Hague, for providing the chemical formulae.

CONTENTS

FOREWORD

If any apology be needed for devoting this first monograph on 'Drug–Induced Disorders' to the liver, then it must surely start from the fact that the liver is and remains a fundamental, fascinating mystery, for the toxicologist and the physician no less than for the layman. Its very name is in many a language tied to that of life itself, but without a full understanding of the role which it actually plays in sustaining that life or its involvement in disease. *'Meum fervens difficili bile tumet jecur'* ('My liver is in a tumult, burning not to be restrained'), wrote Horace, viewing the liver as the seat of the passions (1). The Dutchman who has 'something on his liver' merely has a problem which he needs to discuss. For the ancients, the state of the liver of a slaughtered animal served as an omen, and for centuries after that the human liver was reputed to be the seat of courage. Much of these beliefs persists somewhere in the languages of Europe, mixed with metaphor and misunderstanding. The Frenchman who has 'les foies' is in a dilemma; but the Englishman who proclaims himself 'liverish' and hastens to take his daily dose of 'liver salts' is in all likelihood merely constipated by an indigestible diet.

As medical knowledge has advanced, the solution of one mystery surrounding hepatic structure and function has as a rule merely exposed several others, with the liver's enzymatic chemistry alone now filling entire volumes. The writer of an elementary handbook of physiology who once described the organ as a 'chemical factory of vast complexity' (and left it at that) put the matter in a nutshell in which some, in their bafflement, are only too content to leave it.

Because so little has been understood of the functions of the liver, there has been a corresponding lack of understanding of its dysfunction, despite a wealth of careful observation. 'In cases of jaundice,' wrote Hippocrates in the fifth century before Christ, 'it is a bad symptom when the liver becomes indurated' (2). Twenty–five centuries later with microscopy to hand, Friedrich Theodor von Frerichs (1819–1885) in his *Clinical Treatise on Diseases of the Liver* was able to provide a detailed picture of the morbid changes in that organ in a wide range of disorders: '...the cirrhosis which occurs in syphilitic patients is often accompanied by amyloid degeneration of the spleen and kidneys, and sometimes of the liver and the mucous membranes of the intestines. The cachexia attains a high grade at an early period. In addition to this, the remains of syphilitic inflammation are found in the liver; the gland is divided into lobes by bands of areolar tissues penetrating more or less deeply into its sub-

stance, whilst the cirrhotic induration is restricted to isolated masses...
In cases where chronic inflammation, originating in the capsule or in the
diaphragm, attacks the glandular substance, I have observed the portal
vein or the hepatic vein implicated to a great extent, the glandular parenchyma at different places uniformly indurated, and the outer surface
lobulated...' (3).

It is not entirely clear when the adverse effect of a drug on the liver
was identified for the first time; it may well have been in a report by Bang
who in 1774 first hinted at the possibility of a link between arsenic – then
much in vogue both as a drug and a cosmetic – and chronic liver disease
(4). In 1860 a case of severe fatty liver was ascribed to intoxication with
phosphorus and a range of previously published cases was reviewed.
Nevertheless, such observations remained incidental and they were
hardly followed up. Though fatal chloroform poisoning was recognized
in 1847, when Sir James Young Simpson published his classic description
of its anesthetic properties (5), another half century was to pass before
it was shown that in fact hepatic complications could occur. Many of the
hepatotoxic effects of drugs in use in the first half of the twentieth century long remained unrecognized, though incidental discoveries continued
to be made; in 1923, Worster–Drought first described idiosyncratic hepatic injury in a patient who had taken cinchophen (6), whilst the first cases
of drug–induced intrahepatic cholestasis (involving arsphenamine) were
reported in 1940 (7). On the other hand, oxyphenisatine was in use as a
popular laxative for 4 decades and on a massive scale before a report
from Reynolds and his colleagues in 1971 (8) provided a clue that its use
could lead to chronic active hepatitis; by an odd quirk of circumstance,
'Carter's Little Liver Pills' – long based upon oxyphenisatine – thus finally came to merit their name, though perhaps not in the manner contem-
plated by their originators.

The detection of such problems remains almost as problematical as it
ever was. In the early 1960s there was much reason to think that reports
of hepatic dysfunction were heralding the untimely end of the oral contraceptives, but the dimensions of the problem proved – perhaps fortun-
ately – to be less than was first supposed. By contrast, the lamentable
history of benoxaprofen (9) serves as a reminder that even with current
methods of drug regulation and adverse reaction monitoring we are not
capable of predicting even serious liver damage in subpopulations,
detecting it rapidly enough when it occurs, or even agreeing after the
event on what has actually happened. There is no reasonable doubt that
the community is going to be faced with analogous problems again and
again, particularly where special risk groups or interactions are concerned.

The widespread and largely unrecorded use of herbal preparations, often alongside prescribed medicines, introduces a new element of risk
which it proves extraordinarily difficult to measure or define; certainly
the plant world is a rich source of hepatotoxins, some of which have
found their way into the herbalist's shop; a number of such preparations

have also been found to contain inorganic arsenic and mercury, thus reintroducing two ancient problems which orthodox medicine wisely set aside long ago. In a community in which the understandable desire for freedom in self–treatment and self–indulgence inevitably involves risks which escape any form of organized surveillance, one will have to be prepared for unpleasant surprises from time to time. Just as we still know too little about the hepatotoxicity of many traditional remedies and mixtures thereof, so we are largely in the dark as to the extent to which these may render a liver more susceptible to damage by prescribed drugs. Precisely the same problem arises with respect to other hepatotoxic influences to which society chooses to expose itself, notably alcohol. The effects of various patterns of alcohol intake on the liver are extremely well known, but the pattern of alcohol intake – now an increasing social problem in both East and West – has changed drastically in the course of 20 years; the degree to which these sometimes delectable but inevitably noxious habits will accentuate or alter the hepatotoxicity of newer or older drugs is still a matter for debate and study.

Since the predictive value of animal experiments and short–term human studies in matters of safety is limited, there is now a trend to slow the further growth of pre–marketing regulatory requirements, laying greater weight on effective post–marketing surveillance for drug safety. What this in practice means is that after a drug has been released for sale, one will have to follow carefully the reactions to it in a large sample population as well as in various subpopulations. Particular attention will have to be bestowed on those possible risks suggested by animal or early human studies; in the case of possible hepatotoxicity one will also need to examine carefully all that happens in the very young, the very old, and patients with a history of prior liver disease or secondary risk factors.

We cannot ignore the fact that the nature of the risks to which the liver is exposed during drug treatment is changing, and that those risks may alter quite dramatically within the next decade. There was a time, not so very long ago, when virtually every drug in the pharmacopeia acted by virtue of the fact that it was a toxin, inhibiting one system or another and generally several at the same time. With the advent of antibiotics, substitution therapy and releasers we have in part escaped from that situation, but at the same time society has become less hesitant to tinker with much more subtle processes which it claims to understand. The difficulty is, of course, that we do not understand any of them fully. As we proceed to inhibit enzymes, manipulate genes and influence bodily processes in a host of other ingenious ways we are bound to create unpleasant surprises, and the liver is too involved in life processes to escape risk.

The watcher for adverse reactions is not by nature a pessimist or yet the scaremonger who he is sometimes made out to be; whether he likes the description or not, he is really something of a guardian angel. Like Janus, he must look both backwards and forwards. The authors of *Drug–Induced Hepatic Injury* have looked backwards very carefully, re–evaluating what has been written before in this field, so as not to perpetuate mere myths and misinterpretations; but they are also very deliberately looking forwards, providing a tool with the help of which it should become simpler to record, disseminate and study more efficiently each new suspicion of drug–induced injury. In that way we may be enabled to distinguish facts from mere fears more effectively, to detect new forms of drug–induced injury earlier before irrevocable harm is done, and to create a rather more solid base of knowledge for the study of this field in the future.

M.N.G. DUKES

Oudaen, Breukelen, The Netherlands
August, 1984

(1) Horatius: *Odes, Book I, 13*. (2) Hippocrates: *Aphorisms, VI, 42*. (3) Von Frerichs (1858) *Klinik der Leberkrankheiten*. (4) Cited by Zimmerman (1978) *Hepatotoxicity*. Appleton–Century–Crofts, New York. (5) Simpson (1847) *Account of a New Anaesthetic Agent as a Substitute for Sulphuric Ether*. (6) Worster–Drought (1923) *Br. Med. J., 1*, 148. (7) Hanger et al (1940) *J. Am. Med. Assoc., 115*, 263. (8) Reynolds et al (1971) *N. Engl. J. Med., 285*, 813. (9) Dukes (Ed) (1984) In: *Side Effects of Drugs, Annual 8*, p xvii. Elsevier, Amsterdam.

INTRODUCTION

Reports of symptomatic drug–induced hepatic injury often concern idiosyncratic reactions experienced during treatment with therapeutic doses. These may occur at any place and tend to be published at random all
over the world. Whereas large and well–designed clinical trials of new
drugs – designed to determine their therapeutic effects – are most commonly performed in well–reputed clinics and find their way into prominent medical journals, subsequent reports of idiosyncratic reactions to
these same drugs, however well–documented, often appear in secondary
journals and inaccessible languages. Some are recorded but not published at all.

On a smaller scale, one of us (B.H.Ch.S.) experiences this problem in
his daily work at the Netherlands Center for Monitoring of Adverse Reactions to Drugs. The first and clearest reports of hitherto unknown adverse reactions often originate from small rural hospitals, recalling the
old saying that the finest pearls may be found in small and unspectacular
shells.

Because of the unpredictability and rarity of many instances of drug–
induced hepatic injury our knowledge must often be derived from a small
number of well–documented case–histories. Any book on this subject
therefore has to devote close attention to a relatively small collection of
reports per drug and per group of drugs. In each of these instances, the
presence or absence of a causal relationship will have to be carefully assessed, since the pattern is rarely so specific that other causes (e.g. viral
hepatitis) can readily be ruled out.

Various iatrogenic epidemics, e.g. hepatic injury due to oxyphenisatine and more recently due to tienilic acid and benoxaprofen, clearly demonstrate that early detection of adverse reactions involving the liver is
of the utmost importance. It is an ongoing process which will never cease
in view of the continuing flow of new drugs and the increase in experience with those already in use. This book will therefore be updated regu-
larly. It will include mostly published but, where necessary, also unpublished data; both types of data will naturally only be considered for
inclusion if they are well–documented.

It is hoped that all those who find this book of value will assist the authors in collating new data by reporting to them cases of suspected drug–
induced hepatic injury which may merit inclusion. Such reports should
be as well–documented as possible, and we would suggest that they be
submitted at the same time to the National Adverse Reaction Monitoring

Center in the physician's country of residence. A form of the type used for such reports – but in this instance including a number of specific entries for matters related to hepatic injury – is reproduced at the end of this volume. Reports submitted to the authors will be regarded as confidential unless and until the reporting physician agrees to the form in which it is to be included in this book. They should be addressed to:

The Authors of *Drug–Induced Hepatic Injury*
Netherlands Center for Monitoring of Adverse Reactions to Drugs
c/o B.H.Ch. Stricker, Medical Officer
P.O. Box 439
2260 AK Leidschendam
The Netherlands
Telephone 070–996929

I. PATTERNS OF DRUG–INDUCED HEPATIC INJURY

Generally speaking, patterns of drug–induced hepatic injury are not very specific, showing characteristics identical to those of non–drug–related injury. However, there are important exceptions to this rule (see Section III: 'Diagnosis and Analysis of Drug–Induced Hepatic Injury').

A short description of known patterns is given below. It is based on the assumption that the reader is familiar with the indications and interpretation of diagnostic procedures. Table 1 gives an overview of the patterns.

Mild and transient elevation of serial liver enzyme levels without

TABLE 1 *Patterns of drug-induced hepatic injury*

Acute

    Hepatocellular   A. Steatosis
                         B.1. Degeneration
                               2. Necrosis
                         C. Granulomas

    Cholestatic   A. Pure cholestasis
                         B. Cholestatic hepatitis

Chronic

    Hepatocellular   A. Steatosis and fibrosis
                         B. Lipid storage disease
                         C. Chronic persistent/active hepatitis
                         D. Cirrhosis

    Cholestatic   A. Chronic intrahepatic cholestasis
                         B. Biliary cirrhosis

Vascular disorders

                       A.1. Veno-occlusive disease
                               2. Occlusion of large hepatic veins
                       B. Sinusoidal dilatation/peliosis hepatis
                       C. Hepatoportal sclerosis, perisinusoidal fibrosis

Tumors

                       A. Hepatocellular adenoma
                       B. Hepatocellular carcinoma
                       C. Cholangiocarcinoma
                       D. Angiosarcoma

---

symptoms and histological signs of injury is not uncommon after starting drug therapy. It is uncertain whether this reflects minimal injury to the hepatocyte or enzyme leakage without injury. Although usually without clinical significance, a follow–up in such cases is advised since it may precede symptomatic hepatic injury in a number of patients.

ACUTE

HEPATOCELLULAR

A. Steatosis (e.g. methotrexate, tetracycline, alcohol, valproic acid etc.)

Fatty change of hepatocytes involves either small droplets without displacement of the nucleus (microvesicular, e.g. tetracycline, valproic acid) or large globules displacing the nucleus to the cell border (macrovesicular, e.g. methotrexate). Inflammatory cells are often scanty but may be present when necrosis coexists. Steatosis may predominate in the centrilobular (e.g. alcohol) or periportal (e.g. ethionine) region. Sometimes fatty cells coalesce to form fatty cysts, resulting in lipogranulomas.

Biochemical alterations depend on the degree of steatosis and (if present) necrosis. Aminotransferase and alkaline phosphatase levels may be normal but are mildly/moderately raised in most cases of acute toxic steatosis. Hypolipemia and hypocholesterolemia are present. Acute steatosis may present with acute hepatic failure (coagulation disorders etc.).

Symptoms may show the same spectrum of severity as in necrosis (see below). Immunoallergic manifestations are absent. Acute steatosis may have a rapidly fatal course (e.g. tetracycline).

B.1. Degeneration (e.g. many hepatotoxic drugs in low doses)

Hepatocellular unrest is seen with bi/trinucleation, mitotic figures, ballooning and acidophilic bodies; there is minimal infiltration, mainly by mononuclear cells.

Mild elevation of liver enzymes (ALAT/ASAT, alkaline phosphatase etc.) may occur.

Clinical symptoms are usually absent; sometimes there are vague, non–specific complaints.

B.2. Necrosis (many drugs, e.g. paracetamol, methyldopa, halothane, isoniazide etc.)

Necrosis varies in severity (focal/massive) and pathogenesis (toxic/idiosyncratic) determined by type of drug, status/localization of metabolizing enzymes and individual susceptibility. Necrosis is mainly zonal, but rarely massive in the toxic form. In the idiosyncratic form, necrosis is

2

diffuse (immunoallergy?) or zonal (metabolic variant?). Necrosis may also vary in localization: although mostly centrilobular (Zone III, Rappaport; e.g. paracetamol), necrosis may predominate in the midzonal (furosemide overdose, rats) or periportal region (e.g. $FeSO_4$). Severe necrosis may cause bridging (central–central/central–portal/portal–portal) often with collapse of the reticular framework. Massive necrosis is caused mainly by idiosyncrasy, not toxicity. In immunoallergic hepatitis, necrotic sites and portal areas are infiltrated by mononuclear cells, which sometimes have a granulomatous appearance. Toxic injury may give a less densely, more neutrophilic infiltrate. Although eosinophilic infiltration is not highly specific, it is often associated with an immunoallergic pathogenesis. Necrosis around the central vein may result from severe hypotension or congestive heart failure, in the latter accompanied by edema, extravasation of blood and dilated sinusoids.

The extent of necrosis is usually paralleled by an equivalent rise in serum aminotransferase levels, although a sudden decline indicates hepatic failure when accompanied by a sharp rise in serum bilirubin and prolongation of the prothrombin time. Alkaline phosphatase and bilirubin levels in serum are less markedly elevated. Hypoprothrombinemia is frequent. Many other liver enzymes are elevated (e.g. γ–glutamyl transferase, 5–nucleotidase etc.). No markers of viral hepatitis are present. Eosinophilia in the blood may indicate an immunoallergic pathogenesis. In intoxication, blood levels of drug/metabolites confirm a causal relationship.

Symptoms vary depending on severity and susceptibility. They may be absent, mild (malaise, anorexia etc.) or severe (jaundice, bruising). Extrahepatic manifestations may be prominent, both toxic (e.g. renal, CCl_4) and immunoallergic (rash, fever, arthralgia). The latter can also occur as prodromal signs of viral hepatitis, which should be excluded. Sometimes minor hepatic injury is secondary to extrahepatic drug–induced hypersensitivity reactions (e.g. Stevens–Johnson syndrome, myocarditis, pneumonitis). In some cases a picture arises resembling that of infectious mononucleosis with fever, rash, generalized lymphadenopathy and atypical lymphocytes. Mortality of acute hepatocellular necrosis is high. It depends on which drug is responsible and is estimated at 50% for some drugs.

C. Granulomas (e.g. allopurinol, phenylbutazone, sulfonamides)

Drug–induced granulomas usually appear within the first 4 months of therapy, either with mild cellular swelling/cholestasis or without accompanying hepatocellular injury. Occasionally liver injury is more severe. Drug–induced granulomatous hepatitis is often pericholangitic. Granulomas may appear in portal, lobular and pericentral areas invariably accompanied by portal inflammation with lymphocytes, histiocytes, plasma cells and eosinophils; the eosinophils may be very numerous.

Portal granulomas are usually discrete with a surrounding mononuclear infiltrate but may also be part of a diffuse portal inflammation expanding into the lobules. Granulomas are always non–caseating, although occasionally there is central nuclear fragmentation. Giant–cell formation may be marked. Eosinophilic infiltration may be prominent, especially in the early phase. There are no biochemical abnormalities unless hepatic injury is present. The diagnosis can only be made by biopsy.

Granulomas are often non-symptomatic. However, as part of a generalized hypersensitivity reaction, immunoallergic signs and symptoms (e.g. rash, eosinophilia, fever, arthralgia) may be prominent. Disappearance after discontinuation of therapy suggests a drug–induced cause. It is advisable to exclude at least sarcoidosis and infectious causes (especially tuberculosis, schistosomiasis).

CHOLESTATIC

A. Pure cholestasis (e.g. anabolic steroids)

B. Cholestatic hepatitis (e.g. chlorpromazine, erythromycin)

Predominantly centrilobular bile–staining of hepatocytes and bile casts is seen in (sometimes distended) canaliculi. Bile 'lakes' as seen in extrahepatic obstructive jaundice are absent. It may occur without (pure cholestasis) or with minor/moderate hepatocellular unrest/necrosis (cholestatic hepatitis). In the former, inflammatory cells are virtually absent; in the latter there is a mononuclear and eosinophilic infiltrate, rich in the portal zones, moderate at necrotic sites; some bile duct multiplication is often present. A pattern exists characteristic of both acute cholestatic and hepatocellular hepatitis (mixed pattern).

Serum bilirubin, alkaline phosphatase, 5–nucleotidase and γ–glutamyl transferase levels are high while aminotransferase levels are normal or moderately elevated (the latter especially in cases of cholestatic hepatitis). Imaging procedures (e.g. ultrasound, cholegraphic imaging, computed tomography) show normal extrahepatic bile ducts.

Jaundice and pruritus are outstanding features. Cholestatic hepatitis may be accompanied by rash, fever and arthralgia, manifestations that are usually absent in pure cholestasis. Mortality is low (estimated at less than 1%) especially in cases of pure cholestasis. Occasionally, recovery from cholestasis takes a long time ($> {}^1/_2$ year).

CHRONIC

HEPATOCELLULAR

A. Steatosis and fibrosis (e.g. methotrexate, alcohol etc.)

The same pattern is seen as for acute steatosis. If however accompanied

4

by necrosis, prolonged administration of the responsible hepatotoxin will eventually lead to fibrosis and cirrhosis. In some patients, prolonged administration of a hepatotoxin causes a sudden exacerbation into an acute hepatitis (alcohol!) which may present either a hepatocellular or cholestatic pattern.

All liver enzyme levels may be elevated, mostly mildly; signs of metabolic dysfunction occur (e.g. hyperlipemia, hyperuricemia, hypoglycemia etc.). If necrosis starts early and fibrosis and cirrhosis develop, hepatic dysfunction (hypoalbuminemia, hyperammonemia etc.) may occur.

Often there are no symptoms or only non–specific complaints (malaise, anorexia etc.), unless acute necrosis or cholestasis is present.

B. Lipid storage disease (e.g. 4,4′–diethylaminoethoxyhexestrol, amiodarone, perhexiline)

Drug–induced lipid storage disease usually consists of phospholipidosis although ganglioside accumulation has also been mentioned in the literature (e.g. perhexiline). Hepatocytes, Kupffer cells, endothelial and biliary epithelial cells but also extrahepatic cells, e.g. blood and nerve cells and lung tissue, are involved.

Liver cells are enlarged and have a foamy appearance. Electron microscopy reveals multilamellated ('fingerprint') and crystalloid lysosomal inclusion bodies. In advanced cases, fibrosis and cirrhosis may ensue. The lysosomal inclusions resemble those seen in Niemann–Pick's and Fabry's disease, but the clinical setting differs.

Biochemical abnormalities are usually absent, but elevation of liver enzyme levels after prolonged treatment may reflect severe chronic hepatic injury. Hypertriglyceridemia and elevation of free fatty acids may present early. Lysosomal inclusion bodies in peripheral blood lymphocytes may be indicative and diminish the need for a biopsy.

Symptoms are usually absent but extrahepatic manifestations may indicate toxicity (e.g. neuropathy due to perhexiline or amiodarone, skin discoloration by amiodarone). Immunoallergic signs are absent. Malaise and hepatosplenomegaly, weight loss and hypoglycemia may precede or accompany liver damage.

C. Chronic persistent/active hepatitis (CPH/CAH) (e.g. oxyphenisatine, methyldopa, nitrofurantoin etc.)

Periportal rosette–formation and 'piece–meal' necrosis is seen with a rich portal and periportal infiltrate of lymphocytes and plasma cells. A more active state may be reflected by mild/moderate necrosis and infiltration around the central vein. Bridging necrosis occurs, connecting portal areas. Periportal fibrosis develops and may eventually progress to cirrhosis. In chronic persistent hepatitis (a less aggressive form), inflammatory cells in the portal area do not cross the limiting plate so that necrosis is absent.

5

Most liver enzyme levels are elevated, but are occasionally normal. Serum gammaglobulin levels are elevated, especially IgG. Immunological tests are positive, especially smooth muscle antibodies. If progressive, signs of severe hepatic dysfunction develop.

Symptoms may be absent or non–specific; they may arise suddenly or insidiously. In advanced cases, jaundice, portal hypertension with ascites and hepatic failure are present. Prognosis is good after discontinuation of the causative agent unless damage is too advanced and cirrhosis develops. Since immunoallergic symptoms usually lead to early discontinuation of the causative drug, these symptoms are uncommon in cases of chronic (> 6 months) drug–induced hepatic injury.

D. Cirrhosis (e.g. CCl_4, alcohol etc.)

Diffuse fibrosis occurs with nodules of hepatocytes, alteration of the normal lobular structure, regeneration and necrosis. Either small (micronodular) or large (macronodular) nodules are present. Drugs capable of producing chronic active hepatitis (see above) or any other chronic form of hepatic injury may eventually lead to cirrhosis. 'Cardiac cirrhosis' is not a usual type of cirrhosis but a pericentral fibrosis with 'reversed lobulation' caused by prolonged hepatic venous congestion. Theoretically, it may be induced by drugs aggravating congestive heart failure, but this is probably not of much practical significance.

Liver enzyme levels are elevated and amino acid patterns are changed. Hepatic failure occurs with hypoalbuminemia, hypoprothrombinemia, hyperammonemia etc.

Ascites, splenomegaly, jaundice etc. supervene. Defective coagulation, metabolic disturbances, encephalopathy, portal hypertension with esophageal varices and gastrointestinal blood loss present the main therapeutic problems. They are not present in every patient, however. Portal hypertension may be seen without cirrhosis in hepatoportal sclerosis (e.g. inorganic arsenicals).

CHOLESTATIC

A. Chronic intrahepatic cholestasis

B. Biliary cirrhosis (e.g. chlorpromazine, testosterone)

Centrilobular, midzonal and periportal cholestasis are seen with bile staining of hepatocytes, bile casts and duct dilatation, periductal inflammation and fibrosis. Interlobular and septal bile ducts finally disappear with periportal necrosis and fibrosis, ending in biliary cirrhosis. According to some authors, the drug–induced form of biliary cirrhosis has more scanty portal inflammation and bile duct destruction than primary biliary cirrhosis.

High levels of alkaline phosphatase and cholesterol are found in the serum, but bilirubin and aminotransferase concentrations are moderately elevated. Antimitochondrial antibodies, present in almost every case of primary biliary cirrhosis, were often not assessed in the older reports of drug–induced cases of biliary cirrhosis so that few data are available. Serum IgM may be elevated.

Jaundice, pruritus etc. and dermal xanthomata are found. The prognosis is better than in primary biliary cirrhosis, since discontinuation of treatment in the early stages is often followed by improvement. Nevertheless, some fatal cases have been described. The data, however, are based on very few cases.

VASCULAR DISORDERS

Although the Budd–Chiari syndrome is often used as a synonym for thrombosis of the large hepatic veins, any obstruction of venous outflow, including veno–occlusive disease, causes this syndrome.

A.1. Veno–occlusive disease (e.g. urethane, pyrrolizidine alkaloids, tioguanine, dacarbazine)

Occlusion of the centrilobular and sublobular hepatic veins occurs due to disruption and edema of the venous wall and surrounding tissue (acute) or to fibrotic tissue (chronic). There are no lesions or thrombosis of larger veins. Congestion is found in surrounding dilated sinusoids with hemorrhagic necrosis of hepatocytes. There is collapse of the reticular framework around the central vein and fibrosis. Collateral vessels develop in the surrounding parenchyma.

There is elevation of bilirubin and liver enzyme levels in the serum depending on the extent and number of obliterated veins.

The onset of painful hepatomegaly and ascites is sudden, sometimes with circulatory shock. Collateral abdominal veins may be prominent. Occasionally there is mild jaundice. Mostly prompt clinical recovery occurs unless the drug is continued. Some cases develop recurring ascites, finally developing into cirrhosis.

A.2. Occlusion of large hepatic veins (e.g. contraceptive steroids)

This may lead to the Budd–Chiari syndrome resulting from occlusion of the main hepatic veins or their smaller branches (v. sushepatica) or of the inferior vena cava, mostly caused by thrombosis. There is centrilobular necrosis and congestion, sinusoidal dilatation and extravasation of blood; there are secondary thrombi in different stages of organization. Chronic cases show centrilobular fibrosis and periportal regeneration.

Serum albumin, alkaline phosphatase, bilirubin and aminotransferase levels are moderately elevated. Scintigraphy may show reduced uptake, with maximum uptake in the caudate lobe. Arteriography may show multiple space–occupying areas resembling metastases. Venography shows obstruction and a lace–like pattern in the liver.

Abdominal pain, hepatomegaly, gross ascites and sometimes mild jaundice occur; collateral veins may be visible on the abdomen; the onset may often be insidious. The course may be slow with resistent ascites, portal hypertension, cirrhosis and death from liver failure/gastrointestinal hemorrhage in 3–4 years or rapid with acute hepatic failure in several months.

B. Sinusoidal dilatation/peliosis hepatis (e.g. contraceptive and anabolic steroids)

Dilatation of sinusoids occurs, sometimes resulting in blood pools. There is a phlebosclerotic form with endothelial or fibrous lining, draining into central veins/sinusoids, and a parenchymal type without a lining communicating with sinusoids. Especially the latter is associated with the use of anabolic and contraceptive steroids. Both forms may be present concurrently.

Peliosis hepatis is often secondary to other conditions (e.g. hepatic adenoma) which dominate the clinical and biochemical pattern.

C. Hepatoportal sclerosis, perisinusoidal fibrosis (e.g. arsenicals, vitamin A)

Idiopathic portal hypertension may originate from fibrous thickening of the portal veins and/or perisinusoidal fibrosis. There are varying degrees of portal fibrosis and intimal thickening and sclerosis of portal vein walls. There is often perisinusoidal fibrosis with collagen deposition in the space of Disse and fibers infiltrating between hepatocytes. In cases of vitamin A intoxication there is a marked increase in Ito cells, which may be the only histological feature.

Biochemical values are normal or slightly abnormal unless severe fibrosis and cirrhosis are present. In cases of intoxication, high levels of arsenic or vitamin A in liver tissue are diagnostic; vitamin A has a fluorescent appearance under the microscope.

Although initially without symptoms, prolonged portal hypertension will cause splenomegaly, ascites and collateral venous circulation, often clearly visible on the abdomen. For subsequent cirrhosis and hepatic failure the above–mentioned considerations apply. Extrahepatic manifestations of intoxication may facilitate the assessment of a causal relationship with the suspected agent.

TUMORS

A. Hepatocellular adenoma (e.g. anabolic and contraceptive steroids)

Hepatocellular adenoma is a non–malignant tumor of cells resembling hepatocytes. These cells are arranged in tightly packed trabeculae, 2–3 cells thick, separated by compressed slit–like sinusoids. The cells are slightly larger than hepatocytes and are glycogen–rich, with uniform nuclei and little variation in size and shape; canaliculi are normal, bile ducts absent. The tumor is very vascular with dilated, thin–walled blood vessels which are randomly distributed.

a–Fetoprotein tests are negative. Diagnosis is only possible from the pathology. Liver scanning and ultrasound are helpful. Angiography shows a highly vascularized tumor with an arterial supply originating peripherally with multiple parallel vessels coursing towards the center of the tumor.

Anorexia, nausea and abdominal discomfort occur. The tumor is often palpable. Approximately $1/_3$–$1/_4$ of patients present with hemoperitoneum/rupture of the tumor.

B. Hepatocellular carcinoma (e.g. thorium dioxide, contraceptive steroids?)

Hepatocellular carcinoma is a malignant tumor composed of hepatocyte–like cells, often in combination with cirrhosis of the liver. Local vascular/lymphatic metastases may be present, having a typical appearance ('planet with satellites'). Since there are several variants of the basic trabecular pattern (pseudoglandular, solid, scirrhous, pleomorphic and clear cell), differentiation from other primary hepatic tumors may be difficult. In 'Thorotrast cases' brown–black particles are visible.

Mostly high levels of a–fetoprotein (> 400 ng/ml) are found. High alkaline phosphatase or mildly elevated bilirubin levels in serum may occur but are non–specific. Elevated liver enzymes may reflect underlying cirrhosis. Angiography, ultrasound, isotopic scanning and computed tomography may be helpful by showing a rich arterial supply with clusters of bizarre tumor vessels and focal defects. Proline hydroxylase and chorionic gonadotropin levels may be elevated. Erythrocytosis and dysfibrinogenemia are rare. HbsAg is negative in drug–induced cases.

Abdominal pain and weight loss occur; symptoms may reflect cirrhosis with portal hypertension/(bloody) ascites. Hemoperitoneum by rupture may occur.

C. Cholangiocarcinoma (e.g. thorium dioxide)

Cholangiocarcinoma is a malignant tumor of cells resembling biliary epithelium. It is a firm grayish tumor growing along neighboring bile ducts in an otherwise normal liver. There are glandular mucus–secreting structures with much fibrous stroma or there is a papillary form. If a trabecular pattern is present, the tumor may be indistinguishable from hepatocellular carcinoma. However, a–fetoprotein is usually normal. In 'Thorotrast cases', brown–black particles are present.

Functional hepatic impairment occurs late in course. Diagnosis is from the pathology. Angiography usually shows a less vascularized tumor than in cases of hepatocellular carcinoma, although intermediate forms are not uncommon. Ultrasound and liver scanning are helpful.

Patients may present with obstructive jaundice and weight loss or may have symptoms mimicking hepatocellular carcinoma.

D. Angiosarcoma (e.g. thorium dioxide, inorganic arsenicals)

Angiosarcoma is a malignant tumor of spindle–shaped cells lining vascular spaces. Multiple hemorrhagic nodules and blood–filled cysts are seen. Growth is tectorial on the surface of the liver cells. The tumor cells are elongated with ill–defined borders and with hyperchromatic nuclei varying in size and shape. There is an abundance of reticular fibers in the sinusoids. There is hematopoiesis. In 'Thorotrast cases', brown–black particles are demonstrable.

There are non–specific liver function abnormalities and hematological abnormalities. Angiography, ultrasound or computed tomography are useful for localization of the tumor.

There is progressive hepatomegaly, with hematological abnormalities (pancytopenia, hemolytic anemia, disseminated intravascular coagulation and terminal jaundice). Occasionally the tumor may rupture. The course is rapidly fatal.

II. MECHANISMS OF DRUG–INDUCED HEPATIC INJURY

There are basically 7 mechanisms of hepatic injury. The therapeutic agent or a metabolite may:

1. Interfere with metabolic processes in the hepatocytes (cholestasis, steatosis/necrosis)
2. Destroy the cells through a toxic effect on essential structures (necrosis)
3. Destroy the cells through induction of an immunological reaction (necrosis)
4. Have a carcinogenic/mutagenic action
5. Interfere with the blood supply to the hepatocytes
6. Transmit infection
7. Aggravate underlying disease

1. Interference with metabolic processes in the hepatocytes

It is well known that drugs (or their metabolites) can influence the function of the hepatocytes. One of the best–known examples is the induction of the mixed–function oxidase system by which drugs may influence their own breakdown or that of other drugs.

If it is realized that every drug with a physiological effect also has a toxic potential and that many of these drugs are metabolized in the liver where they can attain considerable concentrations, then it is not surprising that many of them have some measurable effect on liver function. In most cases, however, therapeutic doses of a drug will not cause a clinically significant adverse effect on the liver. Most drugs that do so will be abandoned before they come into widespread clinical use. Some of these drugs may be used as experimental hepatotoxins and demonstrate a selective ability to disturb certain biochemical processes that are essential to cellular function such as uptake, transformation, production and excretion. Bilirubin metabolism, for instance, may be inhibited by impairment of transport of the unconjugated form from the sinusoid into the hepatocyte (e.g. by rifampicin and flavispidic acid), by inhibition of transformation into the conjugated form by glucuronyltransferase (e.g. novobiocin) or by inhibiting the excretion of conjugated bilirubin (e.g. novobiocin, rifampicin). This can lead to hyperbilirubinemia in an otherwise healthy patient.

More serious is interference with bile flow, resulting in cholestasis. In-

11

terference with bile flow has been suggested to be caused by many mechanisms, some of them occurring simultaneously: (a) disturbance of bile flow due to a lack of cellular ATP; (b) injury to the hepatocanalicular membrane; (c) formation of insoluble precipitates in or around the canaliculus, thereby leading to obstruction; (d) impairment of bile–salt–dependent flow by blocking the synthesis of bile acids or their transcanalicular transport; (e) impairment of bile–salt–independent flow by inhibition of $(Na^+ + K^+)$–ATPase; (f) interference with the formation of normal micelles in the bile; (g) increase in membrane viscosity by alteration of lipid composition; (h) abnormal reabsorption or secretion of water and electrolytes along the course of the ductules; (i) injury to the bile ducts. One should realize, however, that not all these mechanisms have been equally well demonstrated by experiments.

Most serious is interference with biochemical processes that are essential to the life of the cell. Histologically, this often leads to steatosis, mostly without infiltrate, but necrosis may occur in cases of severe disturbance. Steatosis can be caused in several ways. Metabolic interference may lead to increased synthesis of lipids in the cell. Alcohol, for instance, may enhance lipogenesis by increasing the NADH/NAD ratio. Increased delivery of fatty acids to the liver due to enhanced mobilization of lipid depots by drugs may also play a role in steatosis in addition to the important influence of dietary lipid intake. A decrease in the rate of oxidation of fatty acids by drug–induced mitochondrial damage is another important cause of steatosis. Some drugs inhibit the formation and/or secretion of very–low–density lipoproteins (VLDL) from the hepatocyte to the blood and thereby account for accumulation of fat. Usually several mechanisms are involved simultaneously (e.g. alcohol), but generally they all reflect either an increased synthesis/uptake or a decreased output/metabolism of lipid constituents by the hepatocyte, either alone or in concert. Necrosis may occur in cases where there is severe interference with metabolic processes either quantitatively or qualitatively. An example of the latter is deficiency of an essential precursor in the synthesis of plasma membrane components such as the relative uridine triphosphate deficiency caused by the administration of galactosamine.

Of course, there can be an overlap between the first and second mechanism, mentioned above. Irreversible destruction of an essential metabolic structure resulting in cell death may be regarded as intermediate between the two groups.

There are several theories for the mechanism of drug–induced phospholipidosis. When amphiphilic cationic drugs (apolar ring structure, polar side–chain) form complexes with phospholipids, they prevent the effect of phospholipase with subsequent complex accumulation and engorgement of lysosomes. Others favor a two–step approach. Firstly, inhibition of phosphotidate phosphohydrolase changes the balance of glycerolipid biosynthesis with subsequent accumulation and abnormal pattern of lipids. Subsequently, this unusual substrate impairs degradation by phospholipase, with accumulation and engorgement.

12

2. Destruction of cells due to a toxic effect on essential structures

The second mechanism of drug–induced hepatic disease comprises the direct toxic action of a drug or (probably more often) one of its metabolites on essential structures, sometimes leading to necrosis within several hours; the extent and time interval depend on whether the drug or one of its metabolites is toxic, on the dose, the metabolic spectrum, protective mechanisms (e.g. glutathione, superoxide dismutase), individual susceptibility, enzyme induction (alcohol) etc. Few therapeutic agents lead to clinical manifestations through this type of injury unless they are taken in excessive amounts. The site of injury with the most far–reaching consequences seems to be the liver cell membrane, either directly due to chemical rupture or change in its physicochemical structure or indirectly due to defective synthesis of membrane components. Subsequent leakage of electrolytes and enzymes will disturb the intracellular environment and result in lysis of the cell. Damage to mitochondria, lysosomes, endoplasmic reticulum and other cell organelles plays an additional pathophysiological role. In less severely injured cells, defective organelles may account for the steatosis which often surrounds necrotic areas.

It is not known how injury takes place, but increasing evidence points to the importance of the formation of free radicals, epoxides, ion radicals, and alkylating, arylating and other highly reactive intermediates of drug metabolism. It is plausible that in these cases the primary site of injury is the endoplasmic reticulum where reactive intermediates of drugs may be formed in very high quantities. It is certainly incorrect to hold the non–synthetic enzymes (e.g. oxidative/reductive enzymes) exclusively responsible since conjugating enzymes may also produce very reactive substances. The reactive metabolites may inactivate vital enzymes, bind to ATP, NADPH and other important micromolecules, attack double bonds in lipids, proteins and nucleic acids, and change biological properties. Radicals may remove a hydrogen atom from a polyunsaturated fatty acid, initiate lipid peroxidation and subsequently damage membranes. Although highly reactive substances usually have a short half–life, they may induce damage to more distant structures by the production of active byproducts. The trichloromethyl radical (CCl_3), a metabolite of carbon tetrachloride, is an example of a very active and rapidly reacting substance that indirectly creates secondary and tertiary active products that escape from the endoplasmic reticulum and damage structures at a distance, due to their longer lifespan.

Two observations are compatible with an important pathogenetic role of toxic metabolites. The first is that the high concentration of cytochrome P450 in the centrizonal hepatocytes is in accordance with the usually predominant localization of necrosis in this area. Secondly, induction of cytochrome P450 may enhance necrosis, as shown in phenobarbital–treated animals with paracetamol–induced hepatic lesions. Although many well–designed studies have been performed on chemically reactive metabolites, one should realize that these were mainly performed in animals or in vitro and thus lack many elements which are relevant to the situation in man. But even if a relationship is shown between a demonstrated metabolite and hepatic toxicity, this does not prove that it is the primary cause. Also, little is known about the cellular site of injury. Hence, interpretation of many experimental studies remains speculative.

An interesting but poorly demonstrated aspect of hepatotoxicity is 'metabolic idiosyncrasy'. It originates in the observation that some drugs cause hepatic injury in only a small and unpredictable minority of patients who do not show signs of a hypersensitivity reaction. Moreover, in some patients the readministration of the drug after complete normalization of all laboratory values results, after only several weeks, in a recurrence of hepatic damage. It may be speculated from these observations and from its infrequent occurrence that an individual metabolic variant in combination with induction of breakdown to an aberrant toxic metabolite is responsible for this delayed effect. Such a qualitative difference in metabolism, however, has never been proven as a cause of hepatic injury and is merely speculative. More probably there is a quantitative difference, yielding a higher–than–usual proportion of toxic byproducts in the susceptible individual. Subsequent to the accumulation of toxic metabolites to a certain level, liver damage ensues.

Experiments in animals have established multiple forms of cytochrome P450 with differing molecular weight and substrate specificity; increasing evidence suggests the same in man. It may be expected that the existence of multiple forms of cytochrome P450 with a different, partly overlapping, substrate specificity combined with individually varying, genetically and environmentally determined enzyme induction, will create a mosaic metabolic pattern with individually differing vulnerability.

3. Destruction of cells due to induction of an immunological reaction

Although the evidence for an immunological type of idiosyncratic hepatic injury seems more concrete, proof of its existence rests heavily on circumstantial evidence such as concomitant rash, fever or eosinophilia. In cases where these extrahepatic manifestations are absent, the accelerated (<3 days) recurrence of hepatic damage after readministration of the drug is compatible with an immunological mechanism.

Another argument is provided by the striking analogy in the clinical and histological pattern between acute and chronic drug–induced parenchymatous hepatitis and acute and chronic viral hepatitis, the latter of which is definitely immunologically mediated. Important differences between the toxic and idiosyncratic pattern are given in Table 1.

It should be emphasized that individual factors determine not only whether one will develop this type of reaction but also which pattern will emerge. While some patients react with an acute parenchymatous/cholestatic hepatitis, others develop chronic active hepatitis/chronic intra-

14

TABLE 1 *Differences between toxic and idiosyncratic pattern of hepatic injury*

| | Toxicity | Idiosyncrasy | |
		Metabolic	Immunoallergy
Onset	rapid, first few days	variable, 1 week to 1 year or more	variable but often within first 6 weeks
Reaction to rechallenge	rapid, first few days	delayed (1–2 weeks)	rapid, first few days
Incidence	high	low	low
Dose-effect relationship	+	+(?)/−	−
Reproducible in animals	+	−	−
'Hypersensitivity' features	−	−	+/−
Every individual susceptible	+	−	−

hepatic cholestasis.

Immunological studies of drug–induced hepatic injury concentrate on one or more of 4 important questions: (a) Are there indications for the immunological nature of the injury? (b) Is it fully responsible for the liver damage both quantitatively and qualitatively? (c) What is the precise mechanism? (d) What are the most sensitive and specific diagnostic tests?

The major problems with these studies are: Firstly, because of the infrequency and unpredictability of the idiosyncratic reactions it is difficult to collect relevant material at the right time. In addition, many of the collected cases have not been proven to be drug–induced (e.g. by rechallenge) so that a negative result of the tests is equivocal, indicating either a wrong test or a wrong diagnosis. It is very difficult to collect a sufficient number of proven cases of a particular drug–related hepatic reaction, to take serum at the same stage of illness and to test it at the same time with the same technique. Secondly, the interpretation of tested cases, scattered throughout the world, is difficult because different tests have been used, because different techniques have been used for the same test, and because most tests are non–specific. If positive, they prove that a drug is 'immunologically recognized' but not that it has caused hepatic injury. Examples of the latter are the lymphocyte stimulation test and

15

the macrophage inhibition test. The more recently introduced drug–mediated cytotoxicity assays with isolated hepatocytes appear to be more specific.

There are two important hypotheses on the immunological mechanism of idiosyncratic drug–induced hepatitis. The first suggests that a drug or metabolite may bind to the liver cell membrane or to another structure in the cell and yield an immunogenic stimulus, resulting in destruction of the hepatocyte. It seems unlikely, however, that a completely intact cell can be destroyed merely by binding to a hapten. More probably, an immunological response is superimposed on an underlying alteration or damage to essential cell structures due to a toxic effect of the drug or a metabolite. This is in accordance with the observation that many drugs established as a cause of this idiosyncratic form of hepatic injury may also cause a minor and often transient rise in the serum concentrations of aminotransferases in a considerable number of patients. In this toxic–immunological theory, immunological destruction occurs, for example, through antibody–dependent K–cells attacking a cellular protein–hapten complex.

Drug–induced liver injury secondary to the precipitation of circulating antigen–antibody complexes ('innocent bystander' reaction) is probably rare. Kupffer cells are thought to be efficient in clearing these complexes. Nevertheless, some drugs (e.g. p–aminosalicylic acid, phenytoin) produce a clinical pattern resembling that of serum sickness.

The second hypothesis suggests that by influencing the immunoregulatory mechanisms, a drug may be responsible for an autoimmune hepatitis. In recent years, increasing attention has been paid to the absolute and relative number of T–helper and T–suppressor lymphocytes. A lower T–suppressor/T–helper ratio might result in enhanced autoimmunological reactivity by deregulation of antibody production. Unfortunately, the same observations have been made in non–drug–related hepatic injury and they therefore lack specificity. The same lack of specificity concerns autoantibodies such as antinuclear antibodies (ANA) and smooth muscle antibodies (SMA) which may appear as an expression of diminished tolerance to autoantigens caused by an effect on the immunoregulatory system of drugs or their metabolites, but they also occur in non–drug–related forms. Interesting are the more recently discovered antimitochondrial antibodies of the M3 (several drugs) and M6 (iproniazid) type which may be more specifically drug–related. The same applies to the liver/kidney Type 2 microsomal antibodies which seem to be specific for tienilic–acid–induced hepatic injury.

Little is known about a relationship between HLA–types and drug–induced liver injury. One may speculate that persons with a relatively inefficient suppressor–cell response (e.g. HLA–DR3) are more vulnerable to a drug which further reduces suppressor–cell activity and thereby causes increased cellular and humoral responses to a wide variety of antigens including the drug itself, autoantigens and combinations thereof.

At the present time, it is impossible to say which of these mechanisms

16

is the more important. It is certainly possible that additional theories will be developed in the near future. There are many drugs and it could be that several mechanisms are involved, alone or concurrently.

4. Carcinogenic/mutagenic action

Many chemical agents, but relatively few drugs, have been incriminated as hepatocarcinogenic. Natural agents such as aflatoxins and pyrrolizidine alkaloids and synthetic compounds such as the aromatic amines, azo–compounds, aliphatic and aromatic chlorinated compounds, hydrazines, nitrosamines and polycyclic hydrocarbons have all been demonstrated to be hepatocarcinogenic in animals. Some have been used in industry (e.g. vinylchloride), as pesticides in agriculture (e.g. DDT) or as medicinal agents (e.g. chloroform). Most are used only for experimental purposes.

For obvious reasons, human experiments are limited. Hence, more recently developed drugs have been tested in animals before being used in man. Although this makes it possible to unmask notorious carcinogens, it does not *guarantee* the safe use in man of drugs which have successfully passed these tests.

No currently used drug has been proven to be hepatocarcinogenic, but some are suspected. The problem is that for a given drug in a particular patient a causal relationship is impossible to prove because of the non–specificity of the tumor, the obscure temporal relationship and the impossibility of excluding other (unknown) causes. Epidemiological studies can show a relationship but can never *prove* a *causal* relationship. Moreover, it is difficult to match a large group of persons with appropriate controls and to follow them up for many years, which would be necessary if a drug appears to be a carcinogen of low potency.

It is assumed that most hepatocarcinogens are produced by metabolization in the hepatocyte. The cytochrome–P450–dependent mono–oxygenase system in particular is held responsible in most cases for the production of the ultimate carcinogen; other Phase I reactions are probably less involved. With some exceptions, Phase II reactions do not produce carcinogens but rather eliminate them. The result of induction of the mixed–function oxidases will depend entirely on their substrate specificity; if the carcinogen is a product of their activity, induction of the corresponding enzyme increases formation and may increase the risk of carcinogenesis. However, this is not necessarily the case. An agent is transformed into several metabolites and it is the relative amount of these formed that is of importance. In addition, several other factors are crucial, such as the number of detoxifying biomechanisms, the nature of the carcinogen, its life–span, the absolute amount formed etc. Induction of Phase II enzymes usually enhances excretion and reduces the carcinogenic potential. Of course, there are several other individual and environmental factors of importance.

Carcinogens are considered to cause tumors either directly (initiation) or indirectly (promotion). Initiators probably have one thing in common, namely they have strong electrophilic centers which react with cell structures with electron–rich components. This may result in arylation or alkylation with a fundamental change in structure or in the production of secondary and tertiary free radicals, thus producing a cascade of radical–induced lesions. If the resulting products are formed in small quantities, protective mechanisms (e.g. catalase, glutathion, a–tocopherol, superoxide dismutase) will succeed in eliminating them without adverse effects. Large quantities may overwhelm the system and exert an effect at many cell sites. The crucial step may be binding to and mutagenic change of nuclear DNA and RNA (many mutagens are also carcinogens but not necessarily so). If nucleases or other repairing enzymes are unable to restore the molecule and if the cell is still viable, it may be the start of a tumor. To undergo carcinogenic evolution a cell must be capable of successful proliferation and resist immunological and other suppressive reactions by the environment. At this stage, promoting agents will play a crucial role: e.g. by impairment of host defences, by altering the surface membrane, thus facilitating the escape of dormant tumor cells, by causing deficiencies, or by the stimulation of liver cell regeneration.

5. Interference with the blood supply to the hepatocytes

A drug–induced decrease in the blood supply to the hepatocytes may be produced in several ways. There may be occlusion of hepatic vessels, either primary or secondary to hepatic injury. There may however also be a deficit in the blood supply without occlusion, either local (e.g. cirrhosis) or systemic (e.g. cardiac failure, shock). Anoxia occurs especially in the centrilobular area. Since the centrilobular hepatocytes (Zone III, Rappaport) are the last cells to receive oxygen and other nutrients from the blood, they are probably more vulnerable. Moreover, the liver cells in Zones I and II may increase their oxygen uptake and aggravate the oxygen deficit in Zone III.

Some therapeutic agents interfere with hepatic blood flow in a negative way but apparently without adverse effects (e.g. propranolol). It can be hypothesized that such drugs should be used with caution in patients with an already impaired blood supply to the liver, either because of a hypoxic effect or because of a reduction in the hepatic clearance of other drugs.

Congestive heart failure precipitated by a negative effect of drugs on myocardial contractility may theoretically cause hepatic venous congestion. In practice, this will only present a problem when there is already congestive heart failure without use of the drug, in which case administration of a negative inotropic agent is usually avoided.

The following vascular lesions have been associated with the use of drugs. With the exception of veno–occlusive disease the causal relationship varies from the probable to the obscure:

18

The Budd–Chiari syndrome is the result of occlusion of venous outflow. This may be secondary to veno–occlusive disease or to thrombosis of large hepatic veins. The course may be acute or chronic depending upon the degree of occlusion and on the rapidity of its occurrence. Drugs that enhance blood coagulability (e.g. estrogens) have been associated with thrombosis of large hepatic veins. Thrombosis of the portal vein or hepatic artery is rare but has also been associated with the use of oral contraceptives.

Veno–occlusive disease is a non–thrombotic, progressive, concentric occlusion of the small hepatic venules by loose connective tissue, invariably associated in advanced cases with centrilobular necrosis. So far, it seems to be caused almost exclusively by drugs or by radiation. Although the mechanism is unknown, it is thought to be secondary either to venous alteration caused by necrosis around the central vein or to a primary lesion of the vascular wall caused by the drug or one of its metabolites.

Sinusoidal dilatation has been associated with the long–term use of oral contraceptives. Mainly the periportal sinusoids are dilated. It is often asymptomatic and discovered by chance. According to recent experiments in rats receiving estrogens, sinusoidal dilatation predominated in Zone I (Rappaport) whereas the volume of Zone III was decreased. Increased sinusoidal pressure in Zone I following constriction in Zone III was suggested.

Peliosis hepatis There are several hypotheses on the mechanism of peliosis hepatis. First, a selective toxic effect on the sinusoidal wall is supported by an experimental study in rats, fed with oxymetholone, which showed endothelial cell injury. According to a second hypothesis, focal cell necrosis produces a cyst by destruction of the reticular framework which is filled with blood from neighboring sinusoids. Third, raised intrasinusoidal pressure and distension could follow blockage of sinusoidal blood flow due to fibrosis of centrilobular vein walls or to prolapse of hyperplastic hepatocytes into small hepatic veins.

Perisinusoidal fibrosis consists of collagen accumulation in the space of Disse. It is often accompanied by portal and periportal fibrosis. Its mechanism is unknown, but increased synthesis of collagen by Ito cells has been suggested. It produces non–cirrhotic portal hypertension but will ultimately end in cirrhosis.

6. Transmission of infection

It is well known that therapeutic interference may result in the transmission of infectious diseases. Some therapeutic agents may be responsible for the transmission of hepatotropic viruses, especially cytomegalovirus and one or more (?), still undemonstrable, viruses, collectively known as 'non–A, non–B viruses'. Transmission occurs invariably through agents derived from human blood (e.g. clotting factors), in particular the highly concentrated products extracted from the blood of sometimes several thousands of donors. Recent progress in vaccine production by recombinant DNA techniques seems promising in this respect.

7. Aggravation of underlying disease

Some drugs are responsible for the precipitation of hepatic porphyrias, in particular acute intermittent porphyria and porphyria cutanea tarda (e.g. barbiturates, anticonvulsants, sulfonamides). Induction of the enzymes involved in heme synthesis increases the amount of porphyrins and/or their precursors.

A negative effect of drugs on an unstable cardiac function may result in congestive heart failure and hepatic venous congestion, as mentioned above.

Drugs that usually have no adverse effect on hepatic tissues and function may sometimes be harmful when used in a patient with severely impaired hepatic function. Since the spontaneous course of an underlying liver disease often fluctuates, it is difficult to know whether the drug or the underlying disease is responsible for the impairment of liver function.

Immunoregulating agents may have an indirect effect on hepatic tissues. In cases of chronic active viral hepatitis, immunostimulants (e.g. levamisole) may enhance necrosis. Immunosuppressive agents (corticosteroids) decrease the necrosis in chronic active (viral) hepatitis but may facilitate viral replication.

III. DIAGNOSIS AND ANALYSIS OF DRUG–INDUCED HEPATIC INJURY

Roughly speaking, the evaluation of drug–induced hepatic injury occurs in two stages. Firstly, clinical, biochemical and other features of a particular case are gathered and a diagnosis is made. Such a procedure may resemble the algorithm shown in Figure 1. Several analogous diagnostic schemes, however, have been published in the past and since the reader of this book will probably be familiar with the more common diagnostic procedures, this algorithm is not discussed in detail.

Secondly, when several reports of suspected drug–induced hepatic injury incriminate a particular drug, monitoring centers will usually perform an in–depth analysis of such cases. To guarantee a consistent approach to the assessment of a causal relationship between hepatic injury and drug use, an analytical scheme may be used (see Fig. 2). Such an approach may be useful as a tentative strategy for decision–making and categorization. It should be realized, however, that such schemes are based on *current* knowledge and need regular updating. *Moreover, a scheme should never be so rigid or so rigidly interpreted that completely new patterns are discounted as unlikely when these do not conform to current knowledge.*

An explanation of the schema shown in Figure 2 is given below.

AN ANALYTICAL SCHEMA FOR DRUG–INDUCED HEPATIC INJURY

The analytical schema is based on 3 points:
1. *Specificity* of the clinicopathological pattern *and* its course
2. The *temporal relationship* between intake/discontinuation of the suspected drug and onset/disappearance of the hepatic injury
3. The *exclusion of other possible causes* for the observed patterns. This is complementary to the specificity. The less specific a pattern is, the more important does this factor become

The clinicopathological pattern is defined as the combination of clinical, histological, biochemical, immunological, toxicological, experimental and other variables by which the pattern may be specified.

The model assesses the degree of certainty of a causal relationship between hepatic injury and the intake of a drug. There are several levels. A and B (see Fig. 2) represent the highest degree of certainty because of a highly specific pattern/course and course/temporal relationship ('posi-

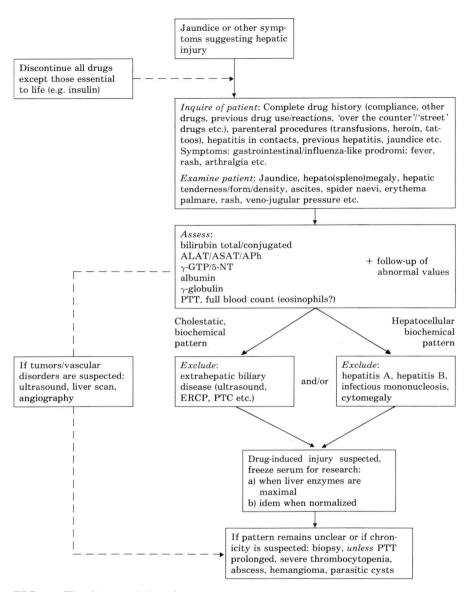

Jaundice or other symp-
toms suggesting hepatic
injury

Discontinue all drugs
except those essential
to life (e.g. insulin)

Inquire of patient: Complete drug history (compliance, other
drugs, previous drug use/reactions, 'over the counter'/'street'
drugs etc.), parenteral procedures (transfusions, heroin, tattoos), hepatitis in contacts, previous hepatitis, jaundice etc.
Symptoms: gastrointestinal/influenza-like prodromi; fever,
rash, arthralgia etc.

Examine patient: Jaundice, hepato(spleno)megaly, hepatic
tenderness/form/density, ascites, spider naevi, erythema
palmare, rash, veno-jugular pressure etc.

Assess:
bilirubin total/conjugated
ALAT/ASAT/APh
γ-GTP/5-NT   + follow-up of
albumin   abnormal values
γ-globulin
PTT, full blood count (eosinophils?)

Cholestatic,   Hepatocellular
biochemical   biochemical
pattern   pattern

If tumors/vascular
disorders are suspected:
ultrasound, liver scan,
angiography

Exclude:
extrahepatic biliary   and/or
disease (ultrasound,
ERCP, PTC etc.)

Exclude:
hepatitis A, hepatitis B,
infectious mononucleosis,
cytomegaly

Drug-induced injury suspected,
freeze serum for research:
a) when liver enzymes are
    maximal
b) idem when normalized

If pattern remains unclear or if chronicity is suspected: biopsy, *unless* PTT
prolonged, severe thrombocytopenia,
abscess, hemangioma, parasitic cysts

FIG. 1 *The diagnostic 'tree'.*

FIG. 2 *Analytical procedure for cases of suspected drug-induced hepatic injury.
If hepatic injury is probably or definitely drug-induced but 2 or more drugs are
equally suspected, a causal relationship* per drug *is possible.*

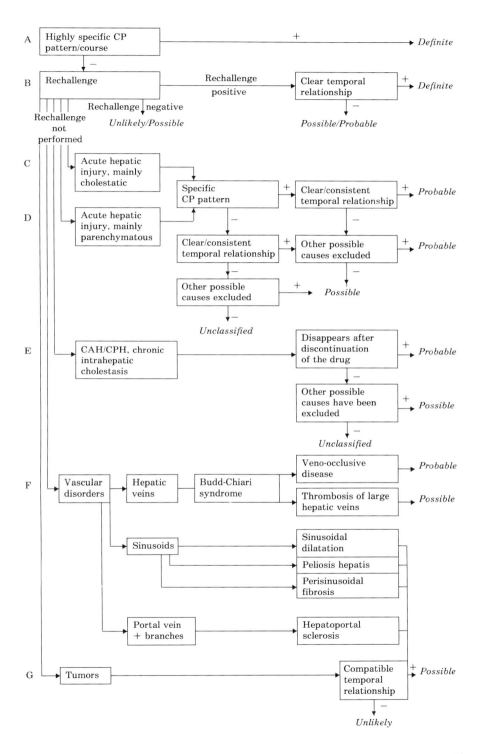

A   Highly specific CP pattern/course   +   → *Definite*

    −

B   Rechallenge   Rechallenge positive   Clear temporal relationship   +   *Definite*

     Rechallenge negative   −

Rechallenge not performed   *Unlikely/Possible*   *Possible/Probable*

C   Acute hepatic injury, mainly cholestatic

Specific CP pattern   +   Clear/consistent temporal relationship   +   *Probable*

    −

D   Acute hepatic injury, mainly parenchymatous

Clear/consistent temporal relationship   +   Other possible causes excluded   +   *Probable*

    −   −

Other possible causes excluded   +   *Possible*

    −

Unclassified

E   CAH/CPH, chronic intrahepatic cholestasis

Disappears after discontinuation of the drug   +   *Probable*

    −

Other possible causes have been excluded   +   *Possible*

    −

Unclassified

F   Vascular disorders   Hepatic veins   Budd-Chiari syndrome

Veno-occlusive disease → *Probable*

Thrombosis of large hepatic veins → *Possible*

Sinusoids   Sinusoidal dilatation

Peliosis hepatis

Perisinusoidal fibrosis

Portal vein + branches   Hepatoportal sclerosis

G   Tumors   Compatible temporal relationship   +   *Possible*

    −

Unlikely

23

tive rechallenge') respectively. This makes it easy to differentiate from non–drug–related causes. C, D, E, F and G represent less certain situations in which the causal relationship is assessed on the basis of a combination of (relative) specificity, temporal relationship and the exclusion of other possible causes. These levels are discussed below.

LEVEL A

A clinicopathological pattern and/or course is highly specific when it has unique features which make it possible to differentiate it from other causes. This may be by demonstration of the responsible agent in toxic amounts or of a unique histological pattern, but also a characteristic course in combination with a proven history of chronic intoxication (Table 1).

LEVEL B

Renewed hepatic injury after (often unintentional) rechallenge. There is an obvious temporal relationship between the intake of the drug and the occurrence of hepatic injury, especially a prompt recrudescence after re-challenge. Between challenge and rechallenge, liver enzyme levels (especially serum aminotransferases) should have returned to normal. The latter is necessary to help differentiate it from fluctuating non–A, non–B viral hepatitis. When a rechallenge is positive but a clear temporal relationship is absent, the causal relationship may be termed 'probable', or 'possible' if it is suspected to be coincidental (e.g. with a flare–up of underlying illness).

A negative rechallenge suggests that a causal relationship is unlikely;

TABLE 1 *Highly specific pattern/course*

Histology	In a certain age-group	Phospholipidosis in adults (e.g. 4,4'-diethylaminoethoxyhexestrol) (Coralgil) (1), amiodarone (31,32)
	Deposits at site of injury	Thorium dioxide (Thorotrast) (33) Polyvinyl pyrrolidone (30)
	Specific combination with extrahepatic lesion	Phenacetin pigmentation (2) and renal papillary necrosis
Demonstrable agent		Toxic blood-levels of hepatotoxins (e.g. paracetamol) (3); residue in stomach of hepatotoxins in combination with a characteristic course (e.g. *Amanita phalloides,* phosphorus, ferrous sulfate poisoning) (4)
Unique course		Well-documented case of prolonged intoxication (e.g. alcoholic hepatitis/cirrhosis)

however, it may be a false–negative because of 'desensitization' (immun-oallergic type), the use of a lower dose (toxic type) or too short a challenge period (metabolic idiosyncratic type). In these cases a causal relationship may still have been present.

LEVELS C AND D

Here, the clinicopathological pattern is called 'specific' when its most characteristic cause is an adverse reaction to a drug. Because a specific pattern does not constitute proof of a drug–induced cause (in which case it would be *highly* specific), it needs a clear or consistent temporal relationship to produce a 'probable' causal relationship. One should realize that the following clinical signs are not specific *per se*, but in combination with hepatic injury and drug use. Moreover, even when the observed pattern is specific for a drug–induced cause, it will remain necessary to exclude other – less likely – causes.

Specific patterns (Levels C and D)

Clinical

Rash and hepatic injury (e.g. allopurinol (5), para–aminosalicylic acid (6))

Rash should *accompany* hepatic injury. The latter is important since rash may be a prodromal sign of viral hepatitis and it subsides when the hepatic injury reaches full expression, i.e. jaundice. In drug–induced injury, however, the rash, when present, remains even after jaundice has appeared. The pattern of rash and serious hepatic injury without an abnormal blood picture and/or preceding pharyngitis is easy to differentiate from infectious mononucleosis. Rash may occur in the immuno-allergic form of drug–induced hepatic injury in adults. In children, this form seems less frequent and, if present, has a wider differential diagnosis.

Peripheral eosinophilia and hepatic injury (e.g. phenytoin (7), erythromycins (8))

Significant eosinophilia of the blood ($\geqq 7\%$ eosinophils) should *accompany* hepatic injury and drug intake and should have been demonstrated on at least 2 successive occasions. This is relatively rare in viral hepatitis and is characteristic of the immunoallergic form of drug–induced injury, especially in combination with a prominently eosinophilic infiltration of the portal area and parenchyma. Helminthic infections should be excluded.

Fever and hepatic injury (e.g. methyldopa (9), nomifensine (10))

Hepatic injury *in combination* with high fever ($> 39°C$) in the absence of sepsis is fairly specific of a drug–induced cause. An elevation in temperature may precede viral hepatitis but is usually mild and it subsides when jaundice appears. Fever should have a close temporal relationship to the intake of the suspected drug and it usually persists even after jaundice appears. There are, of course, other causes to be considered (e.g. acute cholangitis, alcoholic hepatitis).

Hepatic injury and other extrahepatic manifestations

Occasionally, hepatic injury is accompanied by blood disorders (e.g. hemolytic anemia – methyldopa (9), agranulocytosis – chlorpromazine (11)), renal disorders (e.g. methoxyflurane (12)) or pulmonary disorders (e.g. nitrofurantoin (13)), myocarditis (e.g. methyldopa (14)), parotitis (e.g. phenylbutazone (15)), vasculitis (e.g. allopurinol (5)) or Lyell syndrome/Stevens–Johnson syndrome (e.g. ibuprofen (16)).

N.B. A pattern with rash, fever, lymphadenopathy and atypical lymphocytosis seen with some drugs (e.g. sulfasalazine (17), phenytoin (7)) is less specific and should at least be differentiated from infectious mononucleosis.

Histological

Pure cholestasis (e.g. C–17 alkylated steroids (6))

Intrahepatic cholestasis is seen, with bile staining of hepatocytes and bile casts in the canaliculi without parenchymal necrosis/infiltration. There is no portal infiltrate. Cholestasis predominates in the centrizonal area but may extend into the midzonal and periportal areas when the drug is continued. This pattern strongly suggests a drug reaction but may be seen in other conditions (e.g. postoperative cholestasis).

Zonal necrosis

Necrosis predominates in the centrizonal (e.g. paracetamol, CCl_4 (4)), midzonal (e.g. furosemide (31)) or periportal area (e.g. ferrous sulfate (4)) often surrounded by steatosis. There is little (mainly neutrophilic) or no infiltration.

Cholestatic hepatitis with eosinophilic infiltration (e.g. chlorpromazine (18))

The pattern is the same as that of pure cholestasis but with a prominently eosinophilic portal infiltrate and minimal parenchymal inflammation and necrosis. Especially the combination with blood eosinophilia strongly suggests drug–induced cholestasis.

26

Granulomatous hepatitis with eosinophilic infiltration (19)

Portal and/or lobular non–caseating granulomas with a prominently eo-sinophilic infiltrate are fairly specific of a drug–induced cause, especial-ly if combined with peripheral eosinophilia and portal eosinophilic infil-tration. Parasitic diseases should however be excluded. Sarcoidosis and tuberculosis may easily be excluded.

Experimental

Hepatic injury + a positive lymphocyte stimulation test (LST) (20, 22)

The LST usually yields inconsistent results and is insignificant when negative because of many possible interfering factors. However, when a well–performed and controlled LST is positive only if the drug or a meta-bolite is added, it may be regarded as fairly specific. Although a positive LST in this situation only means that the drug is immunologically recog-nized (which may be compatible with almost any immunological form of drug–induced injury), it may be regarded as specific if it is combined with an intake–related course of hepatic injury, especially if the LST becomes negative after recovery. Analogous considerations apply to comparable in–vitro techniques (e.g. leukocyte–migration inhibition)(21).

Hepatic injury + miscellaneous techniques

Less experience has been gained with some newer techniques which promise to develop into specific assessment methods, such as the demon-stration of drug/metabolite–dependent antibodies by indirect immunof-luorescence, drug/metabolite–dependent cytotoxicity assay (23) or possi-bly the demonstration of drug/metabolite in circulating immune–complexes (24) in the serum–sickness–like form of hepatic injury.

Temporal relationship (Levels C and D)

The temporal relationship between the intake of a suspected drug and the onset of hepatic injury should be *obvious,* e.g. promptly after the in-take of toxic agents in overdose and within 6 weeks after initial intake of immunoallergic agents. *Or* the reaction should be *consistent* with a well–known pattern and/or course of the particular drug. Isoniazid, for instance, usually produces hepatic injury after a longer latent period (1 to several months) (25) and the temporal relationship should be compati-ble with this characteristic. The usual onset will depend on the patho-genesis (see Table 2). It is important to emphasize that an usually long latent period does not mean that a causal relationship is unlikely, but merely that the probability is more difficult to establish. In that case, 'probable' may become 'possible' but certainly not 'unlikely'.

Very rapid recovery after discontinuation of the suspected drug strongly favors a drug–related cause. The sudden disappearance of anti-

TABLE 2 *Usual temporal relationship*

1–3 days	Acute toxicity
1–6 weeks	Immunoallergy, metabolic idiosyncrasy
>6 weeks	Metabolic idiosyncrasy, chronic toxicity

gen may even suggest a faster recovery than with non–drug–related causes. Of course, this is not always true since recovery also depends upon regenerative ability, the pharmacokinetics of the drug (some drugs remain in the body for a very long time) and the reversibility of the lesion. Especially jaundice due to prolonged cholestasis may take a long time to disappear.

Exclusion of other possible causes (Levels C and D)

If no specific pattern is present, other possible causes should be excluded. Attention should be paid to the criteria shown in Table 3.

LEVEL E

Disappearance of chronic inflammatory hepatic injury after discontinuation of the suspected drug is highly suggestive of a causal relationship. It constitutes *no proof* because spontaneous remissions may occur (e.g. chronic active hepatitis). No normalization after discontinuation does not prove *the absence* of a causal relationship because the process may be irreversible in some cases and at some stages.

TABLE 3 *Criteria for assessment of cholestatic and parenchymatous patterns of hepatic injury*

Mainly cholestatic pattern
Normal bile ducts, gallbladder and pancreas
No pregnancy, *no* recent operation
No history of cholestasis/jaundice without the use of drugs, *no* underlying liver disease
No malignancy (e.g. Hodgkin's lymphoma!), *no* sepsis, *no* alcohol abuse

Mainly parenchymatous pattern
Viral causes excluded. At least HAV, HBV, Epstein-Barr virus and cytomegalovirus
No lymphadenopathy/lymphocytosis
No recent operation, *no* transfusions, *no* parenteral exposure (e.g. tattoos, heroin), high-risk sexual practice or other suspected exposure to viral hepatitis
No preceding hypotension/cardiac failure
No sepsis, *no* malignancy, *no* underlying liver disease
No alcohol abuse, *no* professional or other exposure to toxic substances (e.g. paraquat, 'glue sniffing')

In cases of suspected drug–induced vascular disorders, the exclusion of other possible causes yields too little additional information to have a decisive effect on the causal relationship, mostly because there are too many unknown factors. Veno–occlusive disease is always chemically induced and/or iatrogenic (e.g. alcoholism (26), pyrrolizidine alkaloids (27), cancer chemotherapy (28), irradiation (29)), so that the causal relationship is always probable.

The causes of large hepatic vein thrombosis, like veno–occlusive disease leading to the Budd–Chiari syndrome, are often unknown and it is therefore impossible to exclude them all.

Both may present acutely or after a prolonged period. Accordingly, the temporal relationship plays a less decisive role in the causality assessment. The other vascular disorders arise largely after long–term use. The temporal relationship between initial intake and appearance should be compatible in these cases. Especially a latent period which is too short (e.g. 1 month) suggests that the abnormalities were already present before the intake of the suspected drug. The same applies to hepatic tumors.

(1) Lüllman et al (1975) *CRC Crit. Rev. Toxicol.*, *4*, 185. (2) Altmann (1982) In: Grosdanoff (Ed), *Zur Problematik der Arzneimittelbedingten Hepatotoxicität*, p 110. Dietrich Reimer Verlag, Berlin. (3) Prescott (1983) *Drugs*, *25*, 290. (4) Zimmerman (1978) *Hepatotoxicity*, p 279. Appleton–Century–Crofts, New York. (5) Al–Kawas et al (1981) *Ann. Intern. Med.*, *95*, 588. (6) Zimmerman (1963) *Ann. NY Acad. Sci.*, *104*, 954. (7) Mullick et al (1980) *Am. J. Clin. Pathol.*, *74*, 442. (8) Funck–Brentano et al (1983) *Gastroentérol. Clin. Biol.*, *7*, 362. (9) Rodman et al (1976) *Am. J. Med.*, *60*, 941. (10) Dankbaar et al (1980) *Ned. T. Geneeskd.*, *124*, 2184. (11) Cheongvee et al (1967) *Br. J. Clin. Pract.*, *21*, 95. (12) Joshi et al (1974) *Ann. Intern. Med.*, *80*, 395. (13) Klemola et al (1975) *Scand. J. Gastroenterol.*, *10*, 501. (14) Seeverens et al (1982) *Acta Med. Scand.*, *211*, 233. (15) Speed (1982) *Aust. NZ J. Med.*, *12*, 261. (16) Sternlieb et al (1978) *NY State J. Med.*, *78*, 1239. (17) Losek et al (1981) *Am. J. Dis. Child.*, *135*, 1070. (18) Ishak et al (1972) *Arch. Pathol.*, *93*, 283. (19) McMaster et al (1981) *Lab. Invest.*, *44*, 61. (20) Namihisa et al (1975) *Leber Magen Darm*, *5*, 73. (21) Vergani (1978) *Lancet*, *2*, 801. (22) Berg et al (1979) In: Eddlestone et al (Eds), *Immune Reactions in Liver Disease*, p 247. Pitman Medical, London. (23) Vergani et al (1980) *N. Engl. J. Med.*, *303*, 66. (24) Wands (panel discussion) (1979) In: Eddlestone et al (Eds), *Immune Reactions in Liver Disease*, p 266. Pitman Medical, London. (25) Mitchell et al (1976) *Ann. Intern. Med.*, *84*, 181. (26) Goodman et al (1982) *Gastroenterology*, *83*, 786. (27) Bras et al (1954) *Arch. Pathol.*, *57*, 285. (28) Zafrani et al (1983) *Arch. Intern. Med.*, *143*, 495. (29) Fajardo et al (1980) *Arch. Pathol. Lab. Med.*, *104*, 584. (30) Kanetaka et al (1973) *Acta Pathol. Jpn.*, *23*, 617. (31) Lim et al (1984) *Br. Med. J.*, *288*, 1638. (32) Poucell et al (1984) *Gastroenterology*, *86*, 926. (33) Salinger et al (1975) *Gastroenterology*, *68*, 799.

IV. INDIVIDUAL AGENTS

INTRODUCTION

The following section of the book provides a review of the clinical experience which has been obtained so far with drug–induced hepatic injury. The data are listed per individual agent.

There are some important points to be made. First, only therapeutically employed agents are discussed which means, for instance, that alcohol–induced hepatic injury is not included. Also, the effects of various experimental hepatotoxins (e.g. thioacetamide, mycotoxins, bromobenzene) are not included. Second, only adverse effects on the liver are included, i.e. signs of injury manifesting clinically, histologically or biochemically. The effects of drugs on enzymes (cytochromes P450 and P448) and their consequences for the metabolism of other exogenous or endogenous substances are mentioned only if considered relevant to a hepatotoxic effect (e.g. rifampicin–isoniazide). Moreover, the hepatic metabolism of drugs in patients with acute or chronic liver disease is considered to be beyond the scope of this book.

The individual agents are divided into therapeutic groups and subdivided therapeutically or chemically, largely according to the *Informatorium Medicamentorum* of the Netherlands Association of Pharmacists who kindly provided the structural formulae. For practical reasons, each drug has been listed only once, although several agents may belong to more than one group. Penicillamine, for instance, is classified in Chapter 2 (Analgesics/Antirheumatics), but is also used as a chelating agent, and phenobarbital, which is listed as a hypnotic, is also used as an anticonvulsant. Each drug, however, can be found in the index at the end of the book.

Chemical structures are included for several reasons, principally because a drug is neither a product name nor a generic name but simply a chemical structure. It is impossible to evaluate adverse effects adequately without paying attention to this aspect. Moreover, even generic names may give rise to serious confusion. This might be expected from different languages, but even within one language (e.g. pethidine, ergometrine and isoprenaline in British English are respectively meperidine, ergonovine and isoproterenol in American English) different generic names are used. This means that attention to the structure is a prerequisite. Most important is the fact that there may be interesting structural analogies between several groups of agents, thereby giving some insight into the expected pattern and mechanism. For instance, isoniazid and the monoamine–oxidase–inhibiting antidepressants are closely similar in their chemical structure. Indeed, their pattern and probably also their mechanism of hepatic injury are very much alike. Another example is the antineoplastic agent, indicine–N–oxide, which, despite the fact that the N–oxides are considered to be less toxic than the pyrroles, may be suspected to cause veno–occlusive disease because it is structurally a pyrrolizidine alkaloid. There are also interesting examples of the opposite. For instance, amineptine, a tricyclic antidepressant, seems to cause more hepatic injury than other tricyclics even though it is not very different in structure. Another example is clometacin, which appears to have led to more reports of hepatic injury in geriatric patients in the French literature than indometacin in the rest of the world despite widespread use. Although one should be careful about the interpretation of case–reports since these do not clarify the incidence, such differences should at least give a strong stimulus to structure–based toxicity research.

Since there is a wide variation in the quality of clinical data, it proved necessary to qualify the probability of a causal relationship between the intake of a drug and the development of hepatic injury. This was done according to the criteria given below (see 'Explanation of Symbols').

Many adverse reactions to drugs in the liver are idiosyncratic. Subtle differences in structure may have serious consequences for the injurious potential of agents within one chemical group, e.g. since seemingly analogous agents are metabolized in a different way – quantitatively or qualitatively – or because they have different antigenic potential. Hence, the causal relationship is based on the *available data per individual agent*. The reader is advised to study not only an individual drug but also the whole group of related compounds, since more data may be available on closely related compounds with which more experience has been gained than with the drug on which information is being sought.

Explanation of symbols regarding the causal relationship

+ + = The drug can *definitely* cause hepatic injury*. Moreover, pattern
and/or frequency are more or less known.
+   = The drug can *definitely* cause hepatic injury*.
o/ + = It is *probable* that the drug may cause hepatic injury*.
o   = None of the above–mentioned qualifications is appropriate. The
causal relationship between hepatic injury and intake of the drug
may range from *possible* via *not impossible* to *unclassifiable*, because of a lack of data. The term *unlikely* or *impossible* is not

---

*Hepatic injury includes symptomless but objective signs of liver involvement, e.g. ALAT/ASAT, bilirubin and APh elevations, in the serum of human subjects treated with therapeutic doses of the drug.

used. For two reasons we consider it unwise to judge the causal relationship between the use of a drug and an unwanted clinical event, reported in the medical literature, as being unlikely or impossible: Firstly, many adverse effects, initially considered as non–drug–related events, have later proved to be caused by drugs. Secondly, a medical doctor who reports a case–history in the medical literature usually has valid reasons for suspecting the drug and for us it is impossible to disqualify at a distance a case as unlikely, i.e. without having seen the patient ourselves.

Comment

The causal qualification 'definite' is used when a well–documented rechallenge – as described in the literature or known to the authors – has demonstrated a causal relationship. When a high frequency of liver enzyme elevations has been observed during a clinical trial, the causal relationship is regarded as 'definite' or 'probable' depending on the quality of documentation and the design of the trial (controls etc.). Less well–documented rechallenges or trials and several well–documented case–histories without rechallenge (but, e.g., with well–performed immunological testing) are considered to indicate a probable causal relationship. Demonstration of hepatotoxicity in animal toxicity tests does not prove a causal relationship between therapeutic drug use and hepatic injury in man, but – if well performed and documented – strengthens the probability of a causal relationship. Since the assessment of the causal relationship between drug intake and hepatic injury may be strongly influenced by the underlying illness (see Section III), this aspect – when relevant – is discussed briefly in each chapter.

Frequently used abbreviations and terms

ASAT = aspartate aminotransferase level in the serum
ALAT = alanine aminotransferase level in the serum
APh   = alkaline phosphatase level in the serum
γ–GT = γ–glutamyl transferase level in the serum
The term 'rechallenge' is used for any readministration, intentional or inadvertent, of the drug.

1. Anesthetics

Introduction

The general effects of a surgical procedure on liver structure and function are minimal in the absence of pre–existing liver disease or operative shock. After major abdominal or thoracic operations, however, transient ASAT/ALAT elevations up to 2–3 times the upper limit of normal may occur within the first 3 days. Serum bilirubin and APh are not significantly elevated (1).

The evaluation of anesthetic–associated liver injury is always complicated by other operative procedures and/or aggravation of underlying illness. These are probably a more frequent cause of severe hepatic injury than the anesthetic agents themselves. The National Halothane Study, for instance, suggested that of 82 cases of histologically confirmed massive hepatic necrosis, 73 could be explained by shock, overwhelming infection, severe and prolonged congestive heart failure or pre–existing liver disease (2). Several causes of postoperative hepatic injury and/or jaundice are listed in Table 1. It is not uncommon for several causes to be acting simultaneously. Moreover, it should be borne in mind that non–anesthetic drugs (e.g. antirheumatics) administered in the weeks before operation may also be responsible for postoperative liver injury.

The hepatic injury caused by anesthetic agents is predominantly hepatocellular. Cholestasis is secondary to cellular injury. Necrosis is centrizonal, although the haloalkanes may also cause a viral–hepatitis–like pattern with diffuse cellular unrest and necrosis.

There are 3 important groups of anesthetics as regards their potential to induce hepatic injury. Firstly, a number of agents with an intrinsic hepatotoxic effect (e.g. CCl_4, $CHCl_3$) may injure the liver when high doses are employed. Their use has been largely abandoned, but they are still used as experimental hepatotoxins in animal studies and cell cultures. Secondly, the haloalkanes (e.g. halothane, methoxyflurane, enflurane) which are widely employed as anesthetics, may cause severe hepatic injury as an idiosyncratic effect, either metabolic or immunoallergic, in a few patients. Mild intrinsic toxicity may be demonstrated in a larger group of patients. There are indications that their potential to induce hepatic injury is related to the extent of their hepatic metabolization: e.g., only 2–3% of enflurane is metabolized as against 15–25% for halothane, and it seems to be less injurious to the liver. Isoflurane, which is not metabolized but is completely expired, has not yet been implicated in unequivocal cases of hepatic injury (3). Thirdly, some agents appear to in-

33

TABLE 1 *Important causes of postoperative liver injury and/or jaundice*

	Usual postoperative latent period		
	1	2	3
Aggravation of underlying illness			
Chronic liver disease	H/M		
Hemolytic anemias	B		
Familial jaundice (e.g. Gilbert's, Dubin-Johnson's syndrome)	B		
Inflammatory bowel disease	M/C		
Congestive heart failure	M		
Operation			
Shock	H		
Transfusions			
Hemolysis (stored blood, artificial valves)	B		
Viral hepatitis			H
Sepsis	M/C		
Trauma			
Hepatic resections	M		
Postoperative pancreatitis	C		
Postoperative cholecystitis	C		
Stricture of bile ducts		C	
Ligation of hepatic artery	H		
Resorption of hematomas		B	
Drugs		H	
Total parenteral nutrition			M/C
Benign postoperative cholestasis	C		

H=mainly hepatocellular pattern (ASAT/ALAT ↑↑, APh ↑, Bil. ↑); C=mainly cholestatic pattern (ASAT/ALAT ↑, APh ↑↑, Bil. ↑↑); M=mixed hepatocellular/cholestatic pattern (ASAT/ALAT ↑ or ↑↑, APh ↑ or ↑↑, Bil. ↑ or ↑↑); B=isolated hyperbilirubinemia (Bil. ↑↑).
1=onset of hepatic injury within the first 3 postoperative days; 2=onset in 3-14 days postoperatively; 3=onset >2 weeks postoperatively.

duce hepatic injury only very rarely or not at all (e.g. ether, nitrous oxide).

Mild liver enzyme elevations or other signs of mild liver injury have been ascribed to several agents, e.g. Althesin (a combination of alfadolone and alfaxalone) (4), ketamine (4, 6), methohexital (7), thiopental sodium (4, 6), etomidate (4) and thiamylal (7). One study noted the highest incidence of abnormalities with Althesin as compared to ketamine, thiopental sodium and etomidate (4).

The mode of administration may be of importance. In a study in children, intravenous administration of succinylcholine was associated with a rise in ASAT/ALAT and LDH, paralleled by a rise in serum myoglobin.

The authors attributed this to muscle damage (5).

Of course, there are also many extrahepatic factors of importance when assessing the risk/benefit ratio of a given anesthetic agent in a given patient, but these are beyond the scope of this book.

(1) Morgenstern (1982) In: Schiff et al (Eds), *Diseases of the Liver, 5th ed*, p 1581. Lippincott, Philadelphia. (2) National Halothane Study (1966) *J. Am. Med. Assoc., 197*, 775. (3) Lewis et al (1983) *Ann. Intern. Med., 98*, 984. (4) Blunnie et al (1981) *Anesthesiology, 36*, 152. (5) Inogaki et al (1983) *Jpn. J. Anesthesiol., 32*, 1079. (6) Dundee et al (1980) *Anesthesiology, 35*, 12. (7) Bittrich et al (1963) *Anesthesiology, 1*, 81.

Bromethol

$CBr_3\text{–}CH_2OH$ *Causal relationship* o/ +

This obsolete anesthetic has been reported to cause hepatocellular injury in both animals (1) and man (2). Its contraindication in cases of underlying liver disease is derived from early studies which showed enhanced sulfobromphthalein (BSP) retention (1, 3). BSP retention is greater when underlying liver disease is present (4).

(1) Bourne et al (1931) *Am. J. Surg., 14*, 653. (2) Little et al (1964) *Anaesthesiology, 25*, 815. (3) Coleman (1938) *Surgery, 3*, 87. (4) Klatskin (1975) In: Schiff (Ed), *Diseases of the Liver, 4th ed*. Lippincott, Philadelphia.

Carbon tetrachloride

CCl_4 *Causal relationship* + +

Formerly used as an anesthetic and vermifuge, CCl_4 is now a standard experimental hepatotoxin. Both animals and man show the same pattern of centrizonal necrosis and surrounding steatosis, the severity of which is dose–dependent. Renal and cardiac failure and pulmonary edema follow hepatic injury within hours or days. For a review, the reader is referred to Zimmerman (1). Despite years of study, the precise mechanism of CCl_4 necrosis remains to be elucidated. Besides covalent binding of CCl_4 cleavage products to cellular constituents, with subsequent lysis, and lipid peroxidation as possible mechanisms, increasing emphasis has been laid in recent years on its disturbing effect on hepatocellular calcium homeostasis (2).

(1) Zimmerman (1978) *Hepatotoxicity*, p 198. Appleton–Century–Crofts, New York. (2) Recknagel (1983) *Trends Pharm. Sci., 4*, 129.

Chloroform

$CHCl_3$ *Causal relationship* + +

Chloroform is an obsolete anesthetic, abandoned in clinical practice because of its toxicity to heart, kidneys and liver. It is still used as an experimental hepatotoxin and, in some parts of the world, for minor procedures. In animals, it causes the same pattern of hepatic injury as in man. Most cases have been reviewed in detail in several textbooks (1, 2). Characteristically, drowsiness and vomiting, followed by jaundice, developed 1–3 days after anesthesia. Convulsions and death due to hepatic or renal failure followed after some days. Histology showed centrizonal necrosis and fatty metamorphosis surrounding necrotic areas. Necrotic cells showed fragmentation and hyaline degeneration. The periportal hepatocytes were reported to remain intact in all cases (1), massive necrosis being absent (2). Fatal cases are overrepresented in the older literature; probably less severe cases remained undetected since sensitive assessment of hepatic injury was impossible at that time. Adults were reported to be more vulnerable than children. Further reported risk factors are multiple exposure (separated by several days only), hypoxia, obesity and high fat or high protein intake. High carbohydrate intake was reported to be a protective factor. The incidence was controversially reported to vary from 1:3500 to 1:30,000, but series of 50,000 chloroform–anesthesias have been reported without hepatic injury. Nevertheless, hepatic toxicity in both animals and man is unequivocal. The drug supposedly acts as a dose–related toxin (1).

(1) Zimmerman (1978) *Hepatotoxicity*, p 370. Appleton–Century–Crofts, New York. (2) Klatskin (1975) In: Schiff (Ed), *Diseases of the Liver, 4th ed*, p 604. Lippincott, Philadelphia.

Cyclopropane

     Causal relationship o

Cyclopropane reduces indocyanine green clearance (1, 2), probably through a change in hepatic blood flow. Only rarely have cases of hepatic injury been ascribed to this anesthetic. One report described 3 cases of hepatitis, with jaundice in 2, within 5 days after anesthesia with cyclopropane. Histology showed a hepatocellular pattern of injury (3). Although generally regarded as being non–toxic to the liver, cyclopropane emerged in the National Halothane Study as the anesthetic with the highest rate of massive hepatic necrosis. This could have been related, however, to the selective use of this agent for patients in shock. It is unknown whether the splanchnic vasoconstriction by this agent increases the probability of shock–induced hepatic injury (4).

(1) Price et al (1965) *Anesthesiology, 26,* 312. (2) Salam et al (1976) *Br. J. Anaesthesiol., 48,* 231. (3) Bennike et al (1964) *Lancet, 2,* 255. (4) National Halothane Study (1966) *J. Am. Med. Assoc., 197,* 775.

Enflurane

$CHF_2-O-CF_2-CHFCl$ *Causal relationship* o/+

Several cases showing a predominantly hepatocellular pattern of injury have been reported (1–12). An extensive review (12) of 24 cases, including literature (1–10), revealed a pattern with striking similarities to halothane(H)– and methoxyflurane(MF)–induced hepatic injury. In 67% there was prior exposure to H, MF or enflurane (E). The mean number of days to the onset of initial symptoms/jaundice was 3/8 after first exposure and 1/6 after multiple exposure. Other signs were fever (79%), eosinophilia (29%), rash (12.5%) and renal failure (12.5%), the latter possibly secondary to hepatic failure (12). The case fatality–rate (21%) seems lower than with H and MF. Biopsy showed necrosis of varying severity, mostly limited to the centrizonal area; ballooning degeneration and steatosis were observed in some cases (12).

The existence of E–induced hepatic injury is still much debated; the problem of evaluation of the cause of hepatic injury in the postoperative period is obvious. The similarity in pattern between H, MF and E favors the existence of E–induced hepatic injury but is no proof. The degree of metabolization (H 25%, MF 50%, E 3%) is possibly related to the potential for causing hepatic injury (12). Ultrastructural signs of toxicity were reported in 1 of 5 patients on E, compared to all of 7 on H, 5 of 6 on fluroxene and 0 of 6 controls (14). A prospective trial showed liver enzyme elevations to be less frequent on E than on H (15).

(1) Van der Reis et al (1974) *J. Am. Med. Assoc., 227,* 76. (2) Sadove et al (1974) *Anesth. Analg., 53,* 336. (3) Denlinger et al (1974) *Anesthesiology, 41,* 86. (4) Tsang (1975) *Ill. Med. J., 148,* 593. (5) Ona et al (1980) *Anesth. Analg., 59,* 146. (6) Kline (1980) *Gastroenterology, 79,* 126. (7) Danilewitz et al (1980) *Br. J. Anaesthesiol., 52,* 1151. (8) Spiegel et al (1980) *Cancer Treatm. Rep., 64,* 1023. (9) White et al (1981) *Dig. Dis. Sci., 26,* 466. (10) Douglas et al (1977) *N. Engl. J. Med., 296,* 553. (11) Mogensen et al (1981) *Ugeskr. Laeg., 143,* 1165. (12) Lewis et al (1983) *Ann. Intern. Med., 98,* 984. (13) Masone et al (1982) *J. Clin. Gastroenterol., 4,* 541. (14) Sindelar et al (1982) *Surgery, 92,* 520. (15) Dundee et al (1981) *J. R. Soc. Med., 74,* 286.

Ether

$C_2H_5-O-C_2H_5$ *Causal relationship* o

Some small studies showed analogous ASAT and/or ALAT elevations after anesthesia with ether and halothane (1, 2), but these were still below the upper range of normal. Ether is probably correctly considered as one of the safest anesthetics as regards the liver.

(1) Scholler et al (1965) *Anaesthesist, 14,* 293. (2) Beckmann et al (1966) *Acta Anaesthesiol. Scand., 10,* 55.

Fluroxene

$$F_3C-CH_2-O-CH = CH_2$$ *Causal relationship* o/ +

Some reports of hepatic injury have suggested the same pattern of centrizonal necrosis as with other haloalkanes (1–3). In one of these cases, massive hemorrhagic centrilobular necrosis was ascribed to the combination of fluroxene with preoperative use of phenytoin and phenobarbital (1); enzyme induction was suggested to be responsible for increased production of a hepatotoxic metabolite (1, 3). That enzyme induction enhances hepatic injury was confirmed in animals (4). Sindelar et al (5) studied pre– and postoperative liver biopsies of patients anesthesized with halothane, fluroxene, enflurane and, as control, a combination of nitrous oxide, fentanyl and thiopental. Five of 6 patients on fluroxene showed toxic changes in more than 25% of cells. In 33% of post–anesthesia cells, as compared to 4% of pre–anesthesia cells, dilatation of both rough and smooth endoplasmic reticulum was seen on electron microscopy. These changes were not present in the control group.

(1) Reynolds et al (1971) *N. Engl. J. Med., 286,* 530. (2) Harris et al (1972) *Anesthesiology, 37,* 462. (3) Tucker et al (1973) *Anesthesiology, 39,* 104. (4) Harrison et al (1973) *Anesthesiology, 39,* 619. (5) Sindelar et al (1982) *Surgery, 92,* 520.

Halothane

$$CF_3-CHClBr$$ *Causal relationship* + +

It is beyond reasonable doubt that halothane can cause hepatic injury. Several cases of recurring jaundice in nurses and anesthetists – directly related to their working situation – are convincing (1–4, 41). This is essential to the causal relationship because in almost every case of halothane hepatitis other postoperative causes of liver injury may be present.

As regards the type of halothane–induced hepatic injury, there are two patterns. It is unclear whether it concerns two types of response or the ends of a continuous spectrum: Firstly, prospective and controlled studies have demonstrated that a relatively large group developed mild to moderate elevations of liver enzymes, mainly serum aminotransferases (5–7). These elevations were symptomless and self–limiting. Repeated exposure resulted in recurrence but not in a more severe reaction (7). Obese persons showed more frequent enzyme elevations (7).

Secondly, a pattern of hepatic necrosis may develop with a high fatality rate. A case fatality rate has been reported ranging from 14% (8) to 71% (9). Inman et al (10) demonstrated a case fatality rate of 35% after 1 exposure rising to 52% after 4 exposures, with an overall rate of 49%. The frequency of this severe type has been estimated at 1:6000–1:20,000 (10) and at 1:7000–1:110,000 (8). There is a female/male ratio of 2:1 (12) and the obese are more likely to develop the reaction (13); children seem less vulnerable (8, 10), but controlled data are lacking. Wark estimated halothane–associated icteric hepatitis at 1:82,000 anesthetized children (37).

Mostly jaundice appears within 14 days after operation. According to a review of 220 cases in the literature (12), approximately 45% occurred between 3 and 7 days, 20% between 8 and 14 days while 10% appeared between 2 and 3 weeks postoperatively. The rest appeared within 2 days postoperatively or later than 3 weeks after operation. In both periods diagnosis is difficult, in the former because of (post)operative complications (e.g. hypoxia, infection) and in the latter because of possible viral infections, transmitted by infusions (e.g. non–A, non–B viral hepatitis). The mean latent period in cases with multiple exposures is shorter than with a single exposure, ranging from 11.4 days after first exposure to 4.1 days after 4 exposures (10).

The incidence of massive hepatic necrosis appeared to increase with multiple exposure (11). Most cases reported in the literature occurred after multiple exposures, varying from 60% (32) to 92% (33) of cases, with a mean of 78% in several studies. In 1 study, 75% of patients were exposed twice or more within 28 days (10). Clinically, jaundice is often preceded/accompanied by fever (75%) and anorexia/nausea (50%); less frequent are chills (30%), myalgia (20%) and rash (10%) (12). Leukocytosis is present in approximately 60%; peripheral eosinophilia has been variously estimated at 20–60% in several studies (12). Histology showed hepatocellular necrosis; according to some authors, the lesion is centrizonal and sharply outlined with scanty infiltration, thereby resembling CCl_4 necrosis (12). Others favor a viral–hepatitis–like pattern with spotty necrosis and mononuclear infiltration in mild cases and (sub)massive necrosis in severe cases (14). Possibly the different patterns reflect different mechanisms of injury, whereby in some cases enhanced production of reductive metabolites produces centrizonal necrosis while others, reacting via an immunoallergic mechanism, develop diffuse necrosis. Chronic active hepatitis and cirrhosis after repeated anesthesia have been noted (35). Granulomatous hepatitis has been reported only rarely (36). Ultrastructural differences with viral hepatitis – mainly concerning mitochondrial damage – were observed by some authors (15, 16), but these results were debatable and were not regarded as significant.

The mechanism of halothane hepatitis has been debated for years. The high incidence of mild enzyme elevation suggests some intrinsic hepatotoxicity, while the rarity of the severe form seems compatible with idiosyncrasy, either metabolic or immunoallergic. Halothane undergoes both oxidative and reductive biotransformation (17). In a 'hypoxic rat model' the usual 3% of reductive metabolism is greatly enhanced by reduced oxygen tension, induction of cytochrome P450, prolonged anesthesia and increased halothane concentration (18). Analogous results were obtained by others (19, 20). Reductive metabolism yields reactive intermediates (e.g. the postulated free radical trifluorochloroethyl) which possibly bind covalently to liver constituents. Histologically, liver cell necrosis was directly related to this induction of reductive metabolism, while cytochrome P450 enzyme inhibition reduced the appearance of liver lesions (18). Animal data cannot be extrapolated without care to man. Nevertheless, the presence of the same enzyme systems in human liver cells and the demonstration of reductive metabolites in plasma and expired air (19) are compatible with the possibility that some genetically vulnerable individuals may form increased amounts of hepatotoxic metabolites and develop hepatic necrosis under adverse circumstances (hypoxia, enzyme induction, prolonged anesthesia with high concentrations of halothane). Indeed, cases of halothane hepatitis in a mother and daughter, 2 sisters and cousins favor genetic vulnerability (21). Studies in rats have also shown genetic differences (22).

Other authors have a different view. Shingu et al (38) suggested that hypoxia per se plays a greater role than the reductive metabolism. Also, Van Dyke et al (39) emphasized the importance of an imbalance of oxygen demand and delivery. They demonstrated that halothane, enflurane, isoflurane, thiopental and fentanyl all caused more centrilobular necrosis in anesthetized rats (10% O_2, 2 h) than in control rats (no anesthesia; 10% O_2, for 2 h). According to the authors, this might have been caused by respiratory depression and a reduction in splanchnic blood flow by anesthesia and is not exclusively caused by halothane (40). However, the fact that even minute amounts in the air of operating theaters suffice to cause hepatitis in healthy medical workers (1–4) strongly suggests that other factors are (co)responsible. Moreover, most cases occur after multiple exposures after shorter latent periods. The presence of a liver–kidney microsomal antibody in 25% of cases (13) suggests sensitization in some of these. In–vitro testing for sensitization to halothane gave conflicting results. Lymphocyte stimulation tests have been positive (23) but mostly negative (24, 25, 34). On the other hand, leukocyte migration inhibition was demonstrated in the presence of halothane in most cases in 2 studies of halothane hepatitis (26, 27). A study with liver homogenate of halothane–pretreated rabbits showed leukocyte migration inhibition in patients whereas there was no reaction in controls (28). A subsequent study with liver cell isolation from pretreated rabbits demonstrated specific antibodies by immunofluorescence; a cytotoxicity assay showed these antibodies to mediate in lymphocyte cytotoxicity (29). These antibodies were not present in patients without abnormalities or in patients with other forms of liver injury and are suggested to be directed against liver membrane components altered by an oxidative metabolite (30). Because these antibodies are of the IgG class, sensitization probably occurred during previous exposure (31). The fact that this antibody was demonstrated in only 50% of patients with massive liver cell necrosis following halothane anesthesia may be explained by the fact that the other half had other possible causes of hepatic injury (31).

(1) Combes (1969) *N. Engl. J. Med., 280,* 558. (2) Klatskin et al (1969) *N. Engl. J. Med., 280,* 515. (3) Belfrage et al (1966) *Lancet, 2,* 1466. (4) Lund et al (1974) *Lancet,*

3, 528. (5) Wright et al (1975) *Lancet, 1,* 817. (6) Trowell et al (1975) *Lancet, 1,* 821. (7) Dundee et al (1981) *J. R. Soc. Med., 74,* 286. (8) Böttiger et al (1976) *Acta Anesthesiol. Scand., 20,* 40. (9) Joshi et al (1974) *Ann. Intern. Med., 80,* 395. (10) Inman et al (1978) *Br. Med. J., 2,* 1455. (11) National Halothane Study (1966) *J. Am. Med. Assoc., 197,* 775. (12) Zimmerman (1978) *Hepatotoxicity,* p 370. Appleton–Century–Crofts, New York. (13) Walton et al (1976) *Br. Med. J., 1,* 1171. (14) Klatskin et al (1975) *Drugs and the Liver,* p 289. Schattauer Verlag, Stuttgart. (15) Klion et al (1969) *Ann. Intern. Med., 71,* 467. (16) Uzunalimoglu et al (1970) *Am. J. Pathol., 61,* 457. (17) Van Dyke et al (1976) *Drug Metab. Disposit., 4,* 40. (18) Sipes (1981) *Drug Reactions and the Liver,* p 219. Pitman Medical, London. (19) Cousins et al (1979) *Anaesthesiol. Intens. Care, 7,* 9. (20) Brown et al (1979) *Anesthesiology, 51, Suppl 239.* (21) Hoft et al (1981) *N. Engl. J. Med., 304,* 1023. (22) Cousins et al (1981) *Br. Med. J., 283,* 1334. (23) Paronetto et al (1970) *N. Engl. J. Med., 283,* 277. (24) Walton et al (1973) *J. Am. Med. Assoc., 225,* 494. (25) Wright (1975) *Br. Med. J., 2,* 69. (26) Jones Williams et al (1972) *Br. Med. J., 4,* 47. (27) Nunez–Gornes et al (1979) *Clin. Immunol. Immunopathol., 14,* 30. (28) Vergani et al (1978) *Lancet, 2,* 801. (29) Vergani et al (1980) *N. Engl. J. Med., 303,* 66. (30) Neuberger et al (1981) *Gut, 22,* 669. (31) Neuberger et al (1983) *Br. J. Anaesth., 55,* 15. (32) Carney et al (1972) *Anesth. Analg. (Cleveland), 51,* 135. (33) Moult et al (1975) *Q. J. Med., 44,* 99. (34) Moult et al (1975) *Br. Med. J., 2,* 69. (35) Kronborg et al (1983) *Digestion, 27,* 123. (36) Shah et al (1983) *Digestion, 28,* 245. (37) Wark (1983) *Anesthesiology, 38,* 237. (38) Shingu et al (1982) *Anesth. Analg. (Cleveland), 61,* 824. (39) Van Dyke (1983) *Clin. Anesthesiol., 1,* 485. (40) Shingu et al (1983) *Anesth. Analg. (Cleveland), 62,* 140. (41) Keiding et al (1984) *Dan. Med. Bull., 31,* 255.

Isoflurane

$CF_3CHCl-O-CHF_2$ *Causal relationship* o

Isoflurane is hardly metabolized and may therefore be a less likely cause of hepatic injury than halothane (1), although it should be realized that relatively few data on safety have been obtained so far with this newer agent. In a study of 6798 patients, 1 case of unspecified postoperative hepatitis occurred in an obese woman with cholecystitis (2). A causal relationship to isoflurane was considered uncertain. Under certain conditions (low O_2 tension, 1.4% isoflurane) ornithine decarboxylase, a sensitive marker of cellular damage, increased in animal tests with isoflurane. Fasted animals exposed to 1.5% isoflurane or enflurane at 10% O_2, developed the same lesions as animals exposed to 0.5% halothane and low O_2 (3).

(1) Lewis et al (1983) *Ann. Intern. Med., 98,* 984. (2) Rehder (1982) *Can. Anaesth. Soc. J., 29,* 544. (3) Van Dyke (1983) *Clin. Anesthesiol., 1,* 485.

Methoxyflurane

$CH_3-O-CF_2-CHCl_2$ *Causal relationship* o/ +

A review of cases of methoxyflurane hepatitis showed that they had largely the same characteristics as halothane (see Table 2). One of the important differences is the renal toxicity of methoxyflurane (2) due to

TABLE 2 *Comparison of features of halothane(H)- and methoxyflurane(M)-associated hepatitis (derived from Joshi et al) (1)*

	H	M
Women	70	67
Prior exposure to H or M	72	54
Fever	75	71
Eosinophilia*	42	38
Rash	7	8
Associated renal disease	0	17
Mortality	71	58

(bar chart with axis 0% — 50% — 100%; legend: □ H, ■ M)

Time to onset fever (days)

	H	M
Total cases	4.1	4.0
Single exposure	6.5	5.5
Multiple exposure	3.0	2.3

Time to onset of jaundice (days)

	H	M
Total cases	7.8	5.8
Single exposure	10.7	8.0
Multiple exposure	6.4	3.5

	H	M
Mean age (yrs)	51	51

* Joshi et al (1) give a percentage of 21 for methoxyflurane. However, 5 of 13 assessed patients had eosinophilia (=38%).

a direct action of the fluoride ion on the renal tubules (3). In fact, this is an important reason for its low popularity nowadays. Several cases of apparent cross–sensitivity between methoxyflurane and halothane have been reported (4–7). Preceding anesthesia with halothane was followed by fever in 4 and hepatitis in 3 patients. Subsequent anesthesia (interval ranging from 11 days to over 3 years) with methoxyflurane resulted in an accelerated reappearance of hepatic injury.

There is probably not much difference from halothane as regards the incidence, but its less frequent use precludes confirmation of this. Nevertheless, occasional cases of methoxyflurane–associated hepatic injury are still reported after its use both as an anesthetic (8, 9) and as an analgesic (10, 11). A peculiar case is that of a gynecologist who repeatedly inhaled a small dose (about 2 ml) almost every day against insomnia (12).

(1) Joshi et al (1974) *Ann. Intern. Med., 80,* 395. (2) Crandell et al (1966) *Anesthesiology, 27,* 591. (3) Tobey et al (1973) *J. Am. Med. Assoc., 223,* 649. (4) Lindenbaum et al (1963) *N. Engl. J. Med., 268,* 525. (5) Judson et al (1971) *Anesthesiology, 35,* 527. (6) Withers (1971) *Am. J. Surg., 121,* 620. (7) Qizilbash (1973) *Can. Med. Assoc.*

J., *108*, 171. (8) Sanchez et al (1980) *Rev. Esp. Anestesiol. Reanim.*, *27*, 481. (9) Zeana et al (1982) *Rev. Roum. Méd.*, *20*, 295. (10) Delia et al (1983) *Int. J. Gynaecol. Obstet.*, *21*, 89. (11) Rubinger et al (1975) *Anesthesiology*, *43*, 593. (12) Okuno et al (1984) *Acta Hepatol. Jpn.*, *25*, 567.

Nitrous oxide

N_2O *Causal relationship* o

This anesthetic has been used for more than a century without being incriminated as a cause of hepatic injury. Although this is not absolute proof, this drug may be regarded as non–toxic to the liver. An occasional case of hepatic injury (1) ascribed to repeated use of this agent may be coincidentally rather than causally related.

(1) Hart et al (1975) *Br. J. Anaesth.*, *47*, 1321.

Thiopental

                                                          Causal relationship +

Hepatic injury after intravenous administration as an anesthetic has been reported only rarely. Occasionally a case of postoperative jaundice has been ascribed to this agent, according to the medical literature. In 1 such case, high fever and jaundice followed operation after 1 day on the 3 occasions that thiopental was used, but not when other anesthetics were used. Biopsy showed slight steatosis and a few areas of focal necrosis (1). See also other barbiturates (Chapter 22).

(1) Hasselstrom et al (1979) *Br. J. Anaesth.*, *51*, 801.

Trichloroethylene

$CCl_2 = CHCl$ *Causal relationship* o/+

Although no longer used as an anesthetic agent, cases of trichloroethylene–induced hepatic injury continue to be reported. It is used as a solvent in spot removers and other cleaning products. Most cases have occurred accidentally (1, 2) or during 'sniffing' (3–6) for their euphoric effect. The pattern of intoxication is largely the same as that of other hydrocarbons such as CCl_4 with neurological, renal and hepatic injury. When used as an anesthetic, however, the incidence is low, possibly because of a more pure form. Indeed, several cases of hepatic and renal injury caused by sniffing were ascribed to 'pollution' with chloroform, CCl_4 and 1,2–dichloroethane (6). Histologically, centrizonal necrosis and

43

steatosis (2, 5), fibrosis (5) and subsequent cirrhosis (1) are prominent after intoxication, either acute or chronic. In some cases, exposure has led to a pattern resembling vinyl chloride disease (7).

(1) Thiele et al (1982) *Gastroenterology, 83,* 926. (2) De Falque (1960) *Clin. Pharmacol. Ther., 2,* 665. (3) Litt et al (1969) *N. Engl. J. Med., 281,* 543. (4) Clearfield (1970) *Dig. Dis. Sci., 15,* 851. (5) Baerg et al (1970) *Ann. Intern. Med., 73,* 713. (6) Conso et al (1982) *Gastroentérol. Clin. Biol., 6,* 539. (7) Rowell (1977) *Practitioner, 219,* 820.

Vinyl ether

$$CH_2 = CH-O-CH = CH_2$$
Causal relationship o/ +

Several cases of massive hepatic necrosis have been ascribed to the use of this anesthetic (1, 2). The picture resembled chloroform–induced hepatic injury. Centrizonal and massive necrosis was also reported in animal toxicity tests in dogs (3, 4) but not in monkeys (4) and depended upon duration of anesthesia, nutritional state and oxygenation. Repeated exposure is suspected to enhance the risk (5).

(1) Little et al (1964) *Anesthesiology, 25,* 815. (2) Schoeffel et al (1965) *South. Med. J., 58,* 198. (3) Orth et al (1940) *Anesthesiology, 1,* 246. (4) Goldschmidt et al (1934) *J. Am. Med. Assoc., 102,* 21. (5) *The Extra Pharmacopoeia, 28th ed,* p 761. Pharmaceutical Press, London, 1982.

2. Analgesics/Antirheumatics

A. Narcotic analgesics
B. Non–narcotic analgesics/antirheumatics
   1. Salicylic acid derivatives
   2. Aniline derivatives
   3. Pyrazole derivatives
   4. Anthranilic acid derivatives
   5. Aryl–alkanoic acid derivatives
   6. Gold compounds
   7. Miscellaneous
C. Drugs against gout

Introduction

Pain, e.g. abdominal pain or headache, may be prodromal symptoms of liver disease. Analgesics used for the relief of such pain may be falsely incriminated as the cause of subsequent hepatic injury.

In the case of antirheumatics there are several factors that should be taken into account. There is more than one relationship between arthritis and liver disease (5). Firstly, arthritis may accompany primary liver disease, e.g. chronic and acute viral hepatitis, hemochromatosis, primary biliary cirrhosis, Wilson's disease. Secondly, in several rheumatoid diseases, the liver may be involved, e.g. rheumatoid arthritis, systemic lupus erythematosus, systemic sclerosis, Felty's syndrome, Still's disease, albeit mildly. Thirdly, intercurrent liver disease may induce remissions in rheumatoid disorders, e.g. rheumatoid arthritis. Fourthly, patients treated for arthritis with analgesics and/or antirheumatics may develop drug–induced hepatic injury. Since several agents are often used concurrently as single drugs or in combination products, the responsibility of one particular agent is often difficult to assess.

It is not known whether drugs potentiate an injurious effect on the liver of underlying rheumatoid disease. Although salicylates have been used as antirheumatics for over a century, comparatively few data are available on serum aminotransferase concentrations in untreated patients with active disease. Since placebo–controlled trials are unethical, one antirheumatic drug always has to be compared with another. In several rheumatoid disorders, high–dose salicylates were associated with an incidence of aminotransferase elevations in up to 70% of cases (1). That

45

TABLE 1 *Probable mechanism of symptomatic hepatic injury by antirheumatics* *

Toxic	Idiosyncratic
Salicylates	Pyrazole derivatives
Anilines (paracetamol)	Anthranilic acids
Pyrazole derivatives (overdosage)	Aryl-alkanoic acids
	Gold compounds
	Most miscellaneous agents

* Several antirheumatics may injure the liver indirectly, e.g. secondary to anaphylactic shock (3) or to aggravation of cardiac failure and hepatic venous congestion due to fluid retention.

these elevations were largely due to salicylates instead of underlying disease was suggested by a double–blind study showing several cases of hepatic injury on aspirin against none on tolmetin in two comparable groups with juvenile rheumatoid arthritis (2). Moreover, up to 30% of patients with non–rheumatoid disease had liver enzyme elevations on high–dose salicylates (1) and a dose reduction in rheumatoid patients led to improvement.

The mechanisms of hepatic injury caused by antirheumatics may differ per group (see Table 1) and data on the adverse hepatic effects of individual agents show a wide variation in quality. Some drugs seem to be incriminated more often than related compounds, e.g. clometacin, although one should be very careful in the interpretation of these data since attention increases recognition and reporting. Despite this variation, it is generally – and probably correctly – assumed that every antirheumatic agent and most analgesics may occasionally cause symptomatic hepatic injury and/or more frequently, non–symptomatic and mild liver enzyme elevations. This applies to the older agents but also to newer ones such as meclofenamate (14), zomepirac (13), isoxepac and amfenac (6), fenoprofen (7) and suprofen (8). Diftalone was withdrawn because of hepatotoxicity and carcinogenicity during toxicological studies (9). Serrapeptase, a proteolytic enzyme used as an anti–inflammatory agent, has been associated with some instances of liver injury with positive lymphocyte stimulation (11) and leukocyte migration inhibition (12) testing.

Narcotic analgesics are almost devoid of adverse hepatic effects, with the exception of dextropropoxyphene which has led to a number of well–documented cases of hepatic injury. Opiates may cause ALAT/ASAT and APh elevations, probably secondary to increased intrabiliary pressure due to spasm of the sphincter of Oddi, although a study in rats suggested that high doses of morphine reduced BSP secretion into bile through a mechanism not involving biliary occlusion (4). We know of 1 case in which a patient immediately responded to several narcotic analgesics, on several occasions, with colicky abdominal pain. Within 12–24 hours liver enzyme elevations followed on each occasion. Porphyria was not present

(10). Unfortunately, the often difficult clinical setting in which these agents are (ab)used (drug abusers, terminal patients) complicates the interpretation of hepatic injury in these patients due to other possible concurrent causes.

Of drugs used in the treatment of gout, allopurinol is the most important, although occasional, cause of hepatic injury. Other agents cause hepatic injury only very rarely when used in therapeutic doses.

(1) Zimmerman (1981) *Arch. Intern. Med., 141,* 333. (2) Levinson et al (1977) *J. Pediatr., 91,* 799. (3) Dux et al (1983) *Br. Med. J., 286,* 1861. (4) Hurwitz et al (1983) *J. Pharmacol. Exp. Ther., 227,* 68. (5) Mills et al (1982) *Ann. Rheum. Dis., 41,* 295. (6) Anonymous (1982) *Scrip, 702,* 9. (7) Danan et al (1984) *Rev. Prat., 34,* 245. (8) Several authors (1983) *Pharmacology, 27, Suppl 1,* 1. (9) Anonymous (1977) *Scrip,* Oct. 15, 22. (10) Van Kersen (1984) Personal communication. (11) Namihisa et al (1975) *Leber Magen Darm, 5,* 73. (12) Morizane (1978) *Acta Hepatol. Jpn., 13,* 281. (13) Ruoff (1980) *J. Clin. Pharmacol., 20,* 377. (14) Lewis (1984) *Clin. Pharm., 3,* 128.

A. NARCOTIC ANALGESICS

Dextropropoxyphene

Causal relationship + +

Jaundice (2–6) or dark urine (1), without (3) or with moderate (1, 2, 4–6) elevation of aminotransferases are consistent with a pattern of cholestatic hepatitis. Less frequently, a mainly hepatocellular pattern is seen (3). Fever (1, 5) and mild eosinophilia (3–5) suggest immunoallergy. Biopsy showed prominent intrahepatic cholestasis without marked necrosis (1, 3). Mild periportal fibrosis after repeated cholestatic bouts has been reported (2).

Rechallenge was positive within 4 days (1–6). In animal toxicity tests, high doses (200 mg/kg) cause ALAT elevations and glutathione depletion (7). Hepatic toxicity in high doses may possibly play some role in drug addicts.

(1) Klein et al (1971) *Dig. Dis. Sci., 16,* 467. (2) Lee et al (1977) *Br. Med. J., 2,* 296. (3) Ford et al (1977) *Br. Med. J., 2,* 674. (4) Van Breukelen et al (1978) *Ned. T. Geneeskd., 122,* 870. (5) Bessard et al (1978) *Nouv. Presse Méd., 7,* 4230. (6) Daikos et al (1975) *J. Am. Med. Assoc., 232,* 835. (7) James et al (1982) *J. Pharmacol. Exp. Ther., 221,* 708.

Nalbuphine

Causal relationship o

A study of 1 week in prior narcotic users (10 mg i.m., 4x daily) showed elevation of ASAT and LDH, conjugated bilirubin and disturbed thymol turbidity (1). The significance of these was questioned because of elevated pre–drug values in most cases (2).

(1) Elliot et al (1970) *J. Med. (N.Y.)*, *1*, 74. (2) Errick et al (1983) *Drugs*, *26*, 191.

Pentazocine

Causal relationship o

A case of cholestatic jaundice was attributed to the intake of pentazocine, with a 'probable' causal relationship (no further specification) (1). Acute intoxication and alcohol abuse was associated with hepatic necrosis (2).

(1) Jick et al (1981) *J. Clin. Pharmacol.*, *21*, 359. (2) Sybirska et al (1980) *Arch. Med. Sadow Kryminol.*, *29*, 309.

Phenoperidine

Causal relationship o

Some cases of cholestatic jaundice have been reported; an in–vitro study showed fatty changes and cell necrosis in cultured human and rat liver cells but not in other cell types (1).

(1) Bewley (1975) In: Dukes (Ed), *Meyler's Side Effects of Drugs, 8th ed*, p 139. Excerpta Medica, Amsterdam.

48

B. NON–NARCOTIC ANALGESICS/ANTIRHEUMATICS

B.1. SALICYLIC ACID DERIVATIVES

Benorilate

Causal relationship +

Benorilate is an ester of paracetamol and acetylsalicylic acid. Salicylism can occur at lower–than–usual total plasma salicylate concentrations, possibly due to interference by benorilate with the binding of salicylate to plasma proteins (1). There are obvious reasons for caution with this type of combination product, which does not have any therapeutic advantage over the individual compounds. Occasional cases of hepatic injury (2, 3) were described with a pattern of injury resembling that of paracetamol rather than that of salicylates, with extensive centrizonal necrosis and minimal infiltration. In a 3–year–old child the paracetamol and salicylate levels were 11 and 35 mg/100 ml, respectively, after a dose increase to 8 g/d. The boy died due to massive necrosis (3). In another case, centrilobular hepatocellular damage after 21 weeks of treatment with benorilate (190 mg/kg/d) and penicillamine was thought to be secondary to an interactive effect on hepatic cysteine (2).

(1) Vanecek (1980) In: Dukes (Ed), *Meyler's Side Effects of Drugs, 9th ed,* p 123. Excerpta Medica, Amsterdam. (2) Sacher et al (1977) *Lancet, 1,* 481. (3) Symon et al (1982) *Lancet, 2,* 1153.

Diflunisal

Causal relationship o

Cholestatic jaundice appeared after 5 days of treatment with diflunisal. Biochemical values suggested a mild hepatitis with a mixed pattern. There was complete resolution in 2 months after discontinuation (1).

(1) Warren (1978) *Br. Med. J., 2,* 736.

Salicylates

Causal relationship +

All salicylates are treated as one group since there is no unequivocal evidence that they have a different tendency to cause liver injury. Most experience has been acquired with acetylsalicylic acid.

Most case–histories of hepatic injury have been recently reviewed (13). There was mostly a mild, often symptomless, hepatocellular pattern of injury; in the majority of cases, serum aminotransferase levels remained below 10x the normal value. Jaundice is rare. In cases where biopsy had been performed, there was mainly focal necrosis, ballooning and degeneration of hepatocytes. Portal and periportal inflammation may be present. Chronic–active–hepatitis–like patterns have been observed. In these cases, discontinuation resulted in improvement or normalization (10, 14, 15).

A high incidence of serum liver enzyme elevations is seen in salicylate–treated patients with connective tissue diseases, e.g. rheumatoid arthritis (11), especially the juvenile form (2, 3, 5, 7–9), rheumatic fever (1, 3, 4) and systemic lupus erythematosus (SLE) (11, 12). It appears to be a dose–dependent type of hepatic injury; discontinuation (3, 12) or reduction (2, 3, 32) of the dose resulted in recovery, although the latter may occur despite continuation at the same dose (5). A correlation between serum aminotransferase levels and salicylate blood level has been observed on several occasions (4, 7, 8). A higher incidence of ALAT/ASAT elevations seems to occur in active juvenile rheumatoid arthritis (7) and SLE (11) than in the inactive form, even at the same salicylate blood level (11). That the underlying illness also plays an important role is illustrated by the fact that untreated patients may also have elevated aminotransferase levels (8, 9). Although there is no absolute margin of safety, 90% of the cases occur at blood levels above 15 mg/100 ml (13). Special attention to age, in 2 studies, demonstrated a higher incidence of aminotransferase elevation in young children, possibly due to a relatively high dose (7, 8). Gitlin (4) observed an inverse relationship between serum ASAT and albumin levels and recommended monitoring of liver enzyme concentrations when albumin is below 35 g/l and the salicylate level exceeds 15 mg/100 ml. These data obviously suggest a toxic mechanism. Immunoallergic signs are almost invariably absent. Eosinophilia seen in 2 studies (16, 17) has not been confirmed by others.

A more controversial issue is the role of salicylates in the development of Reye's syndrome (RS). Since salicylate intoxication (SAL) may mimic RS and may occur in a similar clinical setting (18), a confusing situation may arise. In both cases, vomiting, convulsions, coma, respiratory alkalosis, metabolic acidosis, hypoglycemia and hypoprothrombinemia may be prominent. Microvesicular steatosis, glycogen depletion of hepatocytes without significant necrosis/inflammation and cerebral edema may be present in cases of SAL (18), but it is not clear whether fatty degeneration of other visceral organs, as seen in RS (26), also occurs. Moreover, patients with RS had much lower salicylate blood levels on admission than those with SAL and they showed panlobular fine droplet vacuolization while cases of SAL showed periportal and midzonal mixed droplet vacuolization (31). These studies are small, however, and more histological data will be needed to ensure that the liver histology is really different. Extremely elevated blood levels of ammonia, common in RS, are unusual in SAL (27). Three epidemiological (case–controlled) studies (19–21) demonstrated a higher prevalence of salicylate use in patients with RS than in controls matched for age, sex and race (20, 21), school grade (21), nature of preceding illness (19–21) and febrile response (21). These studies were heavily debated in several medical journals because of potential confounding factors (e.g. 'recall bias'), summarized by Daniels et al (23). Another study of 130 biopsy–proven cases of RS demonstrated a higher serum salicylate level than in varicella controls (22). Partin et al (22) ascribed this to excessive doses or diminished excretion. The latter possibility was confirmed by Rodgers (29), whose method, however, has been criticized (30). Although the end to the RS debate is not yet in sight, it would seem advisable to avoid salicylates in children with influenza or varicella, e.g. by use of other antipyretics or cold sponges. In a recent report (28) of RS, associated with long–term aspirin therapy for connective tissue disease in 2 patients, the causal role is difficult to assess. Both patients had had symptoms of respiratory tract infection in the preceding 2 weeks before they developed the syndrome, which could be compatible with a viral etiology.

(1) Manso et al (1956) *Proc. Soc. Exp. Biol. Med., 93*, 84. (2) Russell et al (1971) *Br. Med. J., 2*, 428. (3) Iancu (1972) *Br. Med. J., 2*, 167. (4) Gitlin (1980) *J. Clin. Gastroenterol., 2*, 281. (5) Athreya et al (1975) *Arthritis Rheum., 18*, 347. (6) Athreya (1976) *Am. J. Dis. Child., 130*, 676. (7) Miller et al (1976) *Arthritis Rheum., 19*, 115. (8) Bernstein et al (1977) *Am. J. Dis. Child., 131*, 659. (9) Rachelefsky et al (1976) *Pediatrics, 58*, 730. (10) Seaman et al (1974) *Ann. Intern. Med., 80*, 1. (11) Seaman et al (1976) *Arthritis Rheum., 19*, 155. (12) Travers et al (1978) *Br. Med. J., 2*, 1532. (13) Zimmerman (1981) *Arch. Intern. Med., 141*, 333. (14) Okumura et al (1965) *Nippon Rinsho, 23*, 1633. (15) Schaffner (1976) In: *Chronic Hepatitis. Proceedings, International Symposium on Problems of Chronic Hepatitis*, p 156. Karger, Basel. (16) Rich et al (1973) *Arthritis Rheum., 16*, 1. (17) Gitlin et al (1977) *S. Afr. Med. J., 51*, 697. (18) Starko et al (1983) *Lancet, 1*, 326. (19) Starko et al (1980) *Pediatrics, 66*, 859. (20) Halpin et al (1982) *J. Am. Med. Assoc., 248*, 687. (21) Waldman et al (1982) *J. Am. Med. Assoc., 247*, 3089. (22) Partin et al (1982) *Lancet, 1*, 191. (23) Daniels et al (1983) *J. Am. Med. Assoc., 249*, 1311. (24) Levinson et al (1977) *Pediatr. Pharmacol., 91*, 799. (25) Daugherty et al (1982) *Hepatology, 2*, 709. (26) Reye et al (1963) *Lancet, 2*, 749. (27) Conn et al (1979) *The Hepatic Coma Syndrome and Lactulose*. William and Wilkins, Baltimore. (28) Young et al (1984) *J. Am. Med. Assoc., 251*, 754. (29) Rodgers et al (1982) *Lancet, 1*, 616. (30) Andresen et al (1982) *Lancet, 1*, 903. (31) Daugherty et al (1983) *Lancet, 2*, 104. (32) Hamdan et al (1983) *Ann. Trop. Paediatr., 3*, 89.

B.2. ANILINE DERIVATIVES

Paracetamol (acetaminophen)

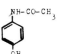

Causal relationship + +

Paracetamol is one of the few proven hepatotoxins still extensively available 'over the counter' for systemic use. Morbidity, however, does not seem to be so high as was previously thought. Two studies in overdosed patients who did not receive specific therapy revealed severe poisoning in only 16% (1, 2). Subsequent severe liver damage occurred in half of this group. Death due mostly to hepatic failure occurred in 0.8 and 3.5%, respectively (1, 2). With some exceptions (see below) therapeutic doses do not cause hepatic damage. In a comprehensive article, Prescott reviewed current knowledge on paracetamol intoxication (1). Acute overdosage (> approx. 125 mg/kg) (20) is mostly followed by nausea and vomiting, starting within 2–24 hours after ingestion (Phase 1). Hepatomegaly and abdominal pain follow, mostly accompanied by aminotransferase elevations and jaundice, usually 1–3 days after ingestion (Phase 2). In some patients, this may progress to hepatic failure with encephalopathy, hypotension, hypoglycemia and coagulation disorders (Phase 3). Cerebral edema may develop in this phase. Central nervous system depression in Phase 1 may be ascribed to concurrent drug inges-

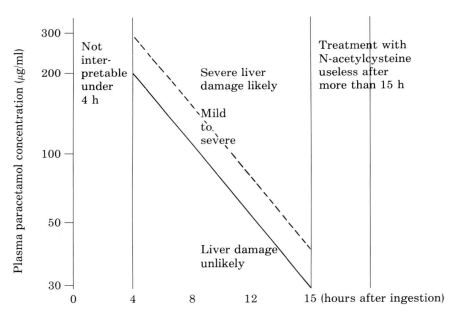

FIG. 1 *Nomogram according to Prescott (1). Relationship between plasma concentration, time after paracetamol overdosage and liver damage. Treatment with N-acetylcysteine according to treatment regimen (shown in Table 2) is indicated above the solid line joining 200 μg/ml at 4 hours and 30 μg/ml at 15 hours (1). Although low plasma concentrations are not interpretable under 4 hours after ingestion, high levels are of course an indication for treatment. It should be emphasized that other authors favor treatment up till 24 hours after ingestion (30). Unfortunately, it is often impossible to know the exact time of intake and the overdose may have been ingested over a period of several hours.*

TABLE 2 *Regimen of intravenously administered N-acetylcysteine (according to Prescott (1))*

N-Acetylcysteine dose (mg/kg)*	Volume of 5% dextrose**	Duration of infusion
150	200	15 min
50	500	4 h
100	1000	16 h

* Total dose 300 mg/kg in 20 h 15 min.
** Reduced in proportion to body weight in children.
150 mg/kg/15 min is followed by 50 mg/kg/4 h and subsequently
100 mg/kg/16 h.

tion, e.g. alcohol, dextropropoxyphene or barbiturates, especially since the half–life of these drugs may be prolonged. Acute renal failure occurs in approximately 10% of severely poisoned patients, usually in association with terminal liver damage, but occasionally without apparent hepatic failure (3–5). In non–fatal cases, recovery is mostly rapid and complete in several weeks. Histology in severe cases shows extensive centrilobular necrosis with reticular collapse and usually little cellular infiltration. Periportal cells are preserved. Children are probably less vulnerable (6, 7), although individual cases have been reported, including 1 case of a neonate whose mother had taken an overdose followed by delivery (8). Although acute alcohol abuse may possibly decrease the chance of liver damage by microsomal enzyme inhibition, as demonstrated in rats (9), long–term intake increases vulnerability (1, 25). Therapeutic doses of paracetamol in patients with chronic liver disease seem to be harmless (24).

The mechanism has been studied extensively during the past decade. Paracetamol is mainly conjugated with sulfate or glucuronic acid. A small proportion is converted to a reactive metabolite which is conjugated with glutathione and ultimately excreted as mercapturic acid and cysteine conjugates (10). In overdose, the amount of toxic intermediate is increased beyond the available tissue level of glutathione, and damage ensues, possibly due to arylation or lipid peroxidation and subsequent increased Ca^{2+} permeability (11).

In the early period after intoxication, i.e. the first 4 hours, gastric aspiration and lavage is important (1). Within the first hour, activated charcoal and cholestyramine may reduce absorption (12). Forced diuresis does not enhance elimination and is contraindicated (1). The treatment of choice is intravenously administered N–acetylcysteine within 10 hours of ingestion, in patients with plasma paracetamol concentrations above the 'treatment line' of the nomogram (see Fig. 1 and Table 2). After 10 hours this treatment is less useful, but some effect may be expected if given within 15 hours (1). According to Rumack et al (30), however, treatment may show some effect even when administered as late as 24 hours after ingestion. The value of charcoal hemoperfusion is controversial since it may be harmful and has not yet proved its value (29). If a patient presents in time, N–acetylcysteine is sufficient. In late cases, it is of dubious value because liver damage starts early.

The role of cimetidine, as an inhibitor of mixed–function oxidases, is still controversial. Critchley et al (21) found no effect on the metabolism of paracetamol, suggesting no protective effect. However, this study was performed in normal volunteers, which clearly differs from the clinical setting of intoxication. Moreover, animal testing demonstrated a protective effect (22, 23, 27). To a lesser extent this was also the case with ranitidine (28).

Besides the well–known 'intoxication pattern', several cases have been reported of hepatic injury during use of (high) normal doses (13–19, 20, 26). If intake–histories are reliable, it could mean that some individuals experience an idiosyncratic reaction, i.e. either metabolic or immunoallergic. All patients, except one, recovered/improved after discontinuation. In 2 cases a rechallenge was clearly positive (14, 16); in some cases mild liver enzyme elevation recurred (15, 25). In some cases a pattern of chronic hepatitis appeared on biopsy (14, 15, 26), whereas in 1 patient cirrhosis was detected after 12 years of daily treatment with paracetamol (20). One patient with acute psittacosis died after ingestion of 5 g/d for 2 days (19); autopsy showed central necrosis and the authors suggested an additive effect.

(1) Prescott (1983) *Drugs, 25,* 290. (2) Hamlyn et al (1978) *Postgrad. Med. J., 54,* 400. (3) Cobden et al (1982) *Br. Med. J., 284,* 21. (4) Emkey et al (1982) *J. Am. Med. Assoc., 247,* 55. (5) Jeffery et al (1982) *Am. J. Hosp. Pharm., 38,* 1355. (6) Meredith et al (1978) *Br. Med. J., 2,* 478. (7) Peterson et al (1981) *Arch. Intern. Med., 141,* 390. (8) Lederman et al (1983) *Arch. Dis. Child., 58,* 631. (9) Sato et al (1980) *Pharmacologist, 22,* 227. (10) Mitchell et al (1973) *J. Pharmacol. Exp. Ther., 187,* 185. (11) Mitchell et al (1981) In: *Drug Reactions and the Liver,* p 130. Pitman Medical, London. (12) Dordoni et al (1973) *Br. Med. J., 3,* 86. (13) Rosenberg et al (1977) *Ann. Intern. Med., 88,* 129. (14) Johnson et al (1977) *Ann. Intern. Med., 87,* 302. (15) Bonkowsky et al (1978) *Lancet, 1,* 1016. (16) Barker et al (1977) *Ann. Intern. Med., 87,* 299. (17) Olsson (1978) *Lancet, 2,* 152. (18) Licht et al (1980) *Ann. Intern. Med., 92,* 511. (19) Davis et al (1983) *Am. J. Med., 74,* 349. (20) Itoh et al (1983) *Hepato–Gastroenterology, 30,* 58. (21) Critchley et al (1983) *Lancet, 1,* 1375. (22) Donn et al (1982) *Clin. Pharmacol. Ther., 31,* 218. (23) Abernethy et al (1982) *Clin. Pharmacol. Ther., 31,* 198. (24) Benson (1983) *Clin. Pharmacol. Ther., 33,* 95. (25) Walker et al (1983) *Toxicology, 28,* 193. (26) De Santa Maria et al (1983) *Rev. Clin. Esp., 168,* 355. (27) Mitchell et al (1981) *Gastroenterology, 81,* 1052. (28) Speeg et al (1984) *Ann. Intern. Med., 100,* 315. (29) Todd (1984) *Lancet, 1,* 331. (30) Rumack et al (1981) *Arch. Intern. Med., 141,* 380.

Phenacetin

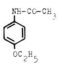

Causal relationship o

Phenacetin is practically non–toxic to the human liver, even after a large overdose (1), although it is partly metabolized to paracetamol, a notorious hepatotoxin. One unspecified case of liver injury with a positive lymphocyte stimulation test (2) may be compatible with rare immunoallergic reactions. However, it should be emphasized that it is difficult to prove or disprove hepatotoxicity in man since phenacetin has been used almost exclusively in combination products. Regular intake may cause lipofuscin deposits in the hepatocytes (3, 4).

(1) Zimmerman (1978) *Hepatotoxicity,* p 544. Appleton–Century–Crofts, New York. (2) Namihisa et al (1975) *Leber Magen Darm, 5,* 73. (3) Abrahams et al (1964) *Lancet, 2,* 621. (4) Faravelli et al (1983) *Pathologica, 75,* 735.

B.3. PYRAZOLE DERIVATIVES

Feprazone

Causal relationship o

Two cases of jaundice, starting 2–4 weeks after initial intake, resolved in 6 weeks after discontinuation (1). Biochemically, a cholestatic and a hepatocellular pattern was seen. Biopsy showed portal and parenchymatous histiocytic granulomas with scanty lymphocytic and eosinophilic infiltration in the former, portal and pericentral infiltration without significant necrosis in the latter.

(1) Wiggins et al (1981) *Rheumatol. Rehabil., 20,* 44.

Kebuzone (ketophenylbutazone)

Causal relationship o/ +

A study of 12 cases (11 females, 1 male) was reported; onset in all cases was with fever and chills, within 4 weeks after first intake. Jaundice developed in 5 cases, eosinophilia in 4. Rash was not mentioned. Normalization occurred within 35 days after discontinuation. Cholestatic hepatitis as well as hepatocellular and mixed patterns were observed, confirmed by biopsy (1).

In 1 clinical trial (6 months) 20 of 75 patients had elevated serum levels of APh or ALAT/ASAT, especially in the first 4 weeks. These were often transient. Two of them developed jaundice (2).

(1) Porst et al (1978) *Dtsch. Gesundheitsw., 33,* 1181. (2) Gibson et al (1971) *Clin. Trials J., 3,* 27.

Mofebutazone

Causal relationship o

A hepatocellular pattern of injury was reported in a patient with rheumatoid arthritis treated with mofebutazone and hydroxychloroquine (1). Biopsy 2 years later showed cirrhosis. No further details were given.

(1) Bjorneboe et al (1967) *Acta Med. Scand., 182, Fasc. 4,* 491.

Oxyphenbutazone

Causal relationship o/ +

Oxyphenbutazone is a hydroxylated metabolite of phenylbutazone. It has the same adverse reaction profile as the latter. Several reports mention hepatic injury (1–4), sometimes even fatal (2), but unfortunately none of these cases has been described in detail. In 1 report, however, a patient with Still's disease was described who developed agranulocytosis, thrombocytopenia, jaundice, fever and convulsions after 3–4 weeks of treatment with oxyphenbutazone. At necropsy, diffuse hepatic necrosis was found (6). A lymphocyte stimulation test was negative with the drug (4) but positive in a patient with hepatitis caused by dipyrone (novaminsulfon), a related pyrazole derivative (4). In another study, the lymphocyte stimulation test was positive with metabolite–containing serum (3). Histology showed non–specific hepatitis without cholestasis (1). Granulomatous hepatitis has also been reported with oxyphenbutazone (5).

(1) Popper et al (1965) *Arch. Intern. Med., 115,* 128. (2) Cuthbert (1974) *Curr. Med. Res. Opin., 2,* 12. (3) Namihisa et al (1975) *Leber Magen Darm, 5,* 73. (4) Kato et al (1979) *Gastroenterol. Jpn., 14,* 216. (5) Ludwig et al (1983) *Dig. Dis. Sci., 28,* 651. (6) Gaisford (1962) *Br. Med. J., 2,* 1517.

Phenazone (antipyrine)

Causal relationship o

Since phenazone is metabolized primarily in the liver by the microsomal

56

mixed–function oxidase system, it has been widely used for drug metabolism studies. Changes in its half–life in the body are used as a test of the
effect of other drugs on the activity of hepatic drug–metabolizing enzymes. As an agent for the prevention of neonatal jaundice, its use is still
experimental (1). Phenazone–induced hepatic injury is seldom reported.
In 1 such case, jaundice coincided with fever, rash, leukocytosis and hy-
pergammaglobulinemia. An unspecified phenazone–antibody was found
in the serum by passive hemagglutination. Biopsy showed cholestasis
with follicular infiltration of lymphocytes in the portal triads (2). The
structurally related compound, aminophenazone, has been associated occasionally with intrahepatic cholestasis, as noted in a 12–year–old girl
with agranulocytosis (3).

(1) Lewis et al (1979) *Lancet, 1,* 300. (2) Kanetaka et al (1973) *Acta Pathol. Jpn.,*
23, 617. (3) Scholz et al (1972) *Dtsch. Gesundheitswes., 27,* 205.

Phenopyrazone

Causal relationship o/ +

Phenopyrazone is part of a mixture of horse chestnut and plant glycos-
ides (Venocuran) which was held responsible for over 100 cases of pseu-
dolupus syndrome, mainly in the Federal Republic of Germany and Switzerland (1, 2). Fever and pulmonary, cardiac and musculoskeletal
symptoms predominated. In some cases a reactive hepatitis with periportal round–cell infiltration was seen (3); a lymphocyte stimulation test
with metabolite–containing serum was positive (3). Phenopyrazone
seems to be responsible (3, 4). Antimitochondrial antibodies are present
in a high percentage (1) and are of the M_3–type (4).

(1) Guardia et al (1977) *Nouv. Presse Méd., 6,* 2873. (2) Walli et al (1981) *Schweiz.*
Med. Wochenschr., 3, 1398. (3) Berg et al (1979) In: *Immune Reactions in Liver Dis-*
ease. Pitman Medical, London. (4) Berg et al (1981) In: Davis et al (Eds), *Drug*
Reactions and the Liver, p 105. Pitman Medical, London.

Phenylbutazone

Causal relationship +

There are two mechanisms by which phenylbutazone may injure the liver. Firstly, intoxication, often reported in young children, is associated
with bone marrow depression, duodenal perforation, renal failure, acido-

57

sis, convulsions, coma and jaundice with hepatocellular injury (1–3). Secondly, when taken in therapeutic doses, the drug is occasionally associated with an idiosyncratic type of hepatic injury. A review of the literature and a study of 23 cases were made by Benjamin et al (4). In 67 and 70%, respectively, hepatic injury appeared within the first 6 weeks of therapy. Hypersensitivity signs (fever and/or rash) were present in 50 and 48%, respectively. There was no sex preponderance. In 28 and 22% the reaction was fatal. Histopathology in the 23 cases revealed moderate to marked hepatocellular injury in 14 cases, 4 of whom had spotty panlobular changes (ballooning, acidophilic bodies, focal necrosis) and 10 severe centrilobular necrosis (some with bridging). Nine of the 14 cases had moderate to marked cholestasis. The remaining patients had non–caseating granulomas, mainly portal/periportal, composed of epithelioid or giant cells with a predominantly eosinophilic infiltrate in 5 patients. In 1 patient the pattern was indistinguishable from primary biliary cirrhosis.

More recent reports largely confirm the above–mentioned features. Romeo et al (5) described a generalized hypersensitivity reaction with granulomas, while in the case of Van der Merwe et al (6) a causal relationship between the intake of phenylbutazone and intrahepatic cholestasis was proven by a prompt reaction to rechallenge. Speed et al (7) described 7 patients with a generalized systemic reaction with parotitis/sialadenitis, fever, rash, conjunctivitis, pericarditis, pleurisy and jaundice or mild hepatic enzyme elevation. The reaction started after 1–2 weeks of therapy and was firstly ascribed to mumps.

Although intrinsic toxicity seems to play an important role in overdosage, the second type clearly shows immunoallergic signs, although not in every patient. It seems possible that in these cases an immunoallergic reaction superimposed on a mild intrinsic toxic effect predominates. A positive patch test (8) suggests a delayed type of reaction in some cases. Bien (9) demonstrated that pyrazole derivatives may decrease the reduced glutathione content in the liver of rats and suggested that this might be one of the primary events in the development of liver damage.

(1) Svihovec (1980) In: Dukes (Ed), *Meyler's Side Effects of Drugs, 9th ed*, p 141. Excerpta Medica, Amsterdam. (2) Prescott et al (1980) *Br. Med. J., 281*, 1106. (3) Berlinger et al (1982) *Ann. Intern. Med., 96*, 334. (4) Benjamin et al (1981) *Hepatology, 1*, 255. (5) Romeo et al (1981) *Progr. Med., 37*, 674. (6) Van der Merwe et al (1981) *Digestion, 22*, 317. (7) Speed et al (1982) *Aust. NZ J. Med., 12*, 261. (8) Goldstein (1963) *Ann. Intern. Med., 59*, 97. (9) Bien (1983) *Biomed. Biochim. Acta, 5*, 561.

B.4. ANTHRANILIC ACID DERIVATIVES

Mefenamic acid

Causal relationship o

One report has been made of 9 cases of severe bridging necrosis of which 1 was caused by mefenamic acid. Recovery was uneventful. Eight cases were confirmed by rechallenge, one by in–vitro testing. No further details were given (1).

(1) Imoto et al (1979) *Ann. Intern. Med., 91,* 129.

Nifluminic acid

Causal relationship +

Acute hepatitis with biochemical evidence of a mixed pattern of hepatic injury was reported in a patient with rheumatoid arthritis. Onset occurred within 3 days of therapy, recovery in 2 weeks after discontinuation. A rechallenge was followed by a relapse within 24 hours (1). Another case was mentioned by Danan et al (2); a rechallenge was positive in this case, but no further details were given (2).

(1) Van Berge Henegouwen et al (1974) *Ned. T. Geneeskd., 118,* 1229. (2) Danan et al (1984) *Rev. Prat., 34,* 245.

Tolfenamic acid

Causal relationship o/ +

A case has been described of hepatocellular injury starting insidiously in the first 6 months of therapy and disappearing after discontinuation. Readministration was followed by a relapse. Biopsy showed 'piecemeal' necrosis but also intralobular, focal and confluent necrosis, with portal infiltration (1). Danan et al (2) briefly mentioned 1 case with a relapse after readministration.

(1) Mickley et al (1981) *Ugeskr. Laeg., 143,* 2036. (2) Danan et al (1984) *Rev. Prat., 34,* 245.

B.5. ARYL–ALKANOIC ACID DERIVATIVES

Benoxaprofen

$$HOOC-\underset{\underset{CH_3}{|}}{CH}-$$

Causal relationship o/ +

The pattern, as reported in the medical literature, is mainly that of cholestatic hepatitis (1–5, 8) and renal failure; occasionally a hepatocellular pattern predominates (6). It has been reported almost exclusively in women over 60 (1–3, 5, 6) with rheumatoid arthritis (2, 3, 5, 6) or osteoarthritis (1, 2). There is a high fatality rate (1–6). Jaundice is seen after a mean treatment period of 5 months (range 1.5–12 months). Immunoallergic signs were absent. Biopsy showed severe hepatocellular/canalicular cholestasis, mild cellular degeneration/necrosis and infiltrate (1–5, 8) or extensive necrosis (6). Most patients used many other drugs concurrently. In a group of 158 patients, 4 developed renal dysfunction and hepatic injury of a mainly cholestatic pattern (8). One of these patients died and 1 patient had to be dialyzed, whereas in the other 2 patients hepatic and renal function returned to normal after discontinuation.

Based on these reports and analogous unpublished cases (60 deaths), this drug was withdrawn from sale in 1982. These cases are unusual since cholestatic hepatitis is rarely fatal and concurrent renal failure is uncommon. Benoxaprofen has a prolonged half–life (7) in geriatric patients and may exceed 100 hours. It has been suggested that an accumulation of toxic intermediates directly damages liver and kidneys with even further inhibition of metabolism as a consequence.

A recent study (9) by the Drugs Surveillance Research Unit of the University of Southampton compared benoxaprofen (15,052 patients; mean treatment: 6.2 months; mean follow–up 12.6 months), fenbufen (6125 patients; mean treatment 7.3 months; mean follow–up 12.9 months) and zomepirac (9416 patients; mean treatment 4.2 months; mean follow–up 4.7 months). The rate of hepatic and biliary events was 6, 2 and 2 per 1000 patient–years in the respective groups and for many of the individual cases non–drug–related causes were found. None of these figures was 2 or more times greater than the expected rate. Although this seems fairly reassuring, it should be noted that as long as the response rate in these studies remains below 100%, these rare idiosyncratic reactions may be missed and their incidence be underestimated.

(1) Goudie et al (1982) *Lancet, 1,* 959. (2) McTaggart et al (1982) *Br. Med. J., 284,* 1372. (3) Prescott et al (1982) *Br. Med. J., 284,* 1783. (4) Fisher et al (1982) *Br. Med. J., 284,* 1783. (5) Firth et al (1982) *Br. Med. J., 284,* 1784. (6) Duthie et al (1982) *Br. Med. J., 285,* 62. (7) Hamdy et al (1982) *Eur. J. Rheumatol. Inflam., 5,* 69. (8) Elling et al (1984) *Ugeskr. Laeg., 146,* 660. (9) Inman et al (1984) *PEM News, 2,* 4.

Carprofen

Causal relationship o/ +

This propionic acid derivative has led to a number of photosensitivity reactions, especially in females. This was brought to the attention of doc-
tors in the Federal Republic of Germany by the Medicines Commission.
Another worrying side–effect appears to be hepatotoxicity of the drug.
In one double–blind study over 4 weeks in patients with osteoarthrosis
9 out of 16 patients developed ASAT, APh and/or bilirubin elevations
versus none in the control group on aspirin (1). Others have also noted
a relatively high incidence of liver enzyme elevations (2).

(1) Stein et al (1983) *Curr. Ther. Res.*, *33*, 415. (2) Jensen et al (1980) *Curr. Ther.
Res.*, *28*, 882.

Diclofenac

Causal relationship o/ +

Liver enzyme and bilirubin assessment in Japanese hospitals revealed
mild elevations in 2–3% of patients on diclofenac, but unfortunately few
details were given about the design of the study (1).
   The symptomatic cases of hepatic injury which have been described in
the literature are compatible with a hepatocellular pattern of injury (1–
3), although a mixed pattern has also been recorded (3). The appearance
of jaundice after 5–7 months of therapy (1, 2), and in a case of rechallenge
(1) after 5 weeks, favors metabolic idiosyncrasy. On the other hand, positive lymphocyte stimulation, macrophage migration inhibition and/or
leukocyte migration inhibition testing (1, 3, 4) are compatible with an immunoallergic mechanism.
   In 1 patient hepatic injury was probably secondary to diclofenac–induced anaphylactic shock (5).

(1) Anonymous (1976) *Jpn. Med. Gaz., April 20th*, 12. (2) Dunk et al (1982) *Br.
Med. J.*, *284*, 1605. (3) Mizoguchi et al (1980) *Gastroenterol. Jpn.*, *15*, 14. (4) Morizane (1978) *Gastroenterol. Jpn.*, *13*, 281. (5) Dux et al (1983) *Br. Med. J.*, *286*, 1861.

Fenbufen

Causal relationship +

Abnormal liver function tests have been reported in up to 25% of patients in some studies (1, 2, 4), both in patients with osteoarthrosis and rheumatoid arthritis. One study mentions a patient who developed rash and biochemical evidence of severe hepatitis (ASAT 1437 U/l, ALAT 454 U/l) which normalized within 10 days after discontinuation (3). In an other study, liver enzyme elevations reappeared after rechallenge (4).

(1)Brogden et al (1981) *Drugs, 21*, 1. (2) Buxton et al (1978) *Curr. Med. Res. Opin., 5*, 682. (3) Kawamura et al (1977) *Kiso to Rinsho, 11*, 171. (4) Becker et al (1980) *J. Int. Med. Res., 8*, 333.

Fenclofenac

CH$_2$-COOH
Cl
Cl

Causal relationship o

In an open multicenter trial 229 of 412 patients experienced 1 or more side–effects. In 79 of these the drug was withdrawn in 4 of whom because of elevated aminotransferases (1).

(1) Smith (1977) *Proc. R. Soc. Med., 70, Suppl 6,* 46.

Fenclozic acid

Cl
S
HOOCH$_2$C   N

Causal relationship o/ +

During clinical trials hepatic injury occurred in up to 10% of recipients (1), which led to withdrawal of the drug. Dudley Hart et al (2) described 8 cases of hepatic injury, 4 of which with jaundice. According to the biochemistry in these cases there was a cholestatic to mixed pattern of injury. Jaundice appeared in the 4 patients after 17–35 days of treatment.

(1) Editorial (1970) *Lancet, 1,* 662. (2) Dudley Hart et al (1970) *Ann. Rheum. Dis., 29,* 684.

Flurbiprofen

CH$_3$-CH-COOH
F

Causal relationship o

Jaundice was reported in a patient with rheumatoid arthritis, starting after 2 months of treatment. A high ASAT level (1200 U/l) was accompanied by fever and facial and palatal rash. Histology showed mild cellular degeneration, acidophilic bodies and moderate portal infiltration with lymphocytes and eosinophils. The condition resolved in 7 weeks after discontinuation (1). Some analogous cases have been reported to the manufacturers, in 1 of which there was a positive reaction to rechallenge (1).

(1) Kotowski et al (1982) *Br. Med. J., 285,* 377.

Ibufenac

CH_3
CH_3 $CH-CH_2$— ⟨ ⟩ —CH_2-COOH

Causal relationship o/ +

Liver enzyme levels, especially ALAT/ASAT, were elevated in 30–40% of patients (1, 2) starting mostly after 3 months or more (2). In jaundiced patients, biochemistry suggested a hepatocellular pattern of injury, which disappeared within 3 months after discontinuation of treatment (1, 2). Immunoallergic signs were absent.

Cuthbert (3) mentions 7 fatal cases with cholestatic jaundice but gives no details. Ibufenac was withdrawn from the market following many reports of hepatic injury to the British Committee on Safety of Medicines.

(1) Thompson et al (1964) *Ann. Rheum. Dis., 23,* 397. (2) Dudley Hart et al (1965) *Ann. Rheum. Dis., 24,* 61. (3) Cuthbert (1974) *Curr. Med. Res. Opin., 2,* 600.

Ibuprofen

$CH_3-CH-COOH$
CH_2-CH CH_3
CH_3

Causal relationship o/ +

Occasionally, cases of hepatic injury have been reported (1–4) showing both a cholestatic/mixed (1, 2) and a hepatocellular pattern (3). Concurrent fever (2, 3), Stevens–Johnson syndrome (2) and lymphopenia (2) have been observed; onset was within 3 weeks after first intake (2, 3), in 1 case after an increase in dose (3). Most patients had connective tissue disease (1, 3, 4). One case was reported of fatal fatty change of the liver with 90% of hepatocytes replaced by fat and minimal portal inflammation (4).

According to Cuthbert's figures (5), hepatic injury was seldom reported to the British Committee on Safety of Medicines in comparison with other reactions to ibuprofen during a 5-year period (5).

(1) Gasparetto (1974) *Minerva Pediatr., 26,* 531. (2) Sternlieb et al (1978) *NY St. J. Med., 78,* 1239. (3) Stempel et al (1977) *J. Pediatr., 90,* 657. (4) Bravo et al (1977) *Ann. Intern. Med., 90,* 657. (5) Cuthbert (1974) *Curr. Med. Res. Opin., 2,* 600.

Pirprofen

CH₃-CH-COOH

During a meeting of the FDA's Arthritis Advisory Committee the results of clinical trials showing severe hepatic injury to this agent were discussed (1). Nevertheless, published studies do not demonstrate more adverse hepatic effects with this drug than with other non–steroidal anti–inflammatory agents. The percentage of liver function abnormalities was estimated by Roth et al (2) at 0.6%.

(1) Anonymous (1982) *Scrip, 702,* 9. (2) Roth et al (1982) *Nouv. Presse Méd., 11,* 2517.

B.6. GOLD COMPOUNDS

Gold–induced hepatic injury is occasionally reported. It is less common than the other important side–effects, e.g. skin reactions and renal injury. Howrie et al (1) reviewed several cases from the literature: both adults and children were affected. Onset was mostly within 5 weeks of starting treatment. Jaundice was most frequent (90%), followed by rash (42%), fever (32%) and abdominal complaints (32%). Thrombocytopenia and/or eosinophilia occurred infrequently in these cases. Histology showed mainly a cholestatic pattern. The predominantly cholestatic pattern has been confirmed by several recent reports (2–4, 7–9, 11) with mainly the same features, although fatal hepatic necrosis has occasionally been attributed to the use of gold compounds (12). One report mentions a combination of pulmonary infiltration, hepatomegaly and lymphadenopathy (5).

The histology, reviewed by LeBodic et al (3), showed mainly centrilobular cholestasis. Necrosis was mostly absent but occasionally focal. Ballooning occurred in 50%. Infiltration (mainly portal) was mononuclear (3). The mechanism is supposed to be immunoallergic based on an intrinsic toxic effect (3). However, cholestasis after an overdose (7) suggests that in some cases toxicity predominates. A recent study indicated that liver toxicity, as well as other side–effects, is more prevalent in patients possessing HLA–DR3 (6). In the above–mentioned cases, gold was administered intramuscularly. One study suggested a higher incidence of liver function disturbances with the recently introduced oral form (auranofin) (10). However, several controlled clinical trials did not demonstrate a significant difference (12).

(1) Howrie et al (1982) *J. Rheumatol., 9,* 727. (2) Chalès et al (1980) *Sem. Hôp. Paris, 56,* 1787. (3) LeBodic et al (1981) *Arch. Anal. Cytol. Pathol., 29,* 98. (4) Weyer-

64

brock (1982) *Akt. Rheumatol., 7,* 138. (5) Prichanond et al (1978) *Ann. Intern. Med., 88,* 579. (6) Gran et al (1983) *Ann. Rheum. Dis., 42,* 63. (7) Jaeger et al (1980) *Toxicol. Lett., 6,* 65. (8) LeBodic et al (1982) *Sem. Hôp. Paris, 58,* 547. (9) Frigero et al (1981) *Minerva Med., 72,* 1941. (10) Gottlieb et al (1980) *Rhumatologie, 32,* 245. (11) Edelman et al (1983) *J. Rheumatol., 10,* 510. (12) Reinicke (1984) In: Dukes (Ed), *Side Effects of Drugs, Annual 8,* p 221. Elsevier, Amsterdam.

B.7. MISCELLANEOUS

Clometacin

CH$_2$—COOH

CH$_3$O—

N

CH$_3$

CO

Cl

Causal relationship +

Hepatic injury with jaundice (1–4, 6, 8–10, 12) has been reported so far almost exclusively in women older than 60 years, which may be partly related to frequent use in this group rather than to susceptibility. A hepatocellular pattern predominated. Onset was within 3 weeks of initial intake (1, 2) although the majority had been using the drug for more than half a year (1, 3, 4, 6, 7, 9), sometimes for up to several years (3, 4, 10). Eosinophilia (1–4, 6, 8, 12), rash (1, 3, 12), thrombocytopenia (4, 6, 8), interstitial nephritis (8, 13), positive in–vitro immunology tests (1, 3, 4, 8) and an elevated IgE level in 1 patient (8) suggest immunoallergy, although overdosage (3.9 g/d) related hepatic injury also suggests intrinsic toxicity (3). Biopsy showed hepatocellular damage (1–3), chronic active hepatitis (1–3, 7, 9) and cirrhosis (1, 3). Death was reported in some cases (3). Other reports mentioned a pattern of cholestatic hepatitis (12) and portal granulomas with pericholangitis (10).

Rechallenge was positive within 2 weeks (1–3, 6, 9, 13) to 1.5 months (1, 3). Antibodies to double–stranded DNA were found in 4 patients with clometacin–associated chronic active hepatitis and the authors suggested that the presence of circulating antibodies to anti–double–stranded DNA in patients with HBsAg–negative chronic active hepatitis could be a pointer to drug–induced liver damage (5).

(1) Lenoir et al (1978) *Nouv. Presse Méd., 7,* 3035. (2) Manigand et al (1979) *Nouv. Presse Méd., 8,* 213. (3) Mamou et al (1981) *Nouv. Presse Méd., 10,* 2719. (4) Seigneuric et al (1982) *Nouv. Presse Méd., 12,* 106. (5) Caruana et al (1983) *Lancet, 1,* 776. (6) Goldfarb et al (1979) *Gastroentérol. Clin. Biol., 3,* 537. (7) Pointrine et al (1983) *Gastroentérol. Clin. Biol., 7,* 99. (8) Spreux et al (1981) *Thérapie, 36,* 293. (9) Chagnon et al (1983) *Gastroentérol. Clin. Biol., 7,* 556. (10) Hillion et al (1983) *Gastroentérol. Clin. Biol., 7,* 1038. (11) Martin et al (1983) *Ouest Méd., 36,* 415. (12) Chavanet et al (1983) *Lyon Méd., 250,* 407. (13) Monnin et al (1984) *Gastroentérol. Clin. Biol., 8,* 264.

Difenamizole

CH₃–CH–CO–NH– [pyrazole/phenyl structure]
   |
   N(CH₃)₂

Causal relationship o

In a report of 9 cases of severe bridging necrosis, 1 was ascribed to use of difenamizole. Recovery was uneventful. Eight cases were confirmed by rechallenge, one by in–vitro testing; however, no further details were given (1).

(1) Imoto et al (1979) *Ann. Intern. Med., 91,* 129.

Etodolac

[chemical structure: H₅C₂, H, C₂H₅, CH₂–COOH on indole-pyranone ring system]

Causal relationship o

One study of 298 patients with rheumatoid arthritis revealed mild and mostly transient liver enzyme elevations in 4% of recipients (1).

(1) Ryder et al (1983) *Curr. Ther. Res., 33,* 948.

Fentiazac

HOOC–CH₂ [thiazole ring with S, N, phenyl]
Cl– [chlorophenyl]

Causal relationship o

In a double–blind study comparing fentiazac (300 mg/d) and indometacin (75 mg/d) in rheumatoid patients, 7 of 20 patients on fentiazac developed slight ASAT and/or APh elevations versus 3 of 20 patients on indometacin (1). During a long–term tolerance study, reversible signs of hepatic injury developed in 3 of 33 patients on fentiazac (2).

(1) Katona et al (1979) *Curr. Med. Res. Opin., 6, Suppl. 2,* 71. (2) Bunde et al (1983) *Curr. Med. Res. Opin., 8,* 310.

Glafenine

CO–O–CH₂–CHOH–CH₂OH
[quinoline structure with NH]
Cl

Causal relationship +

Glafenine is an analgesic with a 4–aminoquinoline structure, related to chloroquine. However, its adverse reaction profile is different. Ocular deposits are not known, but anaphylactic reactions, often with shock, are frequent. Glafenine also shows some structural resemblance to cinchophen and indeed the, often severe, necrosis is common to both agents. Several cases of hepatocellular necrosis have been attributed to the use of this analgesic (1–7), although 1 case of acute hemolysis and renal failure, accompanied by liver enzyme and conjugated bilirubin elevations, showed a histological pattern of pure cholestasis (8). Usually icterus appeared 1 month (1–3, 6) to several months (1–4, 5, 7) after starting therapy. Fever (3, 7) and peripheral eosinophilia (1, 5–7) have been observed, but rash was not reported. One patient had concurrent signs of pulmonary involvement (7). In another patient, arthralgia, fever, mild liver enzyme elevations and renal dysfunction accompanied by diffuse intravascular coagulation developed in several hours after the intake of 1 tablet (9). A lymphocyte stimulation test performed in 1 case was negative (6). A rechallenge performed in several cases was positive (1, 2, 6, 7). Histology showed mostly extensive confluent centrilobular or massive necrosis (1–5) but also chronic hepatitis with beginning or advanced cirrhosis (1, 3, 7). One report mentioned significant infiltration with eosinophils (1), whereas others noted their presence (3, 7) amid a predominantly mononuclear infiltrate, both lobular and portal.

In view of the malicious nature of the hepatic injury and of the high incidence of anaphylactic reactions, the usefulness of this drug for uncomplicated and transient pain may be seriously doubted.

(1) Ypma et al (1978) *Lancet, 2,* 480. (2) Stricker et al (1979) *Ned. Tijdschr. Geneeskd., 123,* 1807. (3) Brandt et al (1979) *Ned. Tijdschr. Geneeskd., 123,* 1798. (4) Lekkerkerker (1979) *Ned. Tijdschr. Geneeskd., 123,* 1800. (5) De Vries (1979) *Ned. Tijdschr. Geneeskd., 123,* 2193. (6) Brissot et al (1982) *Gastroentérol. Clin. Biol., 6,* 948. (7) Verhamme et al (1984) *Neth. J. Med., 27,* 35. (8) Pinta et al (1983) *Thérapie, 38,* 701. (9) Ducroix et al (1984) *Presse. Méd., 13,* 1220.

Indometacin

Causal relationship o/ +

Several cases of hepatic injury have been reported, either mainly hepatocellular (2–4, 8, 9) or cholestatic (1, 5). The reaction appeared in one (1, 9) to several months (2, 4, 8) after starting treatment. Immunoallergic symptoms were absent in these cases. One patient had biliverdinemia (1). In some reports the course was fatal (2, 4, 9). Biopsy performed in some patients showed extensive hepatic necrosis (2, 4, 9) and centrilobular cellular degeneration with bile stasis (1). One report mentioned many eosinophilic granulocytes in the infiltrate (4). Morizane found a positive leukocyte migration inhibition in the presence of the drug and serum, the drug and liver homogenate, but also in the presence of liver homogenate alone (7).

In a presentation of reports to the Committee on Safety of Medicines Cuthbert compared the adverse reaction profiles of several analgesic and antirheumatics (6). According to his figures, approximately 3–5% of 1261 cases comprised liver toxicity, which accounted for approximately 5–10% of the 114 fatal cases ascribed to indometacin.

(1) Fenech et al (1967) *Br. Med. J.*, *2*, 156. (2) Kelsey et al (1967) *J. Am. Med. Assoc.*, *199*, 586. (3) Opolon et al (1969) *Presse Méd.*, *77*, 2041. (4) De Kraker–Sangster et al (1981) *Ned. Tijdschr. Geneeskd.*, *125*, 1828. (5) Driessen et al (1971) In: *Pathologie van Lever en Galwegen*. Thoben Offset, Nijmegen. (6) Cuthbert (1974) *Curr. Ther. Res. Opin.*, *2*, 12. (7) Morizane (1978) *Gastroenterol. Jpn.*, *13*, 281. (8) Iwaoka et al (1982) *Jpn. J. Med.*, *21*, 29. (9) Jacobs (1967) *J. Am. Med. Assoc.*, *199*, 182.

JPC–80   *Causal relationship* o

JPC–80 is a new, slow–acting antirheumatic. Elevated liver enzymes were found in 1 patient, reversible on withdrawal, during a trial in 12 patients (300 mg/d) for up to 12 weeks (1). This drug is related to pyritinol (see below).

(1) Norton et al (1982) *J. Rheum.*, *9*, 951.

Lonazolac

HOOC–CH_2

Cl

Causal relationship o

In a study of 152 patients this arylacetic acid derivative has been reported as the possible cause of 2 cases of cholestatic hepatitis appearing within 4 weeks after starting therapy (1).

(1) Nobbe–Balogh et al (1983) *Z. Allgemeinmed.*, *59*, 94.

Naproxen

CH_3
CH—COOH
H_3CO—

Causal relationship o

Some cases of jaundice have been described, attributed to the intake of naproxen (1–4). In another case, mild ASAT and APh elevations accompanied the development of pulmonary infiltrates with complaints of malaise, cough, fever and eosinophilia after 2 weeks of treatment (5). Biochemically, the jaundiced cases were mainly of the cholestatic (1, 4) or hepatocellular (2, 3) type. Symptoms appeared from 1 to 8 weeks after starting treatment. In some cases a biopsy was performed showing mild steatosis with scattered foci of portal and parenchymal mononuclear infiltration (3) and centrilobular cholestasis with mild cellular unrest (4).

According to Krogsgaard et al (4), 19 cases of hepatic injury, of which 3 were fatal, were reported from the U.S.A. to the manufacturer in the period 1978–1979.

(1) Bass (1974) *Lancet, 1,* 998. (2) Law et al (1976) *N. Engl. J. Med., 295,* 1201. (3) Victorino et al (1980) *Postgrad. Med. J., 56,* 368. (4) Krogsgaard et al (1980) *Ugeskr. Laeg., 142,* 450. (5) Buscaglia et al (1984) *J. Am. Med. Assoc., 251,* 65.

Penicillamine

$$H_3C - \underset{\underset{HS}{|}}{\overset{\overset{CH_3}{|}}{C}} - \underset{\underset{NH_2}{|}}{CH} - COOH$$

Causal relationship +

Penicillamine is a degradation product of penicilline used as a chelating agent (e.g. in Wilson's disease and primary biliary cirrhosis) and antirheumatic. It is far more toxic than its parent compound. Penicillamine–induced hepatic injury is less common than its other side–effects. Data about the frequency are conflicting. Weiss et al (1) saw no hepatotoxicity in a study of 63 patients with rheumatoid arthritis while another study demonstrated liver enzyme elevations in 6% of patients on 250–750 mg/d for rheumatoid arthritis, which were reversible after discontinuation (2). Biopsies showed focal necrosis in 2 and fibrosis in 1 patient. Renal dysfunction, thrombocytopenia and rash occurred concurrently in some cases. As appeared from a review of the literature (3), most reported cases show biochemically a cholestatic pattern of injury. The onset varied from 10 days to 21 weeks (mean: 41 days) after starting treatment for rheumatoid arthritis, scleroderma, Wilson's disease or systemic lupus erythematosus. Concurrent rash, fever and/or eosinophilia were reported in 20–30% of these cases. Only 1 case ended fatally secondary to renal failure. Most biopsies showed intrahepatic cholestasis (3). Several additional reports have appeared of cholestasis, often with jaundice (4–11). One of these cases had rash, granulomatous parotitis and a pulmonary reaction as extrahepatic manifestations and granulomatous hepatitis (4). A rechallenge, performed in some cases, was mostly positive (2, 3, 12) but in one without recurrence of abnormalities (11). One patient showed a positive reaction to intradermal administration (13), but in another case this test and a lymphocyte stimulation test were negative (11). At least 2 patients had a history of hypersensitivity to penicillin, suggesting cross–sensitivity between these agents. Patients who are allergic to penicillin are more prone to develop a hypersensitivity reaction to penicillamine and evidence of sensitization to penicillamine was obtained by several tests in half the penicillin–allergic patients (13). However, penicillin–induced hepatic injury is less frequent.

(1) Weiss et al (1978) *Am. J. Med., 64,* 114. (2) Wollheim et al (1979) *Scand. J. Rheumatol., Suppl 28,* 100. (3) Seibold et al (1981) *Arthritis Rheum., 24,* 554. (4) Crickx et al (1979) *Nouv. Presse Méd., 8,* 212. (5) Jensen (1981) *Ugeskr. Laeg., 143,* 347. (6) Multz (1981) *J. Am. Med. Assoc., 246,* 674. (7) Peters et al (1982) *Ugeskr. Laeg., 144,* 1924. (8) Job–Deslandre et al (1982) *Nouv. Presse Méd., 11,* 2356. (9) Weyerbrock (1982) *Akt. Rheumatol., 7,* 138. (10) Grauer et al (1983) *Presse Méd., 12,* 1997. (11) Wozel et al (1982) *Dtsch. Z. Verdau.–Stoffwechselkr., 42,* 85. (12) Rosenbaum et al (1980) *Ann. Rheum. Dis., 39,* 152. (13) Meyboom (1975) In: Dukes (Ed), *Meyler's Side Effects of Drugs, 8th ed,* p 529. Excerpta Medica, Amsterdam.

Piroxicam

Causal relationship o/ +

Mild and transient ALAT/ASAT and APh elevations have been recorded during clinical trials at approximately the same rate as for other antirheumatics. In some cases it led to withdrawal from treatment (1, 2), while readministration caused a recurrence (1). Of 102 fatal adverse reactions ascribed to piroxicam, 4 were secondary to hepatitis (3). Mitnick et al (4) noted interstitial nephritis, hepatitis and nephrotic syndrome, appearing after 1 week of treatment. They ascribed this reaction to altered hemodynamics or to a change in cellular or humoral immunity, related to prostaglandin synthesis inhibition. Despite discontinuation of piroxicam and treatment with prednisone the nephrotic syndrome persisted. Although it is uncertain how an injurious effect takes place, it has been pointed out that piroxicam has a long half–life, especially in the elderly (5), and this may be compatible with a toxic mechanism, if cumulation occurs.

(1) Telhag (1978) *Eur. J. Rheum. Inflamm., 1,* 352. (2) Zizic et al (1978) In: *Piroxicam. Proceedings, International Congress and Symposium Series 1,* p 93. Academic Press, London. (3) Moebius (1983) *Arznei–Telegramm, 10,* 89. (4) Mitnick et al (1984) *Arch. Intern. Med., 144,* 63. (5) Woolf et al (1983) *Br. J. Clin. Pharmacol., 16,* 433.

Proquazone

Causal relationship o

Elevated ASAT, APh and bilirubin levels in serum were reported to occur in 1.8% of treated patients with osteoarthrosis and rheumatoid arthritis, compared to 3.1% in aspirin–treated patients (1). No further details were provided. Fluproquazone, the parent compound, caused hepatic injury including jaundice in 14% of patients and proved too hepatotoxic for clinical use (2).

(1) Anonymous (1983) *Scrip, 796, 13.* (2) Lewis (1984) *Clin. Pharm., 3, 128.*

Pyritinol

Causal relationship +

Pyritinol has a sulfhydryl–group, thereby showing some resemblance to penicillamine. Cholestatic hepatitis has been reported with jaundice, appearing within 1 month after first intake (1, 2). No immunoallergic symptoms were noted, but a lymphocyte stimulation test was positive (1). A rechallenge was followed by signs of serious hepatocellular injury (1), whereas histology showed hepatocellular degeneration and portal inflammation. A pattern of centrilobular cholestasis (1, 2) with minimal infiltration has also been noted. Imoto et al (3) noted severe bridging necrosis in a patient on pyritinol but gave no further details.

(1) Valat et al (1982) *Nouv. Presse. Méd., 11,* 1875. (2) Gouet et al (1983) *Rev. Rhum. Mal. Ostéo–articulaires, 50,* 167. (3) Imoto et al (1979) *Ann. Intern. Med., 91,* 129.

Sudoxicam

Causal relationship o/ +

Mild ALAT elevations were observed in 1.2% of 1000 patients during a clinical trial; an additional 0.6% was jaundiced (1 fatal case). Biopsy showed centrilobular focal necrosis; there was 1 case of extensive necrosis (1).

(1) Zimmerman (1978) *Hepatotoxicity,* p 428. Appleton–Century–Crofts, New York.

Sulindac

Causal relationship +

Mild to moderate liver enzyme elevations (3, 8, 9) and jaundice (1, 2, 5–7,

10, 11, 13) have been noted, the latter as a symptom of a mainly mixed to cholestatic pattern of injury. Hepatocellular injury, however, may occasionally predominate (10). The reaction usually started in the first 6 weeks of therapy (2–4, 7, 10, 12), but sometimes after several months (1, 8, 14), and was almost invariably accompanied by signs of generalized hypersensitivity such as rash (2, 4, 8, 10), fever (2–5, 7, 8, 10–12, 14), Stevens–Johnson/Lyell syndrome (9, 10, 12), pneumonitis (3), arthralgia (10), blood disorders (9, 11) and lymphadenopathy (11). In cases where a rechallenge was performed, relapse occurred within 3 days (3–8, 10). In only some of the cases was a biopsy performed, showing 'toxic hepatitis' (1), centrilobular cholestasis, casts and dilated bile ducts, and scattered areas of mononuclear infiltration without (6) or with minimal necrosis (7). Some reports mentioned mild patchy necrosis with mononuclear infiltration of portal and necrotic areas without marked cholestasis (10, 14). Fagan et al (14) noted marked eosinophilic infiltration.

(1) Wolfe (1979) *Ann. Intern. Med., 91,* 656. (2) Anderson (1979) *N. Engl. J. Med., 300,* 735. (3) Smith et al (1980) *J. Am. Med. Assoc., 244,* 269. (4) Dhand et al (1981) *Gastroenterology, 80,* 585. (5) Kaul et al (1981) *J. Pediatr., 99,* 650. (6) Giroux et al (1982) *Can. J. Surg., 25,* 334. (7) Whittaker et al (1982) *Gut, 23,* 875. (8) ADRAC (1982) *Med. J. Aust., 2,* 191. (9) Levitt et al (1980) *J. Am. Med. Assoc., 243,* 1262. (10) Park et al (1982) *Arch. Intern. Med., 142,* 1292. (11) Anonymous (1983) *Aust. Adverse Drug React. Bull., June.* (12) Klein et al (1983) *J. Rheum., 10,* 512. (13) McIndoe et al (1981) *NZ Med. J., 94,* 430. (14) Fagan et al (1983) *Gut, 24,* 1199.

Tiaramide

Cl —⟨⟩— $N-CH_2-CO-N$ ⟨⟩ $N-CH_2-CH_2-OH$ *Causal relationship* o

Tiaramide has been held responsible for a case of mixed cholestatic and hepatocellular hepatitis (no specification) confirmed by immunological testing (positive lymphocyte stimulation test, macrophage–activating– and migration–inhibitory factor and macrophage–mediated cytotoxicity) (1).

(1) Mizoguchi et al (1980) *Gastroenterol. Jpn., 15,* 14.

Tinoridine

⟨⟩ CH_2-N ⟨⟩ S NH_2 $CO-O-C_2H_5$ *Causal relationship* o

Changes in liver function may occur (1). One unspecified case of hepatic injury was confirmed by a positive lymphocyte stimulation test (2).

(1) *The Extra Pharmacopoeia, 28th ed,* p 234. Pharmaceutical Press, London, 1982.
(2) Namihisa et al (1975) *Leber Magen Darm, 5,* 73.

Tolmetin

Causal relationship o

Tolmetin was evaluated in 171 geriatric patients with rheumatoid arthritis and in 676 with osteoarthritis (1). The average dose was 1141 mg/d and 953 mg/d, respectively. Abnormal ASAT values were reported in 9 (5.3%) and 10 (1.5%), respectively, while APh levels were abnormal in 25 (14.6%) and 10 (1.5%) patients. The high percentage in the first group may be related to the underlying illness itself or to its treatment with higher doses. In a double–blind trial with aspirin and tolmetin in patients with juvenile rheumatoid arthritis, aspirin was associated with a significantly higher incidence of hepatic injury than tolmetin (2).

(1) O'Brien (1983) *J. Clin. Pharmacol., 23,* 309. (2) Levinson et al (1977) *J. Pediatr., 91,* 799.

C. DRUGS AGAINST GOUT

Allopurinol

Causal relationship + +

A predominantly hepatocellular pattern is produced, either mild (2, 5, 7–13) or severe (1, 3, 8, 10, 14). Rash (1, 3, 5, 6, 8, 10, 14–16, 18–20, 23), often exfoliative, fever (1–3, 6, 8–10, 12–16, 18–20, 23), eosinophilia (1–3, 5–8, 10, 11, 13–16, 18–20, 23), leukocytosis (1, 3, 5–8, 10–12, 14), vasculitis (1–3, 5–8, 14, 15) and concurrent renal impairment (1–3, 5–8, 10, 14, 16, 18–20, 23) are frequent; the latter often pre–exists in a mild form. Lymphadenopathy is less frequently mentioned (6, 14–16, 18). Injury starts within 6 weeks (1–12, 14–16, 18–20, 23). A fatal outcome (2, 3, 5, 8, 10, 16, 18) is due to hepatic failure (3), renal failure (5) or sepsis (2, 16). Biopsy shows hepatocellular necrosis of varying severity, massive (3), centrilobular (1, 8, 10) or focal (7, 11). Non–caseating granulomas with giant cells are frequently seen (7, 9, 11–13, 19). In some cases cholestasis predominated (18, 20), in 1 case with eosinophilic cholangitis (18).

Lymphocyte stimulation testing with allopurinol has been both positive (15, 17) and negative (14). In 1 report there was cross–sensitivity to oxypurinol (21). An immunoallergic pattern seems to predominate. However, there is a higher incidence of liver injury in patients with renal impairment than in those with a normal renal function (4). Moreover, most reported cases have renal dysfunction, which suggests that a toxic mechanism may be important. The combination of renal dysfunction and use of diuretics was suggested to play a deleterious role by increasing blood–levels of oxypurinol, the major metabolite (1). Since renal clearance of oxypurinol is directly proportional to renal clearance of creatinine, dose reduction is sufficient to inhibit uric acid production and to reduce side effects (22).

(1) Al–Kawas et al (1981) *Ann. Intern. Med.*, *95*, 588. (2) Kantor (1970) *J. Am. Med. Assoc.*, *212*, 478. (3) Butler et al (1977) *J. Am. Med. Assoc.*, *237*, 473. (4) Lidsky et al (1967) *Arthritis Rheum.*, *10*, 294. (5) Jarzobski et al (1970) *Am. Heart J.*, *79*, 116. (6) Mills (1971) *J. Am. Med. Assoc.*, *216*, 799. (7) Simmons et al (1972) *Gastroenterology*, *62*, 101. (8) Young et al (1974) *Arch. Intern. Med.*, *134*, 553. (9) Espiritu et al (1976) *Am. J. Dig. Dis.*, *21*, 804. (10) Boyer et al (1977) *West. J. Med.*, *126*, 143. (11) Chawla et al (1977) *Arthritis Rheum.*, *20*, 1546. (12) Swank et al (1978) *Arch. Intern. Med.*, *138*, 997. (13) Medline et al (1978) *Br. Med. J.*, *1*, 1320. (14) McKendrick et al (1979) *Br. Med. J.*, *1*, 988. (15) Malé et al (1978) *Schweiz. Med. Wochenschr.*, *108*, 681. (16) Phanichphant et al (1980) *J. Med. Ass. Thailand*, *63*, 155. (17) Namihisa (1975) *Leber Magen Darm*, *5*, 73. (18) Korting et al (1978) *Lancet*, *1*, 275. (19) Ramond et al (1982) *Gastroentérol. Clin. Biol.*, *6*, 138. (20) Bruguera et al (1983) *Gastroenterol. Hepatol.*, *6*, 253. (21) Lockard et al (1976) *Ann. Intern. Med.*, *85*, 333. (22) Hande et al (1983) *Am. J. Med.*, *76*, 47. (23) Raper et al (1984) *Aust. NZ J. Med.*, *14*, 63.

Cinchophen

Causal relationship + +

The use of this uricosuric and analgesic agent has become obsolete since its toxicity outweighs its therapeutic value. It is however of note since cinchophen serves as a prototype of idiosyncratic hepatocellular injury; in fact, it was through this drug that the dose–independent and unpredictable nature of some types of liver damage was recognized for the first time. Whereas the first case was recognized in 1923, over 200 cases had been reported by 1936 (1). The pattern consisted of hepatocellular jaundice with severe parenchymal injury and a high case–fatality rate. The onset was usually within the first 8 weeks but often within the first 2 weeks. Immunoallergic signs were noted in a minority (2). Children and young adults were less vulnerable (1).

Histology showed acute or subacute hepatic necrosis collapse and fibrosis (1).

The mechanism has never been elucidated, but metabolic idiosyncrasy has been considered to be most likely (3).

(1) Zimmerman (1978) *Hepatotoxicity*, p 418. Appleton–Century–Crofts, New York. (2) Weir et al (1933) *Arch. Intern. Med.*, *52*, 685. (3) Palmer et al (1936) *J. Am. Med. Assoc.*, *107*, 760.

Colchicine

Causal relationship o/ +

Besides its well–known effect in the treatment of acute gout this drug has been reported to cause regression of fibrosis and clinical improvement in cirrhotic patients (1, 2). However, this claim is under current investigation and needs to be substantiated.

Colchicine overdosage is associated with gastroenteritis, metabolic acidosis, central nervous system involvement, bone–marrow depression, renal failure, and liver damage (3). As far as we know, no cases have been described of hepatic injury secondary to this drug in therapeutic amounts. However, we have received reports of mild liver enzyme elevation possibly related to its intake. Colchicine impairs bile flow and induces hepatic APh in rats (4); it is likely to have the same effect in man, although without much clinical significance if therapeutic doses are employed.

(1) Rojkind et al (1973) *Lancet, 1*, 38. (2) Kershenobich et al (1979) *Gastroenterology, 77*, 532. (3) Prescott (1975) In: Dukes (Ed), *Meyler's Side Effects of Drugs, 8th ed*, p 207. Excerpta Medica, Amsterdam. (4) Hatoff et al (1983) *Proc. Soc. Exp. Biol. Med., 173*, 227.

Demecolcine

CH₃O— —NH–CH₃
CH₃O—
CH₃O
OCH₃

Causal relationship o/ +

Demecolcine is a derivative of colchicine and has been successfully used in the treatment both of gout and of chronic myelocytic leukemia (1). The drug is no longer very popular because of its toxicity to bone marrow and because better agents are available. Occasionally, cholestatic jaundice has been described in man after administration of therapeutic doses (2). Overdosage caused hepatic necrosis in rabbits (2).

(1) Dittman et al (1959) *Am. J. Med., 27*, 519. (2) Velasco et al (1959) *N. Engl. J. Med., 260*, 1280.

Probenecid

COOH

SO₂–N—C₃H₇
         C₃H₇

Causal relationship o/ +

One case of hepatitis has been described which occurred after 2 years of intermittent therapy. Rechallenge, after recovery, proved fatal with asthma, rash and progressive liver failure. Biopsy showed massive hepatic necrosis and mild portal inflammation (1). Probenecid has been mentioned as a cause of hepatic granulomas (4).

Probenecid interfered with BSP (2) and indocyanine green excretion (3) in a dose–dependent way in animal tests.

(1) Reynolds et al (1957) *N. Engl. J. Med.*, *256*, 592. (2) Goetzee et al (1960) *Clin. Sci.*, *19*, 63. (3) Vogin et al (1966) *J. Pharmacol. Exp. Ther.*, *152*, 509. (4) Demeulenaere et al (1982) *Ziekten van Lever en Galwegen*, p 181. Story–Scientia, Ghent.

3. Antidotes

Introduction

Antidotes are used mainly in the treatment of poisoning by substances such as organophosphorus insecticides, heavy metals, cyanide and arsenic, but they are also employed in methemoglobinemia, Wilson's disease, hemachromatosis, primary biliary cirrhosis and hypercalcemia. The group comprises chelating agents and drug antagonists.

Hepatic injury will be mostly secondary to intoxication, e.g. paracetamol, or the underlying condition, e.g. Wilson's disease, for which the antidote has been given. It is obvious that this will complicate the assessment of the eventual responsibility of the antidote for observed hepatic injury.

Some of these agents (e.g. penicillamine) are discussed elsewhere. Obidoximine and pralidoxime, antidotes used in the treatment of organophosphorous poisoning, have been associated with cholestatic jaundice(1).

(1) Klinge (1979) *Klinische Hepatologie,* p 6.158. Thieme, Stuttgart.

Mercaptamine (cysteamine)

$HS-CH_2-CH_2-NH_2$ *Causal relationship* o

Mercaptamine has been used in the treatment of paracetamol intoxication but has been largely abandoned in favor of N–acetylcysteine. No hepatic injury has been ascribed to its use. Recently a case of veno–occlusive disease was discovered after 22 months of treatment with mercaptamine (10 mg/kg/d increasing to 58 mg/kg/d) for nephropathic cystinosis (1).

(1) Avner et al (1983) *J. Pediatr., 102,* 793.

Tiopronin

$CH_3-CH-CO-NH-CH_2-COOH$
$\quad\ \ |$
$\quad\ \ SH$ *Causal relationship* o

Tiopronin is used in some countries as an adjunct to the treatment of liver and eczematous disorders. Because of its sulfhydryl group it has been claimed to be of use in cystinuria and as an antidote in heavy–metal poisoning.

Several reports of hepatic injury have appeared, especially in the Japanese medical literature (1–5). In most of these, jaundice and/or liver enzyme elevations developed 19–25 days after starting treatment (1, 3). Besides a positive lymphocyte stimulation test (1, 3–5), mild eosinophilia was reported once (1) but otherwise immunoallergic signs were uncommon. Biochemically, the pattern varied from a mainly cholestatic (1) to a mixed or mainly hepatocellular pattern of injury (1, 2, 4). Recovery may be prolonged (1, 4). Histology showed bile plugging (1), residual parenchymal injury (3) and portal zone fibrosis (2, 3), but also large multinucleated cells (1) and fatty liver with giant mitochondria (2). One case showed a pattern resembling primary biliary cirrhosis with destruction of interlobular bile ducts (4).

Although one may suspect that underlying liver disease for which the drug is often given plays an important role, in at least 2 cases the drug was used for non–hepatic disorders (3, 4).

(1) Kusakabe et al (1982) *Acta Hepatol. Jpn., 23,* 432. (2) Koike et al (1982) *Acta Hepatol. Jpn., 23,* 921. (3) Aramaki et al (1982) *Acta Hepatol. Jpn., 23,* 1342. (4) Hattori et al (1983) *Acta Hepatol. Jpn., 24,* 1298. (5) Namihisa et al (1975) *Leber Magen Darm, 5,* 73.

4. Anticonvulsants

A. Hydantoins
B. Succinimides
C. Oxazolidines
D. Miscellaneous

Introduction

Although some hepatic syndromes may be preceded or accompanied by convulsions, e.g. Reye's syndrome, there is no clear association between epilepsy and hepatic disease. The incidence of non–drug–related hepatic disease is probably as high in epileptics as in the general population. However, patients in mental institutions may be exposed to epidemics of viral hepatitis (1), but these may be differentiated from drug–induced liver injury by their explosive character.

Epilepsy is usually treated with several agents concurrently, which complicates the assessment of a causal relationship between hepatic injury and one of the employed agents. This is only one of the many reasons for encouraging monotherapy.

Anticonvulsants are a frequent cause of isolated γ–glutamyl transpeptidase elevation. It is thought that this reflects increased synthesis of the enzyme rather than liver damage (2). It parallels enzyme induction, which may possibly lead to clinically significant interactions with other drugs, e.g. paracetamol and isoniazid. An increase in serum APh is usually accompanied by a change in serum calcium and phosphate, which indicates osteomalacia rather than hepatic damage.

There are studies suggesting that long–term administration of anticonvulsants has an injurious effect on the liver, by demonstrating a significant increase in serum liver enzyme concentrations (3) and minimal focal necrosis (4). Nevertheless, serious toxicity appears to be rare and is attributed mostly to idiosyncratic reactions in vulnerable individuals. With the exception of valproate, which seems to damage the liver as a consequence of metabolic derangement of the hepatocytes, the other anticonvulsants probably damage the liver as part of an immunoallergic reaction. The frequency is unknown but it is estimated to be lower than the 2% incidence of phenacemide–associated hepatic injury (5). Hydantoins and acetylureas seem to be most frequently implicated.

The pattern of injury caused by anticonvulsants is mainly hepatocellular, although mixed cholestatic–hepatocellular patterns also occur.

(1) Koff et al (1982) In: Schiff et al (Eds), *Diseases of the Liver, 5th ed*, p 461. Lippincott, Philadelphia. (2) Rosalki (1976) In: Richens et al (Eds), *Anticonvulsant Drugs and Enzyme Induction*, p 27. Associated Scientific Publishers, Amsterdam. (3) Buch Andreasen et al (1973) *Acta Med. Scand., 194*, 261. (4) Jacobsen et al (1976) *Acta Med. Scand., 199*, 345. (5) Tyler et al (1951) *J. Am. Med. Assoc., 147*, 17.

A. HYDANTOINS

Mephenytoin

Causal relationship o

Occasional cases of hepatocellular jaundice have been reported (1). According to one textbook, hepatitis is more frequently caused by this agent than by phenytoin (2), but it is unclear by which data this claim is supported.

(1) Zimmerman (1963) *Ann. NY Acad. Sci., 104*, 954. (2) *The Extra Pharmacopoeia, 28th ed*, p 1251. Pharmaceutical Press, London, 1982.

Phenytoin (DPH)

Causal relationship + +

A uniform pattern in cases of clinically overt hepatic injury emerges from a literature review (1), a clinicopathological study (2) and a study of 38 cases with a hypersensitivity reaction, 13 of which had hepatic injury (3). Frequently present are fever (90%, 75%, 62%) (respective percentages), rash (90%, 63%, 62%), often exfoliative, leukocytosis (sometimes with atypical lymphocytes) (80–100%) (1, 2) although leuko–/pancytopenia may occur (3, 8, 13, 14), eosinophilia (80%, 80%, 46%), and lymphadenopathy (80%, 60%, 46%). Involvement of other organs, e.g. interstitial nephritis (22–24), is frequent. The pattern may strongly resemble infectious mononucleosis with lymphadenopathy, lymphocytosis and atypical lymphocytes. A malignant lymphoma may be mimicked (18) or possibly caused (20). The reaction starts mostly within 5 (1), 6 (2) or 5 (3) weeks, although some cases take several months. Fatality is reported in 30–40% (1, 2), but is not primarily caused by DPH in every case. This high case–fatality rate concerns the symptomatic form of hepatic injury; since the hypersensitivity reaction may be accompanied by only mild liver enzyme elevations (3), the overall case–fatality rate may be lower. Liver injury varies from almost trivial to massive hepatic necrosis. It is mostly hepatocellular, although cholestasis may predominate (10, 16, 23). One case

80

of prolonged cholestasis followed hepatocellular damage (4).

Recently, several additional cases have been reported with essentially the same features as above (5–10, 14, 16, 25). Biopsy, extensively described by Mullick and Ishak (2), showed many variants (acute and chronic) ranging from spotty necrosis and degeneration to (sub)massive necrosis. A mixed hepatocellular/cholestatic pattern is present in some cases. (Non–caseating) granulomas with or without hepatocellular injury, composed of giant cells and eosinophils, sometimes with arteritis, may be seen. One of their patients had chronic persistent hepatitis while another showed features of reticuloendothelial malignancy involving the liver, which has been observed earlier (11). Besides some reports of mild enzyme elevations, we have received reports of 3 cases with the above–mentioned hypersensitivity syndrome: 2 had abnormal renal function, 1 thrombocytopenia. All patients used DPH and phenobarbital; both drugs might have been responsible (see 'Phenobarbital').

A preponderance has been reported in blacks (1, 2) and adults (1, 2). Rechallenge is usually positive in 24 hours (5, 13, 17, 19, 21), the lymphocyte stimulation test (4, 5, 7, 22, 23) is positive, and antibodies to DPH (12, 22) and a strongly elevated IgE (7) have been demonstrated. A recent study (14) showed enhanced in–vitro toxicity of DPH metabolites to lymphocytes of patients with the generalized hepato–hypersensitivity syndrome. A role was suggested by the authors for increased arene oxide formation, subsequent covalent binding to macromolecules and superimposed immunoallergic reaction.

Mild liver enzyme changes may occur during therapy with anticonvulsants. Drugs such as phenytoin and phenobarbital may increase γ–GT by enzyme induction and APh by interference with vitamin D metabolism. A long–term study with phenytoin demonstrated significantly increased liver enzyme concentrations compared with healthy controls (15).

(1) Zimmerman (1978) *Hepatotoxicity*, p 395. Appleton–Century–Crofts, New York. (2) Mullick et al (1980) *Am. J. Clin. Pathol., 74,* 442. (3) Haruda (1979) *Neurology, 29,* 1480. (4) Campbell et al (1977) *Am. J. Dig. Dis., 22,* 255. (5) Ting et al (1982) *Ann. Allergy, 48,* 331. (6) Cook et al (1981) *Aust. NZ J. Med., 11,* 539. (7) Josephs et al (1980) *J. Allergy Clin. Immunol., 66,* 166. (8) Parker et al (1979) *Neurology, 29,* 175. (9) Koren et al (1980) *Drug Intell. Clin. Pharm., 14,* 252. (10) Spechler et al (1981) *Ann. Intern. Med., 95,* 455. (11) Rausing et al (1971) *Acta Med. Scand., 189,* 131. (12) Kleckner et al (1975) *Ann. Intern. Med., 83,* 522. (13) Dhar et al (1974) *Postgrad. Med. J., 56,* 128. (14) Spielberg et al (1981) *N. Engl. J. Med., 305,* 722. (15) Buch Andreasen et al (1973) *Acta Med. Scand., 194,* 261. (16) Harney et al (1983) *Neurology, 33,* 790. (17) Chaiken et al (1950) *N. Engl. J. Med., 242,* 897. (18) Saltzstein et al (1959) *Cancer, 12,* 164. (19) Pezzimenti et al (1970) *Arch. Intern. Med., 125,* 118. (20) Cuerin et al (1983) *Presse Méd., 12,* 1491. (21) Siegal et al (1961) *J. Allergy Clin. Immunol., 32,* 447. (22) Hyman et al (1978) *J. Pediatr., 92,* 915. (23) Sheth et al (1977) *J. Pediatr., 91,* 438. (24) Michael et al (1976) *J. Am. Med. Assoc., 236,* 2773. (25) Stanley et al (1978) *Arch. Dermatol., 144,* 1350.

Thyphenytoin (phethenylate)

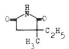

Causal relationship o

Hepatocellular damage was seen in 5 patients with a fatal course in 4, either due to liver failure or secondary to complications (1, 2). Jaundice appeared mostly after 5–6 months (1, 2). There were no concomitant immunoallergic signs. Autopsy in 3 cases showed massive necrosis (1, 2). There had been coadministration of phenobarbital in 3 patients (1, 2).

(1) Butscher et al (1952) *J. Am. Med. Assoc., 148,* 535. (2) Pryles et al (1952) *J. Am. Med. Assoc., 148,* 536.

B. SUCCINIMIDES

Ethosuximide

Causal relationship o

Liver enzyme elevations may occur (1). In a recent report, a 6–month–old boy developed ALAT elevation after 1 month of treatment with ethosuximide (60 mg/kg/d). Discontinuation was followed by significant improvement within 1 week. Other anticonvulsants were not held responsible in this case (2).

(1) *The Extra Pharmacopoeia, 28th ed,* p 1250. Pharmaceutical Press, London, 1982. (2) Coulter (1983) *Arch. Neurol., 40,* 393.

C. OXAZOLIDINES

Trimethadione

Causal relationship o

Hepatitis with jaundice (1, 2), exfoliative dermatitis (1) and erythema multiforme (2) appeared 2 weeks (2) to 4 weeks (1) after starting therapy; recovery was uneventful after discontinuation of the drug. One patient had a leukematous reaction in the bone marrow (1).

Coadministration of phenobarbital may have been responsible in 1 case (2).

(1) Leard et al (1949) *N. Engl. J. Med., 240,* 962. (2) Leblanc et al (1961) *Can. Med. Assoc. J., 85,* 200.

D. MISCELLANEOUS ANTICONVULSANTS

Acetoxyphenacemide (acetoxyphenurone)

Acetoxy derivative of phenacemide   *Causal relationship* o/+

Severe hepatic necrosis with fatal liver failure developed in 4 patients after 1–3 months of therapy (1). There were no immunoallergic signs. Most patients had used other anticonvulsants (phenytoin, phenobarbital) concurrently. Biopsy showed a pattern varying from centrizonal necrosis with surrounding steatosis to submassive necrosis; there was moderate infiltration, mainly by lymphocytes.

Animal toxicity tests proved this drug to be an intrinsic hepatotoxin (1), producing the same histological abnormalities as in the 4 human cases. Coadministration of other anticonvulsants (phenytoin, phenobarbital) was possibly responsible for enhanced toxicity due to enzyme induction.

A related compound, acetylpheneturide, has also been associated with hepatic injury (no further details); a leukocyte migration inhibition test was positive (2).

(1) Schnabel et al (1964) *Zentralbl. Allg. Pathol. Anat., 106,* 42. (2) Morizane (1978) *Gastroenterol. Jpn., 13,* 281.

Carbamazepine

Causal relationship +

A cholestatic to mixed pattern (1, 2, 13–15, 19, 20) as well as a hepatocellular pattern (3, 9, 14) has been observed. In other cases, a granulomatous hepatitis was present with mildly elevated liver enzymes (5, 7, 8). The onset was mostly within the first 6 weeks of treatment (1, 2, 4–9, 13–15), in some cases accompanied by fever (5, 8, 9, 14, 15, 20), rash (sometimes exfoliative) (1, 9, 13, 20), eosinophilia (11, 12, 14, 20), pancytopenia (10), agranulocytosis (4) and thrombocytopenia (13). Two cases resembled glandular fever with rash, eosinophilia, lymphadenopathy and hepatosplenomegaly (11, 12). There was a fatal course in some cases (3, 9). There was a positive reaction to rechallenge (2, 5, 15, 19, 20). In 1 case the transient presence of antimitochondrial antibodies was observed (5). Biopsy showed non–caseating granulomas (5, 7, 8, 14, 15), as well as cholestasis (2, 7, 8) and extensive necrosis (3, 6, 9, 14) with bridging (14). A pattern resembling chronic active hepatitis was observed in 1 case (6), cholangitis in 2 cases (8).

A case was described with a clinical picture resembling intermittent porphyria, possibly induced by carbamazepine via depression of uroporphyrinogen–I synthetase (16). This was debated by others (17) who pointed to a possible interfering effect of depression of 5–aminolevulinic acid dehydratase (17) and to the possible precipitation of latent acute intermittent porphyria (18). In a small study comparing carbamazepine–treated epileptics with controls (other anticonvulsants), Doss et al (21) found no significant difference in uroporphyrinogen–synthetase activity or in urinary excretion of heme precursors.

(1) Spillane (1964) *Practitioner, 192*, 71. (2) Ramsay (1967) *Br. Med. J., 4*, 155. (3) Zucker et al (1977) *J. Pediatr., 91*, 667. (4) Prieur et al (1973) *Ann. Pédiatr., 20*, 909. (5) Levander (1980) *Acta Med. Scand., 208*, 333. (6) Bertram et al (1980) *Am. J. Gastroenterol., 74*, 78. (7) Mitchell et al (1981) *Am. J. Med., 71*, 733. (8) Levy et al (1981) *Ann. Intern. Med., 95*, 64. (9) Hopen et al (1981) *Acta Med. Scand., 210*, 333. (10) Fellows (1969) *Headache, 9*, 92. (11) Taylor et al (1981) *Practitioner, 225*, 219. (12) Lewis et al (1982) *Postgrad. Med. J., 58*, 100. (13) Ponte (1983) *Drug Intell. Clin. Pharm., 17*, 642. (14) Soffer et al (1983) *South. Med. J., 76*, 681. (15) Knudsen et al (1979) *Ugeskr. Laeg., 141*, 3160. (16) Yeung Laiwah et al (1983) *Lancet, 1*, 790. (17) Rideout et al (1983) *Lancet, 2*, 464. (18) Shanley et al (1983) *Lancet, 1*, 1229. (19) Brukker et al (1966) *Ned. T. Geneeskd., 110*, 1181. (20) Davion et al (1984) *Gastroentérol. Clin. Biol., 8*, 52. (21) Doss et al (1984) *Lancet, 1*, 1026.

Phenacemide (phenurone)

$$CH_2—CO—NH—CO—NH_2$$ *Causal relationship* o/ +

This anticonvulsant is rarely used nowadays. Some fatal cases of hepatic injury have been described (3, 4, 7–9) with symptoms usually starting 1–3 months after first intake. In all cases, other anticonvulsants were taken concurrently. Several clinical trials mentioned cases of jaundice (1–3, 5), attributed to phenacemide–induced hepatic damage and an incidence was observed of 1–3% (2, 5, 6). The frequency of mild liver function disturbances was not given. Rash occurs in 3–5% (5, 6) to 9% (2) but is not mentioned in combination with hepatic injury, except in 1 case (4).

(1) Gibbs et al (1949) *Dis. Nerv. Syst., 10*, 47. (2) Carter et al (1950) *Dis. Nerv. Syst., 11*, 139. (3) Davidson et al (1950) *Dis. Nerv. Syst., 11*, 167. (4) Levy et al (1950) *N. Engl. J. Med., 242*, 933. (5) Tyler et al (1951) *J. Am. Med. Assoc., 147*, 17. (6) Livingston et al (1957) *N. Engl. J. Med., 256*, 588. (7) Liversedge et al (1952) *Lancet, 1*, 242. (8) Field et al (1954) *N. Engl. J. Med., 251*, 147. (9) Craddock (1955) *J. Am. Med. Assoc., 159*, 1437.

Valproate

$$C_3H_7—CH—COOH$$
$$\quad\ \ \ \ C_3H_7$$ *Causal relationship* + +

Valproate is sometimes given as valproic acid but mostly as sodium valproate, the latter commonly in a dose of 20–30 mg/kg/d. It is used in various forms of epilepsy. Its mechanism of action is unknown but may involve an alteration of γ–aminobutyric acid levels in the brain. Although marketed in some European countries since 1968, it took a decade before the first case–reports of hepatic injury appeared in the literature. Two studies of 31 (1) and 23 (2) fatal cases and a review article (7) had already been preceded by clinical studies showing liver enzyme (mainly ASAT/ALAT) elevations as high as 44% (3,4) or even 67% (5), but a lower percentage (7%) has also been mentioned (6). These elevations were transient despite continuation or responded to dose reduction. Moreover, several cases of mostly fatal hepatic injury ascribed to the use of valproate were reported in this period (8–20). The above–mentioned studies of fatal cases (1, 2) showed a fairly characteristic pattern. They concerned mostly children who developed prodromal manifestations such as lethargy, anorexia, nausea and abdominal discomfort. Convulsions increased in most patients (2, 7). Subsequently, jaundice, hypoglycemia, bleeding disorders, hyperammonemia, coma and ascites followed in varying frequency. Death was mostly due to hepatic failure. Striking are the absence of immunoallergic signs and the relatively low serum aminotransferases in the majority of cases (1, 2, 7). The onset was mostly at 1–4 months after starting therapy (1, 2, 7). One study mentioned a dose range of 13–71 mg/kg/d (2). In the other study, half of the patients were reported to have hypofibrinogenemia and/or thrombocytopenia, possibly secondary to disseminated intravascular coagulation (1). Important is the apparent absence of preceding influenza–like symptoms, unlike the Reye syndrome which resembles valproate hepatic injury (7). Histology showed microvesicular steatosis in most patients in both studies while in one the localization was mainly centri– and midzonal (1). Whereas in one study the localization of necrosis is mainly centrizonal (1), the other study mentions both centrizonal and non–zonal necrosis (2). Submassive necrosis is present in a minority (1, 2). One study reports mild to moderate cholestasis in all cases (2). Some cases showed cirrhosis (2).

In most cases other anticonvulsants (e.g. phenytoin, phenobarbital, carbamazepine) had been used concurrently and in 1 case symptoms of phenytoin intoxication were the first signs of valproate–associated liver damage (45). Although other anticonvulsants are not known to cause microvesicular steatosis, their enzyme–inducing effect may possibly play a role in the enhanced production of toxic metabolites of valproate.

Several recent reports of fatal hepatic injury confirm the fairly characteristic pattern (21–25, 34) by showing mainly the same clinical and histological features, although necrosis may predominate while steatosis is almost absent (45). In some non–fatal cases a rechallenge was positive (35, 46) but responded to a dose–reduction (46).

In a fatal case, a–antitrypsin deficiency (heterozygous) was suspected of having potentiated valproate–induced hepatic injury (39). In some cases of acute overdosage, severe hepatic injury was absent although microvesicular steatosis (40) and mild hyperbilirubinemia (41) were recorded.

Valproate has several metabolic effects. Hyperglycinemia/glycinuria (26), propionic acidemia (27) and hyperammonemia without hepatic injury (28, 29) have been described. The latter may even be accompanied by encephalopathy and impaired seizure control (36). Inhibition of fatty acid oxidation (30, 31, 43) and synthesis (38) may possibly account for steatosis by impairing fat metabolism.

The precise mechanism of injury is unknown. High doses in rats (750 mg/kg) produced significant microvesicular steatosis (33). Similar changes occurred with lower doses (350 mg/kg) and pretreatment with phenobarbital, while no steatosis was seen with this lower dose without pretreatment. The clinicopathological pattern resembles both Reye's syndrome and Jamaican vomiting disease, although necrosis is more prominent. In the latter, a toxic metabolite of hypoglycin A is held responsible (32). This metabolite resembles both 4–pentanoic acid, a powerful inhibitor of fatty acid oxidation, and 2–propyl–4–pentanoic acid, one of the metabolites of valproate (see formulae). The latter is formed by ω–oxidation, which is responsible for only a small part (5–15%) of metabolism. Indeed, this metabolite was toxic in cultured hepatocytes (37). It seems plausible that this metabolite is at least partly responsible for hepatic injury in some patients, who form increased amounts, e.g. by genetic predisposition and enzyme induction. Another mechanism was suggested by Coulter (44). He postulated that valproate may lower carnitine levels and thereby impair the metabolism of short– and long–chain fatty acids, since carnitine transports fatty acids across mitochondrial membranes (44). Indeed, hypocarnitinemia has been mentioned in some reports (23, 42). Unfortunately, there still are no sensitive methods for the early detection of valproate–induced hepatic injury (7). In severe cases, liver enzymes are often only mildly elevated. Zafrani et al (1) advised that excessive exercise or fasting should be avoided since these may increase ω–oxidation.

1. Hypoglycin A toxic metabolite

$$CH_2=C-CH-CH_2-COOH$$
with CH_2 branch on the C

2. 4–Pentanoic acid

$$CH_2=CH-CH_2-CH_2-COOH$$

3. Valproate toxic metabolite(?)

$$CH_2=CH-CH_2-CH-COOH$$
$$\qquad\qquad\qquad C_3H_7$$

(1) Zafrani et al (1982) *Hepatology, 2,* 648. (2) Zimmerman et al (1982) *Hepatology, 2,* 591. (3) Sussman et al (1979) *J. Am. Med. Assoc., 242,* 1173. (4) Coulter et al (1980) *J. Am. Med. Assoc., 244,* 785. (5) Vining et al (1979) *Am. J. Dis. Child., 133,* 274. (6) Sherard et al (1980) *Neurology, 30,* 31. (7) Stricker (1982) *Ned. Tijdschr. Geneeskd., 126,* 2111. (8) Mathis et al (1979) *Pediatr. Res., 13,* 527. (9) Suchy et al (1979) *N. Engl. J. Med., 300,* 962. (10) Gerber et al (1979) *J. Pediatr., 95,* 142. (11) Ware et al (1980) *Lancet, 2,* 1110. (12) Coeckelberghs et al (1980) *Ned. Tijdschr. Geneeskd., 124,* 1428. (13) Jacobi et al (1980) *Lancet, 1,* 712. (14) Young et al (1980) *Ann. Neurol., 7,* 389. (15) Le Bihan et al (1980) *Lancet, 2,* 1298. (16) Donat et al (1979) *Neurology, 29,* 273. (17) Vanasse et al (1981) *Neurology, 31,* 644. (18) Addison et al (1980) *Dev. Med. Child. Neurol., 22,* 248. (19) Tripp et al (1981) *Lancet, 1,* 1165. (20) Anonymous (1981) *FDA Drug Bull., 11,* 12. (21) Voigt et al (1982) *Rev. Méd.*

Toulouse, 18, 37. (22) Seghieri et al (1982) *Clin. Med., 63,* 610. (23) Böhles et al (1982) *Eur. J. Pediatr., 139,* 185. (24) Höjer et al (1982) *Dev. Med. Child. Neurol., 24,* 846. (25) Rolland et al (1982) *Arch. Fr. Pédiatr., 39,* 723. (26) Jaeken et al (1977) *Lancet, 2,* 617. (27) Schmid (1977) *Clin. Chim. Acta, 74,* 39. (28) Coulter et al (1980) *Lancet, 1,* 1310. (29) Rawat et al (1981) *Neurology, 31,* 1173. (30) Shumate et al (1981) *Ann. Neurol., 10,* 88. (31) Mortensen (1980) *Lancet, 2,* 856. (32) Tanaka (1979) In: *Vinken et al (Eds), Handbook of Clinical Neurology, Vol 37,* p 511. North Holland Publishing Co., Amsterdam. (33) Lewis et al (1982) *Hepatology, 2,* 870. (34) Axelgaard (1982) *Ugeskr. Laeg., 144,* 105. (35) Itoh et al (1982) *Am. J. Gastroenterol., 77,* 875. (36) Zaret et al (1982) *Neurology, 32,* 206. (37) Kingsley et al (1983) *J. Clin. Pharmacol., 23,* 178. (38) Becker et al (1983) *Arch. Biochem. Biophys., 223,* 381. (39) Moore et al (1984) *Lancet, 1,* 221. (40) Schnabel et al (1984) *Lancet, 1,* 221. (41) Karlsen et al (1983) *Acta Med. Scand., 213,* 405. (42) Ohtani et al (1982) *J. Pediatr., 101,* 782. (43) Coude et al (1983) *Biochem. Biophys. Res. Commun., 115,* 730. (44) Coulter (1984) *Lancet, 1,* 689. (45) Palm et al (1984) *Br. J. Clin. Pharmacol.,17,* 597. (46) Ramsay et al (1983) *Ann. Neurol., 13,* 688.

5. Antihistamines and other antiallergic agents

A. H_1–Receptor antagonists
B. H_2–Receptor antagonists
C. Miscellaneous

Introduction

Nausea may be the first symptom of hepatic disease. Antiemetics, e.g. H_1–receptor antagonists, may be falsely incriminated under such circumstances, but in view of the very rare cases in the literature of hepatic injury attributed to these agents, such an association is not often made.

Hepatic injury caused by these agents is very rare. H_1–receptor antagonists are only rarely reported as a cause, which is rather surprising for the phenothiazine derivatives, e.g. promethazine, of this group. The H_2–blockers seem to be a more frequent and better documented cause of hepatic injury, especially cimetidine. However, clinically significant hepatic injury is also rare with these agents.

In a post–marketing surveillance of ketotifen (5), 3 cases of jaundice were reported, but no details were given about pattern or causal relationship.

H_2–receptor antagonists reduce indocyanine green clearance, probably by a decrease in hepatic extraction (1). A reduction in hepatic blood flow, as previously suggested (2, 6), has been discarded by others (3) and does not probably occur, either in normal volunteers or in cirrhotic patients (4). Their inhibition of mixed–function oxidases has been suggested as useful in the early treatment of paracetamol intoxication but is controversial.

(1) Dunk et al (1983) *Br. J. Clin. Pharmacol., 16,* 117. (2) Feeley et al (1981) *N. Engl. J. Med., 304,* 692. (3) Groszmann (1983) *Hepatology, 3,* 1039. (4) Henderson et al (1983) *Hepatology, 3,* 919. (5) Maclay et al (1984) *Br. Med. J., 288,* 911. (6) Feeley et al (1982) *Lancet, 1,* 169.

A. H$_1$-RECEPTOR ANTAGONISTS

Cyclizine

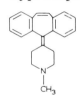

Causal relationship o/ +

Cyclizine is a piperazine antihistamine. One case of jaundice has been reported in a 8–year–old girl treated with 25 mg/d for 5 days (1). Discontinuation was followed by improvement. Readministration caused a relapse. A lymphocyte stimulation test was negative but 'anti–liver' antibodies were noted, a claim which has remained unsubstantiated (1).

A related compound, homochlorcyclizine, has been associated with a case of mixed cholestatic–hepatocellular injury, but no details were provided. A lymphocyte stimulation test and an assay for macrophage–mediated cytotoxicity were both positive (2).

(1) Kew et al (1973) *Br. Med. J., 2,* 307. (2) Mizoguchi (1980) *Gastroenterol. Jpn., 15,* 14.

Cyproheptadine

Causal relationship o

Cyproheptadine bears a structural resemblance to the tricyclic antidepressants. A case of cholestatic jaundice was reported in a 25–year–old woman after 1 month of therapy (1). Discontinuation was followed by recovery. Wortsman et al (2) found no liver function abnormalities in 20 patients treated with 16–32 mg/d for various disorders.

(1) Henry et al (1978) *Br. Med. J., 1,* 753. (2) Wortsman et al (1978) *Br. Med. J., 1,* 1217.

Trimethobenzamide

Causal relationship o

One case has been reported of jaundice, appearing after 5 days of therapy with this agent (1). However, the patient had been operated on for breast cancer in the preceding month and had received radiation therapy. Discontinuation of the drug was followed by almost complete recovery in 3 weeks. Histology showed centrilobular cholestasis, focal necrosis and portal inflammation mainly with neutrophils and mononuclear cells. Occasional wall thickening of vein tributaries was observed but no frank veno–occlusive disease.

(1) Borda et al (1967) *Arch. Intern. Med., 120,* 371.

Tripelennamine

Causal relationship o

A mixed cholestatic–hepatocellular pattern with jaundice (1) has been reported. Recovery was in 7 months after discontinuation. Biopsy showed centrilobular bile staining of hepatocytes, bile thrombi and necrosis. No further details were provided.

(1) Bjørneboe et al (1967) *Acta Med. Scand., 182, Fasc. 4,* 491.

B. H₂–RECEPTOR ANTAGONISTS

Cimetidine

Causal relationship +

Animal toxicity testing in dogs treated with 504 mg/kg for up to 12 months was associated with centrilobular degenerative changes and liver enzyme elevations (1). Early clinical trials also showed liver enzyme elevations (2). Some studies showed ASAT/ALAT elevations in 22–38% of patients on 1200–2000 mg/d (2), which suggests that the drug has a mild hepatotoxic effect. Intrinsic hepatotoxicity is also suggested by the observation of bile acid elevation in 5 children on 20–30 mg/kg/d (3).

Nevertheless, cimetidine–associated hepatic injury is probably rare when therapeutic doses are employed. Occasionally, clinically important cases have been reported of hepatic injury with a mixed cholestatic–hepatocellular pattern (4, 5), while in other cases cholestasis (3, 6) or hepatocellular damage (2, 7) predominated. The appearance of symptoms/signs was varyingly reported from 2 days (6) to more than half a year (5, 7, 8) after starting therapy. In 1 case there was concurrent thrombocytopenia (6), while another patient developed rash simultaneously (4). A rechallenge was positive (4–7), in 2 reports within 3 days (4, 5).

Histology showed focal (4) or zonal necrosis with collapse (7). Cholestasis and mild steatosis predominated in another case (6).

The mechanism is obscure. Mild intrinsic hepatotoxicity seems to be

90

present as suggested by aminotransferase elevations on high doses and in one case (1) a dose–dependent reaction to rechallenge. On the other hand, the accelerated reaction to rechallenge (1, 2), rash, and a positive macrophage inhibition test in 1 patient (8) may be compatible with an immunoallergic component in some cases.

(1) Leslie et al (1977) In: Burland and Simkins (Eds), *Cimetidine. Proceedings, Second International Symposium on Histamine H₂–Receptor Antagonists*, p 24. Excerpta Medica, Amsterdam. (2) Bleumink (1978) In: Dukes (Ed), *Side Effects of Drugs, Annual 2*, p 144. Excerpta Medica, Amsterdam. (3) Lilly et al (1978) *J. Surg. Res., 24*, 384. (4) Lorenzini et al (1981) *Dig. Dis. Sci., 26*, 275. (5) Villeneuve et al (1979) *Gastroenterology, 77*, 143. (6) Züchner (1977) *Dtsch. Med. Wochenschr., 102*, 1788. (7) Ruiz del Arbol et al (1982) *Am. J. Gastroenterol., 74*, 267. (8) Delpre et al (1982) *Am. J. Med. Sci., 283*, 153.

Ranitidine

$$(CH_3)_2 - N - CH_2 \underset{O}{\longrightarrow} CH_2 - S - CH_2 - CH_2 - NH - \underset{\underset{CH-NO_2}{\parallel}}{C} - NH - CH_3$$

Causal relationship o/ +

Occasional cases of hepatic injury have been ascribed to the use of ranitidine but some of these are not very convincing. In 1 such case a biochemical pattern of mainly hepatocellular injury appeared after 2 weeks of treatment but returned to normal despite continuation of therapy (1). In 2 other cases, mild to moderate liver enzyme elevations appeared 2–4 weeks after institution of ranitidine (2, 3). The former (2) was however disqualified by Halparin (4) who gave a more complete description of the same case.

We have received data on a patient who developed a rash to ranitidine which disappeared after discontinuation. After inadvertent rechallenge, the rash reappeared immediately, accompanied by mild ASAT/ALAT elevation (6).

In a case of granulomatous hepatitis appearing after 4–5 weeks of treatment (5), eosinophilic infiltration was seen on biopsy. Liver enzyme levels returned to normal after discontinuation, but a follow–up biopsy was not performed.

Recently a case was reported of mild anicteric hepatitis with slight focal necrosis and mild bile stasis, appearing within 12 days after starting treatment, with fever, chills and nausea. Readministration after recovery was immediately followed by a relapse with very high liver enzyme elevations (7). Black et al (8) reported 3 additional cases, 1 with a pattern of cholestatic hepatitis, appearing 3–5 weeks after initial treatment; not all other causes, however, could be ruled out.

(1) Barr et al (1981) *Med. J. Aust., 2*, 421. (2) Cleator (1983) *Can. Med. Assoc. J., 129*, 405. (3) Proctor (1984) *J. Am. Med. Assoc., 251*, 1554. (4) Halparin (1984) *Can. Med. Assoc. J., 130*, 668. (5) Offit et al (1984) *N. Engl. J. Med., 310*, 1603. (6) Nicolai (1984) Personal communication. (7) Souza Lima (1984) *Ann. Intern. Med., 101*, 207. (8) Black et al (1984) *Ann. Intern. Med., 101*, 208.

C. MISCELLANEOUS ANTIALLERGIC AGENTS

Cromolyn sodium

Causal relationship o

One case of a primary–biliary–cirrhosis–like illness was reported. Onset occurred after 10 months. There was purpura/eosinophilia. Skin biopsy showed vasculitis. The lymphocyte stimulation test was negative and no antibodies to cromolyn could be demonstrated. Purpura/eosinophilia quickly subsided after discontinuation of the drug and treatment with prednisone. Biopsy showed portal expansion, predominantly eosinophilic infiltration, periportal fibrosis and eosinophilic granulomas. A control biopsy showed primary biliary cirrhosis (1), but eosinophilic granulomas and infiltration had disappeared.

(1) Rosenberg et al (1978) *Arch. Intern. Med., 138,* 989.

6. Antihypertensive agents

A. Rauwolfia alkaloids
B. Hydralazines
C. Adrenergic neuron blockers
D. Miscellaneous

Introduction

Diuretics and vasodilators are also used as antihypertensive agents. These are discussed elsewhere (Chapters 18 and 23).

Hypertension is not associated with liver disease. However, it may be associated with congestive heart failure with liver injury secondary to hepatic congestion.

Patients with cardiovascular disease often receive many drugs, which may complicate the assessment of a causal relationship with the suspected drug. Moreover, concurrent illnesses, e.g. diabetes mellitus, may even further complicate evaluation.

The aim of treating hypertension is to restore normal blood pressure, thereby preventing long–term organ damage, without a strong decrease in blood flow to vital organs. This is especially important in geriatric patients who may already have a reduced blood supply. Although the liver can withstand a significant decrease in systemic blood pressure, a serious and rapid reduction may occasionally cause elevations of liver enzyme concentrations, e.g. by precipitation of congestive heart failure (diazoxide!) or reduction of an already impaired blood flow below a critical point. The usual antihypertensive drugs do not cause hepatic injury through their hypotensive effect but more probably through an idiosyncratic mechanism, either metabolic or immunoallergic.

Antihypertensive agents produce a mainly hepatocellular pattern. Most frequently incriminated are methyldopa and the hydralazines; relatively little is known about the absolute incidence, however. Rauwolfia alkaloids, β–adrenoceptor antagonists and adrenergic neuron blockers (with the exception of guanoxan), have only rarely been associated with hepatic injury. Mild liver enzyme elevations, however, have been noted with some agents, e.g. guanoclor (1). β–Adrenoceptor antagonists reduce blood flow. They are employed for the reduction of portal venous pressure in cirrhotic patients but have been associated with a rise in arterial ammonia (2) and with precipitation of encephalopathy (3). Direct liver injury by propranolol has been reported very rarely (4). In a 2–year study abnormal liver function tests were obtained in 8 of 25 patients on meto- prolol as against 2 of 30 patients on methyldopa (5). However, no details were given by the author, which makes the figures difficult to interpret. Practolol has been associated with biliary cirrhosis (9).

Some older drugs which have been implicated are para–aminobenzyl- caffeine and pargyline. The former was withdrawn from trial because it was associated with prolonged intrahepatic cholestasis (6), whereas the latter, a monoamine–oxidase inhibitor without a hydrazine moiety, caus- ed dose–dependent hepatic injury in rats for which the propioaldehyde metabolite was held responsible (7). Chlorisondamine, a ganglion–block- ing agent, decreased ornithine decarboxylase activity in liver tissue of young rats (8); it has not caused hepatic injury in man, as far as we know.

(1) Bayne et al (1980) In: Dukes (Ed), *Meyler's Side Effects of Drugs, 9th ed*, p 317. (2) Van Buuren et al (1982) *Lancet, 2*, 951. (3) Tarver et al (1983) *Br. Med. J., 287*, 585. (4) Iwamura (1973) *Z. Gastroenterol., 11*, 65. (5) Karachalios (1983) *Int. J. Clin. Pharmacol. Ther., 21*, 476. (6) Borges et al (1956) *J. Lab. Clin. Med., 47*, 735. (7) DeMaster et al (1982) *Toxicol. Appl. Pharmacol., 65*, 390. (8) Kuhn et al (1982) *Bio- chem. Pharmacol., 31*, 1798. (9) Brown et al (1978) *Br. Med. J., 1*, 1591.

A. RAUWOLFIA ALKALOIDS

Reserpine

Causal relationship o

Cholestatic hepatitis occurred 1 year after intermittent intake of a com- bination of reserpine, phenobarbital and quinidine; there was eosinophi- lia (1). Intracutaneous testing with reserpine (1:1000) was positive; quini- dine and phenobarbital tests were negative.

The leukocyte migration inhibition test was positive in another unspe- cified case of hepatic injury (2). Animal toxicity tests (hamsters) showed hepatocellular degeneration and necrosis at 3x the therapeutic dose (3).

(1) Möckel (1965) *Med. Klin., 60*, 294. (2) Morizane (1978) *Gastroenterol. Jpn., 13*, 281. (3) Windborn et al (1970) *Lab. Invest., 23*, 216.

B. HYDRALAZINES

Dihydralazine

Causal relationship +

Cases of icteric parenchymatous hepatitis have been reported, starting within about 1 month (8, 16), but mostly after several months (8, 9, 11–13, 16–18), with recovery usually in 2 months. Fever (9), rash and eosinophilia (8) were reported. Biopsy showed extensive necrosis usually with bridging (8, 11–13). There was a resemblance to alcoholic hepatitis in 1 case (8).

Rechallenge was positive (8, 9, 13) within several days (8, 9). Slow acetylator status (8) was suggested to play a causal role (14).

Roschlau (19) presented a study of 20 cases of confluent, predominantly centrilobular, necrosis mostly with central–central bridging. Necrotic areas were surrounded by a dense, mixed mononuclear and granulocytic infiltrate. The periportal area was largely preserved. The reaction appeared after 0.5–11 months of treatment. Rechallenge in 3 patients was positive with a relapse in 2 days to 5 weeks. One patient had a 5th relapse in 10 years of intermittent treatment. Most patients were women (M:F, 1:3). Jaundice was present in 16, whereas immunoallergic signs were absent. An analogous case was described by Pariente et al (18), in whom acute bridging necrosis appeared after 2–5 months of treatment, who improved after discontinuation but relapsed after rechallenge. Fibrotic sequelae were observed on follow–up.

Ecarazine

NH-NH-CO-O-CH$_2$-CH$_3$

Causal relationship o

Mild to extensive hepatocellular necrosis was reported, starting after 1–2 years of use and resolving in several months (5). Biopsy showed focal necrosis in 1 case, submassive necrosis and subsequent fibrosis in another.

Hydralazine

NH-NH$_2$

Causal relationship +

A moderate (2, 3) to severe (1, 4, 5), predominantly hepatocellular pattern of injury has been reported, although cholestatic hepatitis (6) has been observed. An incidental report of associated lupus–syndrome has been made (10). Fever (3, 4, 6, 7, 18), rash (3) and eosinophilia (3, 7, 17) occur. Onset is within days/weeks of initial intake (1, 2, 6, 7, 17) or only after several months/years (3, 4). Biopsy showed extensive bridging necrosis and fibrosis (4, 5), granulomatous hepatitis (7, 17, 18) and centrilobular cholestasis (6).

A rechallenge, performed in some cases, was positive in several days (1) to 2 weeks (4). The mechanism of hepatic injury is unknown. Although immunoallergic signs may be present, it is probably not the mechanism of injury. Hydralazine, ecarazine and dihydralazine, as hydrazine derivatives, may be suspected of causing hepatic injury in individuals with an abnormal metabolism. An enhanced risk for slow acetylators has been suggested (8, 14), but since hepatic injury has also been noted in rapid acetylators (2), the mechanism is probably, like that of isoniazid, more complicated. Noda et al (15) demonstrated hydrazine formation in animal toxicity testing and although it does not prove a pathogenetic role in man, it does favor metabolic idiosyncrasy as a mechanism in patients producing relatively large quantities of toxic intermediates.

(1) Bartoli et al (1979) *Arch. Intern. Med., 139,* 698. (2) Barnett et al (1980) *Br. Med. J., 1,* 1165. (3) Forster (1980) *N. Engl. J. Med., 302,* 1362. (4) Itoh et al (1980) *Dig. Dis. Sci., 25,* 884. (5) Itoh et al (1981) *Hepato–Gastroenterology, 28,* 13. (6) Stewart et al (1981) *Lancet, 1,* 1207. (7) Jori et al (1973) *Gastroenterology, 64,* 1163. (8) Knoblauch et al (1977) *Schweiz. Med. Wochenschr., 107,* 651. (9) Enat et al (1977) *Schweiz. Med. Wochenschr., 107,* 657. (10) Perry (1973) *Am. J. Med., 54,* 58. (11) Roschlau et al (1982) *Dtsch. Gesundheitsw., 37,* 709. (12) Mölleken et al (1980) *Z. Ges. Inn. Med., 35,* 296. (13) Bayer (1984) Personal communication. (14) Paumgartner (1977) *Schweiz. Med. Wochenschr., 107,* 649. (15) Noda et al (1979) *Chem. Pharm. Bull., 27,* 1938. (16) Brücker et al (1983) *89. Tagung der Deutschen Gesellschaft für Innere Medizin, Wiesbaden,* (Abstract). (17) Klatskin (1975) In: Schiff (Ed), *Diseases of the Liver, 4th ed,* p 604. Lippincott, Philadelphia. (18) Pariente et al (1983) *Digestion, 27,* 47. (19) Roschlau (1983) *Zbl. Allg. Pathol. Pathol. Anat., 127,* 385.

C. ADRENERGIC NEURON BLOCKERS

Guanoxan

Causal relationship o/ +

Liver damage was reported in some clinical trials in up to 30% of cases (1, 2), but not in others (3, 4). In 1 study of 96 hypertensive patients, minor and severe abnormalities in liver function were present in 26 (27%) and 10 (10%) cases, respectively. Of the latter cases, 4 had jaundice; 1 of these cases had a fatal course (1). Jaundice appeared after 2–13 months of treatment. The reaction was not dose–related (5). Biopsy showed a pattern resembling viral hepatitis, sometimes of chronic hepatitis. These data led to withdrawal of the drug by the manufacturers.

(1) Cotton et al (1967) *Br. Med. J., 3,* 174. (2) Frohlich et al (1966) *Clin. Pharmacol. Ther., 7,* 599. (3) Vejlsgaard et al. (1967) *Br. Med. J., 2,* 598. (4) Sheps et al (1966) Mayo Clin. Proc., 41, 577. (5) Anonymous (1966) *Drug Ther. Bull., 4,* 15.

Prenylamine

Causal relationship o

Prenylamine is an antianginal agent with quinidine–like effects on the heart. It is a known cause of ventricular tachycardia. An occasional case of nausea and ASAT elevation has been described which disappeared after a dose reduction from 240 mg to 180 mg daily (1).

(1) Cardoe (1968) *Br. J. Clin. Pract., 22,* 299.

D. MISCELLANEOUS ANTIHYPERTENSIVE AGENTS

Captopril

COOH

N-CO-C-CH₂SH
         |
         CH₃

Causal relationship +

The adverse reaction profile of captopril resembles that of penicillamine. Both drugs have a sulfhydryl group. Cases of icteric (1) and non–icteric (2), acute hepatocellular injury have been observed. Another case of cap-topril–associated jaundice showed biochemically a cholestatic pattern with high APh and/or bilirubin levels and mild to moderate ASAT/ALAT elevation (3, 4). Concurrent immunoallergic signs were not reported. The reactions appeared variably after 1–2 months (3, 4), 6 months (1) and 20 (2) months of treatment. In 1 case, a rechallenge was positive (2). Histolo-gy showed cellular degeneration with mild infiltration (2) and in another case pericentral cholestasis with bile plugging (4).

(1) Vandenburg et al (1981) *Br. J. Clin. Pharmacol., 11,* 105. (2) Ryckelynck et al (1982) *Nouv. Presse Méd., 11,* 1950. (3) Zimran et al (1983) *Br. Med. J., 287,* 1676. (4) Parker (1984) *Drug Intell. Clin. Pharm., 18,* 234.

Methyldopa

              CH₃
              |
HO⟨   ⟩-CH₂-C-COOH
  | |
  OH   NH₂

Causal relationship + +

Serum aminotransferase elevations have been reported to range from 1 to 35% (1), but most large studies give an overall incidence of approxi-mately 5% or lower (2). Jick et al (3) estimated methyldopa–induced symptomatic liver disease to occur in less than 0.1%.

Symptomatic hepatitis consists of acute hepatocellular injury, al-though a predominantly cholestatic pattern has been reported occasion-ally (4). Injury appeared mostly within the first 3 months of therapy; less than 10% occurred later (4). There was no dose dependence. Fever oc-curred in approximately one–third of patients, while rash or eosinophilia were infrequent (4). Hemolytic anemia may be present; Coombs' direct antiglobulin test was positive in 43% of the assessed cases (4) as against 15% in the total population (5). Anti–smooth–muscle antibodies were present in one–third of the tested cases, while antinuclear factor was frequently positive. Antimitochondrial antibodies were absent (4). Seventy percent of the reported cases were in female patients. In approximately 9% of the clinically overt cases the course was fatal (4). Histology showed focal patchy necrosis in 48% of performed biopsies while 44% exhibited a more severe pattern with bridging or massive necrosis. Mononuclear infiltration predominated. In chronic cases, periportal 'piecemeal' necrosis and fibrosis and ultimately cirrhosis ensued. Rodman et al (4) concluded that methyldopa hepatitis has the same clinical and histological spectrum as viral hepatitis. Arranto et al (6) distinguished 2 syndromes in their 31 patients with methyldopa hepatitis. Seven patients developed severe acute hepatitis, fatal in 2 of them, within the first 6 months of therapy. Histology ranged from focal to confluent and massive necrosis. The other 24 patients developed symptoms of nausea and abdominal pain after 2 or more years. Biopsy showed chronic inflammation with fatty accumulation, fibrosis, granulomas and vacuolated hepatocyte nuclei.

Two reports suggest that, relative to all known causes of chronic active hepatitis (CAH), methyldopa is frequently incriminated. One report ascribed 5 of 21 consecutive cases of CAH to the use of methyldopa (17), but in a more recent study this drug was held responsible for only 2 of 61 cases (18).

Several more recent reports of acute hepatocellular injury (8–10) or of chronic active hepatitis (7, 10–14) showed largely the above–mentioned features. In one report, several immunological markers and inactivity of T–lymphocytes were demonstrated; autoantibodies (antinuclear factor, smooth muscle antibodies) disappeared after recovery (8). Some cases of CAH were accompanied by hemolytic anemia (11, 24). In another patient, antibodies were demonstrated against endoplasmic reticulum (12).

In a report of 6 cases of granulomatous myocarditis, 4 patients exhibited granulomatous hepatitis and 2 CAH (15). In 4 of these patients, granulomatous pneumonitis was demonstrable. Five patients died secondary to cardiac failure. In an almost identical case, granulomas were demonstrated in heart, liver, lungs, spleen, bone marrow and lymph nodes (16). Both reports mentioned vasculitis. The onset in these cases is not known, but duration of therapy ranged from 1–2 weeks to several years. Histology of the liver showed 'granulomatous hepatitis' (15) and portal and lobular non–necrotizing granulomas (16).

A retrospective analysis of 82 patients with biliary carcinoma suggested a higher–than–usual prevalence of methyldopa consumption (20). However, a correct control group was not included, duration of therapy was unknown, and tests for statistical significance were not performed. Another study comparing the incidence rates of this tumor with methyldopa sales rates failed to show a correlation (21).

The mechanism of methyldopa–induced liver lesions is unknown. The relatively frequent liver enzyme elevations are compatible with an intrinsic toxic effect and indeed a reactive metabolite of methyldopa has been demonstrated (19). On the other hand, a recent study suggested that methyldopa indirectly inhibits suppressor T–cell function, thereby leading to unregulated autoantibody production by B–cells in some patients (5). Because an anamnestic response is probably absent, readministration does not cause the same prompt reaction as is known from the immunoallergic type. Several methyldopa cases exhibited this delayed reaction to rechallenge. Nevertheless, in a number of cases, immunoallergy may play a role as demonstrated by leukocyte migration inhibition or lymphocyte stimulation in the presence of the drug (8, 9, 22). Moreover, some cases seem to experience desensitization after rechallenge (4, 23).

(1) Zimmerman (1978) *Hepatotoxicity*, p 510. Appleton–Century–Crofts, New York. (2) Tester–Dalderup (1979) In: Dukes (Ed), *Side Effects of Drugs, Annual 3*, p 189. Excerpta Medica, Amsterdam. (3) Jick et al (1981) *J. Clin. Pharmacol., 21*, 359. (4) Rodman et al (1976) *Am. J. Med., 60*, 941. (5) Kirtland et al (1980) *N. Engl. J. Med., 302*, 825. (6) Arranto et al (1981) *Scand. J. Gastroenterol., 16*, 853. (7) Balazs et al (1981) *Hepato–Gastroenterol., 28*, 199. (8) Delpre et al (1979) *Am. J. Med. Sci., 277*, 207. (9) Anomymous (1978) *Jpn. Med. Gaz., 15*, 7. (10) Seggie et al (1979) *S. Afr. Med. J., 55*, 75. (11) Shalev et al (1983) *Arch. Intern. Med., 143*, 592. (12) Beaugrand et al (1980) *Gastroentérol. Clin. Biol., 4*, 219. (13) De Oliveira e Silva et al (1982) *Gastroenterol. Endosc. Dig., 1*, 91. (14) Romeo et al (1981) *Prog. Med., 37*, 590. (15) Seeverens et al (1982) *Acta Med. Scand., 211*, 233. (16) Bezahler (1982) *Am. J. Med. Sci., 283*, 41. (17) Goldstein et al (1973) *Dig. Dis. Sci., 18*, 177. (18) Hodges et al (1982) *Lancet, 1*, 550. (19) Dybing et al (1976) *Mol. Pharmacol., 12*, 911. (20) Brodén et al (1980) *Acta Chir. Scand., 500*, 7. (21) Stolley (1982) *J. Clin. Pharmacol., 22*, 499. (22) Morizane (1978) *Gastroenterol. Jpn., 13*, 281. (23) Elkington et al (1969) *Circulation, 40*, 589. (24) Breland et al (1982) *Drug Intell. Clin. Pharmacol., 16*, 489.

7. Lipid–lowering agents

A. Clofibrate and related compounds
B. Ion exchange resins
C. Miscellaneous

Introduction

Nicotinic acid derivatives are also used as lipid–lowering agents but are discussed in Chapter 23.

Most forms of lipoprotein disorders do not show a significantly increased risk of hepatobiliary disease. Mild fatty change, however, is not uncommon, especially not if associated with obesity. Moreover, patients with familial hyperlipoproteinemia, particularly hypertriglyceridemia (Type IV), generally have a relatively high incidence of gallstones (1). Hyperlipidemia may also be a sign of underlying liver disease, in which case therapy–associated injury may be partly ascribed to the underlying condition.

Mild elevation of serum aminotransferase concentrations has been reported during therapy with clofibrate and related compounds such as halofenate (2), ciprofibrate (3), tibric acid (2), clofibride (4), pirinixil (8) and etofibrate (5). Mostly these are minimal and transient and do not present a serious clinical problem unless as part of the muscular syndrome. The agents increase the biliary excretion of cholesterol and enhance the risk of biliary disease, probably through increased gallstone formation secondary to supersaturation of bile. The acute toxicity of these agents is low, but long–term toxicity, related to their shift in lipid spectrum, gives rise to concern. Moreover long–term, high–dose administration of ciprofibrate (7) and related compounds caused liver carcinomas in rats and mice (6). Studies in the USA with nafenopin were stopped following a report of liver nodules in rats (2). Ion exchange resins are not absorbed and probably do not injure the liver directly. There is some reason to believe that they can increase the risk of gallstone formation through a decrease in reabsorption of biliary acids with secondary bile supersaturation.

(1) Tan et al (1982) In: Schiff et al (Eds), *Diseases of the Liver, 5th ed*, p 1507. Lippincott, Philadelphia. (2) *The Extra Pharmacopoeia, 28th ed*, p 412. Pharmaceutical Press, London, 1982. (3) Olsson et al (1982) *Atherosclerosis, 42*, 229. (4) Foucault (1975) *Ouest Méd., 28*, 1387. (5) Scheer (1981) In: Dukes (Ed), *Side Effects of Drugs, Annual 5*, p 401. Excerpta Medica, Amsterdam. (6) Blümcke (1983) *Athe-*

rosclerosis, 46, 105. (7) Rao et al (1984) *Cancer Res., 44,* 1072. (8) Nunes (1982) *Curr. Ther. Res. Clin. Exp., 31,* 193.

A. CLOFIBRATE AND RELATED COMPOUNDS

Bezafibrate

$$CH_3$$
$$H_3C-C-COOH$$
$$O$$

OC-NH-CH$_2$-CH$_2$

Cl

Causal relationship o/ +

Hepatomegaly has been recorded in 5 of 63 patients on 600 mg/d for 12 weeks (1). In a smaller study of 10 patients on 2 g/d mild hepatomegaly occurred in about half the patients (2). Like clofibrate, elevations of aminotransferase concentrations may occur as part of the muscular syndrome (3).

(1) Fellin et al (1981) *Curr. Ther. Res., 4,* 657. (2) Martini et al (1982) *Curr. Ther. Res., 31,* 354. (3) Heidemann et al (1981) *Klin. Wochenschr., 59,* 413.

Clofibrate

$$CH_3$$
$$CH_3-C-CO-OC_2H_5$$
$$O$$

Cl

Causal relationship +

Mild and transient elevation of aminotransferase concentration in serum may occur but is usually of little clinical importance. However, it may be part of the 'muscular syndrome' with myalgia, stiffness and weakness, and with elevated CPK values in the serum (1). When administered in high doses to animals, clofibrate caused hepatomegaly, enlargement of hepatocytes, variable steatosis and an increase in lysosomes (2). Hepatomegaly may also occur in man, and was occasionally reported in up to 50% of the patients (3).

A study of liver biopsies of 40 patients with hyperlipoproteinemia before and after 3 months of therapy did not show significant differences in patients on 500 mg/d. On 1.5 g/d, 6 patients showed improvement and 3 patients deterioration of pre–existing fatty change (4). Symptomatic cases of hepatic injury in man have been seldom reported. In 1 patient granulomatous hepatitis appeared after 3 months of treatment with the

101

drug. Discontinuation led to recovery (5). In another patient, intrahepatic cholestasis was ascribed to this agent (6).

Clofibrate increases the incidence of gallbladder disease (7, 10). Through a decrease in bile acid pool size and synthesis and an increase in cholesterol (8, 12), bile saturation is enhanced. In some patients with primary biliary cirrhosis, clofibrate paradoxically increased cholesterol blood levels (9, 13) and xanthoma formation (13). There is concern about the long–term safety of clofibrate. The WHO cooperative clofibrate trial suggested a reduction in cardiovascular disease but an increased total mortality, mainly secondary to liver and gallbladder complications, intestinal disturbances and malignancies (10). One recent report of a 76–year–old woman who had been treated with clofibrate for 7 years described preneoplastic and other adenomatous hepatocellular lesions (11). These lesions consisted of multiple small hyperplastic (PAS–positive) liver foci and adenomatous noduli in a non–cirrhotic liver. This report, however, is still speculative.

(1) Dukes (1977) In: Dukes (Ed), *Side Effects of Drugs, Annual 1*, p 329. Excerpta Medica, Amsterdam. (2) Zimmerman (1982) *Diseases of the Liver*, p 621. Lippincott, Philadelphia. (3) Martini et al (1982) *Curr. Ther. Res., 31*, 354. (4) Schwandt et al (1978) *Lancet, 2*, 325. (5) Pierce et al (1978) *N. Engl. J. Med., 299*, 314. (6) Valdes et al (1976) *Am. J. Gastroenterol., 66*, 69. (7) Coronary Drug Project Research Group (1977) *N. Engl. J. Med., 296*, 1185. (8) Bateson et al (1978) *Am. J. Dig. Dis., 23*, 623. (9) Summerfield et al (1975) *Gastroenterology, 69*, 998. (10) Committee of Principal Investigators (1978) *Br. Heart J., 40*, 1069. (11) Mori et al (1982) *Acta Pathol. Jpn., 32*, 671. (12) Pertsemlidis et al (1974) *Gastroenterology, 66*, 565. (13) Schaffner (1969) *Gastroenterology, 57*, 253.

Fenofibrate

Causal relationship +

Mild to moderate non–symptomatic elevations of ASAT/ALAT were reported in 9% (2) to 19% of patients (300–400 mg/d). Children seem more vulnerable (1). Cases of mild parenchymatous hepatitis (3, 4, 6), one of which had a positive reaction to readministration after 6 weeks, have been reported. In one of these reports, however, concurrent use of amiodarone or pyridinol carbamate could have been responsible (3). Blümcke et al (5) studied biopsies from 38 hyperlipidemic patients, 28 on fenofibrate and 10 controls. The treatment period varied from 2 months to 3 years. Peroxisome proliferation, as seen in animals, was not present in these patients. Mild changes in mitochondria and endoplasmic reticulum and mild fatty change were not considered to be significantly different from controls (5).

(1) De Gennes et al (1978) *Nouv. Presse Méd., 7*, 2398. (2) Fromantin et al (1981) *Thérapie, 36*, 473. (3) Aron et al (1979) *Nouv. Presse Méd., 8*, 783. (4) Vachon (1980)

Nouv. Presse Méd., 9, 2740. (5) Blümcke et al (1983) Atherosclerosis, 46, 105. (6) Couzigou et al (1980) Thérapie, 35, 403.

Gemfibrozil

Causal relationship o

Gemfibrozil is a new lipid–lowering agent structurally related to clofibrate. It has been tested in several types of hyperlipoproteinemia, usually in a dose of 1.2 g/d. Up till now, adverse effects seem minor. Transiently elevated serum aminotransferases occurred occasionally (1). According to Pickering et al (3) the incidence of liver enzyme elevations above the upper limit of normal was less than 3% in a study of over 400 patients. In a study of 9 patients on long–term treatment (17–27 months) for hyperlipoproteinemia Type IIa, IIb and IV, mild to severe panlobular steatosis was found in 8 patients, both obese and non–obese (2). Liver architecture was preserved. Isolated cell necrosis was found in 4 patients. Both small lipid droplets and large fatty cysts were seen. Kupffer cell hyperplasia with lipid inclusions was present in several cases. Cholestasis was absent. Electron microscopy demonstrated a predominance of small fat droplets in the sinusoidal region of hepatocytes. However, mitochondria and endoplasmic reticulum were mostly of normal shape. Unfortunately, little is known about the liver in untreated patients. Although the obesity in some of these patients may have contributed to steatosis, caution seems warranted with long–term treatment and further study is indicated.

(1) Manninen et al (1982) Acta Med. Scand., Suppl, 82, 668. (2) De la Iglesia et al (1982) Atherosclerosis, 43, 19. (3) Pickering et al (1983) Am. J. Cardiol., 52, 39B.

B. ION EXCHANGE RESINS

Cholestyramine

Chloride of a polystyrene resin with quaternary ammonium groups

Causal relationship o

Occasional elevations in aminotransferase concentrations seem to occur (1), although one may wonder whether this is coincidence since cholestyramine is not absorbed from the gastrointestinal tract. There has been some concern that this type of drug might enhance gallstone formation by decreasing the enterohepatic recirculation of bile acids, thus causing supersaturation of bile (2). A recently published multicenter, randomized, double–blind trial on cholestyramine indeed showed an increase in diagnosis of gallstones and in gallbladder operations, but no statistically significant differences were obtained (3). The mean serum ASAT level was minimally elevated after 1 year in the treated group, but the meaning of this remains obscure.

(1) Scheer (1981) In: Dukes (Ed), *Side Effects of Drugs, Annual 5*, p 401. Excerpta Medica, Amsterdam. (2) Meinertz et al (1978) In: Dukes (Ed), *Side Effects of Drugs, Annual 2*, p 360. Excerpta Medica, Amsterdam. (3) The Lipid Research Clinics Coronary Primary Prevention Trial Results (1984) *J. Am. Med. Assoc., 251,* 351.

Colestipol

Copolymer of diethylenetriamine and
1–chloro–2,3–epoxypropane HCl
(with approximately 1 out of 5 amine
nitrogens protonated)   *Causal relationship* o

Analogous to cholestyramine, colestipol is probably harmless to the liver. Like the former, it has been suspected of increasing bile stone formation, but convincing data are lacking. In a study of 14 patients, one of them with a marked increase in bile lithogenicity was found to have developed (?) gallstones after 3 weeks of treatment. For the group as a whole, no significant change in biliary lipid composition was reported (1).

(1) Grundy et al (1977) *J. Lab. Clin. Med., 89,* 354.

C. MISCELLANEOUS

Dextrothyroxine

Causal relationship o

Above–normal values of direct bilirubin and ASAT were reported in 30.8% and 40.2% respectively of patients (1074 men) on this agent as compared to 20.5% and 32% respectively (2683 men) on placebo at any moment over an average follow–up period of 36 months. Both groups had coronary heart disease (1). The reason for this difference is unknown. The study was discontinued because of an excess number of non–fatal cardiovascular incidents in the treatment group.

(1) The Coronary Drug Project Research Group (1972) *J. Am. Med. Assoc., 220,* 996.

Probucol

The structure of probucol differs from that of other lipid–lowering agents. It is stored in fatty tissue and may still be demonstrated in plasma several months after discontinuation (1). Liver enzyme elevations have been recorded.

(1) *The Extra Pharmacopoeia, 28th ed,* p 414. Pharmaceutical Press, London, 1982.

8. Drugs for gallstone dissolution

Introduction

These agents desaturate the bile by expanding the bile acid pool, thereby facilitating gallstone dissolution in an indirect way. Ursodeoxycholic acid, however, probably also has a directly dissolving effect on gallstones. These agents are used preferably for small radiolucent gallstones in an otherwise normal gallbladder of a non–obese person.

Mild and transient elevations of aminotransferase concentrations in serum are most frequently caused by chenodeoxycholic acid. Serious toxicity seems to be absent.

Chenodeoxycholic acid

Causal relationship +

Chenodeoxycholic acid (CDCA) occurs naturally as one of the primary bile acids formed in the liver from cholesterol. It is further metabolized by intestinal bacteria to lithocholic acid, a proven and experimentally used cholestatic hepatotoxin. Orally administered, it is used for the dissolution of gallstones at a dose of 15 mg/kg/d and up to 20 mg/kg/d in obese individuals. The main adverse effects are diarrhea and serum aminotransferase elevations. The consequences of changes in serum lipids as reported in the National Cooperative Gallstone Study (1) are still unknown. Aminotransferase elevations have been reported in high percentages in some studies depending upon the dose (2) and the capacity to metabolize lithocholic acid, especially by sulfate conjugation (3). Mostly these elevations during the first weeks of therapy do not exceed the normal limit by more than 3 times. A slight elevation in unconjugated bilirubin (4, 5) is probably of little importance. Sinusoidal dilatation, reported by some authors (6), needs further confirmation. In the above–mentioned gallstone study, 8% of patients treated with 750 mg/d, 5% on 375 mg/d and 4% on placebo had ALAT elevations of more than 3 times the normal limit (1). 'Clinically significant' hepatic injury occurred in 3%, 0.4% and 0.4%, respectively, and was reversible after discontinuation. Three patients were withdrawn because of chronic active hepatitis,

2 of whom were from the high–dose group. A rechallenge was positive in most CDCA–treated patients. Concomitant studies of biopsies obtained before and after 9 and 24 months of treatment suggested mild abnormalities. Light microscopy (7) was equivocal: one of the 2 pathologists saw a mild increase of ballooning, binucleation, ductule proliferation, portal expansion and sinusoidal dilatation. Electron microscopy (8) showed ultrastructural evidence of intrahepatic cholestasis in 64% before and in 89% during therapy, independent of the dose. The mechanism inducing a hepatotoxic effect is still unknown. Either CDCA itself has intrinsic toxic potential or it is secondary to the formation of lithocholic acid and the incapacity to metabolize the latter safely; the latter mechanism seems the more probable. According to the results of the National Cooperative Gallstone Study, the agent was recommended for selected patients with radiolucent stones in a radiologically opacified gallbladder, a clinical need for treatment and an increased operative risk (9). Because only a small proportion of patients are candidates, efficacy is low, and recurrence rates are high; since the risk of serious hepatic injury in a larger population is still unknown, CDCA's usefulness has been questioned (10).

(1) Schoenfield et al (1981) *Ann. Intern. Med., 95,* 257. (2) Langman (1984) In: Dukes (Ed), *Meyler's Side Effects of Drugs, 10th ed,* p 699. Elsevier, Amsterdam. (3) Sue et al (1980) *Gastroenterology, 78,* 1324. (4) Thistle et al (1973) *N. Engl. J. Med., 289,* 655. (5) Capron et al (1979) *Gastroenterology, 77,* 121. (6) Levy et al (1978) *Lancet, 1,* 206. (7) Fischer et al (1982) *Hepatology, 2,* 187. (8) Philips et al (1983) *Hepatology, 3,* 209. (9) Schoenfield et al (1983) *Gastroenterology, 84,* 644. (10) Way (1983) *Gastroenterology, 84,* 648.

Ursodeoxycholic acid

Causal relationship o

Liver enzyme elevations are less frequent with ursodeoxycholic acid than with chenodeoxycholic acid (1, 3, 4) but have been reported. Although a study in rhesus monkeys showed the same changes with ursodeoxycholic acid as with chenodeoxycholic acid (2), the hepatotoxicity of the former seems minimal.

(1) Bell (1983) In: Dukes (Ed), *Side Effects of Drugs, Annual 7,* p 358. Excerpta Medica, Amsterdam. (2) Sarva et al (1980) *Gastroenterology, 79,* 629. (3) Fromm et al (1983) *Gastroenterology, 85,* 1257. (4) Gatto et al (1984) *Clin. Trials J., 21,* 135.

7–Ketolithocholic acid   *Causal relationship* o

7–Ketolithocholic acid is mainly metabolized to chenodeoxycholic acid (see above). In a study of 9 patients (400 mg/d), one had an aminotransfer-ase elevation which disappeared after discontinuation (1).

(1) Mazzella et al (1982) *Gastroenterology, 82,* 1236.

9. Antiparkinsonian agents

A. Anticholinergics
B. Dopaminergics

Introduction

Parkinsonism is not associated with an increased incidence of hepatic disease.

Anticholinergic antiparkinsonian agents cause hepatic injury only very rarely or not at all. Of the 6 different pharmacological dopaminergic groups – levodopa, peripheral decarboxylase inhibitors, aporphines, adamantanamines, dopamine–β–hydroxylase inhibitors and polypeptide ergot alkaloids – the latter are most frequently implicated as a cause of hepatic injury. Both bromocriptine in high doses and lergotrile probably have an intrinsic hepatotoxic effect. Pergolide is supposed to be less toxic because of the absence of a cyano–moiety in the 8–β–acetonitrile group (1).

Piribedil, a non–ergot dopamine receptor agonist, has occasionally been associated with a rise in serum APh and/or aminotransferase levels (2, 3).

(1) Teychenne et al (1979) *Gastroenterology, 76,* 575. (2) Sweet et al (1974) *Clin. Pharmacol. Ther., 16,* 1077. (3) Engel et al (1975) *Eur. J. Clin. Pharmacol., 8,* 223.

A. ANTICHOLINERGICS

Trihexyphenidyl

Causal relationship o

Two fatal cases of subacute hepatic necrosis were ascribed to use of this drug; however, no further specification was given (1). Its misuse by drug addicts (2) suggests other possible causes.

(1) Kanetaka et al (1973) *Acta Pathol. Jpn., 23,* 617. (2) Dukes (1980) In: Dukes (Ed) *Meyler's Side Effects of Drugs, 9th ed,* p 213. Excerpta Medica, Amsterdam.

B. DOPAMINERGICS

Bromocriptine

Causal relationship o/ +

Symptomless and transient increases in serum aminotransferase levels, up to 4–fold, occurred in 6 of 92 patients with parkinsonism treated with high doses (50–90 mg/d). Other liver enzymes were normal. In 2 of them the drug had to be discontinued or reduced (1). In another study non–symptomatic APh elevations were observed in 10 of 45 patients (2). One patient developed jaundice after 2 months of treatment. Histology showed necrosis and inflammation 'compatible with viral or toxic hepatitis' (2).

(1) Calne et al (1978) *Lancet, 1,* 735. (2) Lieberman et al (1979) *Neurology, 29,* 363.

Lergotrile

Causal relationship +

Liver enzyme elevations, mainly aminotransferases, were observed in 20–60% of treated patients (1–5). In some of these cases high ASAT/ALAT levels suggested serious hepatocellular damage (3–5) and in 1 case jaundice was reported (1). Immunoallergic signs were absent, although one study mentioned peripheral eosinophilia in 2 patients (5). Histology in 3 patients showed hepatocellular unrest and degeneration and small foci of necrosis. A few lymphocytes and Kupffer cell hypertrophy were seen (5). Other studies mentioned the same pattern of mild hepatocellular necrosis (3, 4).

Although a direct relationship between liver enzyme elevations and dose is not evident (5), these data strongly suggest that lergotrile is an intrinsic hepatotoxin.

(1) Lieberman et al (1979) *Neurology, 29,* 267. (2) Calne et al (1978) *Med. J. Aust., Suppl,* 25. (3) Klawans et al (1978) *Neurology, 28,* 699. (4) Zimmerman (1978) *Hepatotoxicity,* p 544. Appleton–Century–Crofts, New York. (5) Teychenne et al (1979) *Gastroenterology, 76,* 575.

110

Levodopa

Causal relationship o

ALAT/ASAT levels may occasionally be elevated (1). One unspecified case of hepatic injury was reported, confirmed by a positive lymphocyte stimulation test with metabolite–containing serum (2).

(1) Dukes (1980) In: Dukes (Ed) *Meyler's Side Effects of Drugs, 9th ed*, p 219. Excerpta Medica, Amsterdam. (2) Namihisa (1975) *Leber Magen Darm, 5*, 73.

Pergolide

Causal relationship o

One case of moderate ALAT/ASAT elevation and pleural fibrosis was discovered after approximately 2–3 months of therapy, while changing to bromocriptine (1). Recovery occurred after discontinuation of both drugs.

Pergolide lacks the cyano–moiety in the 8–β–acetonitrile group, which is supposed to be the basis of lergotrile hepatotoxicity (2).

(1) LeWitt et al (1983) *Neurology, 33*, 1009. (2) Teychenne et al (1979) *Gastroenterology, 76*, 575.

10. Antithrombotic agents

A. Direct anticoagulants
B. Indirect anticoagulants
   1. Coumarins
   2. Indanediones
C. Platelet aggregation inhibitors
D. Fibrinolytics

Introduction

The clinical setting in which antithrombotic agents are employed can be very complicated. Concurrent drug therapy, preceding operative procedures or cardiovascular complications may be causative in cases where an antithrombotic drug has been suspected of causing hepatic injury.

There are however several ways by which these agents may interfere with normal liver function. Firstly, by impairing vitamin–K–dependent production of clotting Factors II, VII, IX and X, both coumarins and indanediones selectively impair liver function without causing injury. Secondly, all antithrombotic agents may cause hemorrhagic complications. Subcapsular or hepatosplenic hematomas, eventually followed by rupture, have been described subsequent to coumarins as well as to streptokinase (1–3). Thirdly, they may injure the liver directly, either in the form of frequent but transient and mild liver enzyme elevations (heparin), or in the form of a rarely occurring cholestatic or hepatocellular pattern of injury (coumarins, phenindione). Animal toxicity tests have suggested an intrinsic toxic effect of coumarins in high doses (4) with centrizonal necrosis, but therapeutic doses in man rarely cause hepatic injury and probably not by direct toxicity. Hepatic injury by phenindione is probably immunoallergic.

Some analgesics/antirheumatics have been advocated for their platelet–aggregation inhibiting properties but are not discussed here.

(1) Eklöf et al (1978) *Läkartidningen, 75,* 777. (2) Kriesmann et al (1977) *Fortschr. Med., 95,* 858. (3) Roberts et al (1975) *Arch. Surg., 110,* 1152. (4) Rose (1942) *Proc. Soc. Exp. Biol. Med., 50,* 228.

A. DIRECT ANTICOAGULANTS

Heparin

Causal relationship +

Mild to moderate ALAT and ASAT elevations were observed in 89% and 82%, respectively, of a group of 46 patients who had been treated with heparin for 5 days (1). Normalization of values occurred despite continuation of therapy. The elevations were less frequent in patients who had been treated with the lowest dose (5000 IU/8 h i.c.). γ–GT, APh and LDH were less frequently elevated (37%, 15% and 24%, respectively). In another study, serum aminotransferase elevations were observed in 10 of 14 patients treated intravenously with 10,000 IU/8 h. In all cases the elevations occurred in the first 15 days of therapy and disappeared after discontinuation (2). Interference with the determination of serum liver enzymes was excluded (2).

Minar et al (1) suggested that heparin may exert this effect by complex formation with proteins, secondary to its strong electric charge. Subsequent interference with enzymatic reactions should explain the elevations which are transient since induction neutralizes this effect. Other proposed explanations are an increase in enzyme release by a detergent effect of heparin or competition with the clearance of the enzyme by the monocyte macrophage system (3).

(1) Minar et al (1980) *Dtsch. Med. Wochenschr., 105,* 1713. (2) Sonnenblick et al (1975) *Br. Med. J., 3,* 77. (3) Loeliger (1984) In: Dukes (Ed), *Meyler's Side Effects of Drugs, 10th ed*, p 648. Elsevier, Amsterdam.

B. INDIRECT ANTICOAGULANTS

B.1. COUMARINS

Acenocoumarol

Causal relationship o

One case was reported of anicteric, mild cholestatic hepatitis starting 5 years (!) after initial intake and resolving within 3 weeks after discontinuation. Biopsy showed no significant abnormalities (1).

After complete normalization of laboratory values, phenprocoumon

produced recurrence of mild hepatic injury after 1 year of use; eosinophilia was observed during this recurrence (1).

(1) Kreiter et al (1967) *Med. Klin., 62,* 12.

Dicoumarol

Causal relationship o

Liver enzyme elevations, mainly ASAT and ALAT, have been ascribed
to dicoumarol and ethyl biscoumacetate (1, 2). Occasional cases of liver
damage were recorded in the older literature (3).

(1) Wróblewski et al (1958) *J. Am. Med. Assoc., 167,* 2163. (2) Clark (1977) *Adverse
Drug React. Bull., Oct,* 232. (3) Schoen et al (1951) *Münch. Med. Wochenschr., 93,*
22.

Phenprocoumon

Causal relationship +

An icteric hepatocellular pattern of injury (1, 2) has been observed, appearing 2–6 months after starting therapy and recovering in 2–5 months
with (1, 2) or without (1) corticosteroid therapy. Biopsy showed a pattern
'resembling acute viral hepatitis' (1) in 1 case and chronic active hepatitis in the other patient (1). A rechallenge was followed by a relapse (1,
2). One case exhibited mainly cholestatic hepatitis (1).
    In a study of 73 patients who had been treated mostly for more than
1 year, Renschler et al (3) found abnormal ASAT and ALAT levels in 22%
and 37%, respectively. This high incidence has not been confirmed by
others, as far as we know.

(1) Slagboom et al (1980) *Arch. Intern. Med., 140,* 1028. (2) Den Boer et al (1976)
Lancet, 1, 912. (3) Renschler et al (1963) *Dtsch. Arch. Klin. Med., 208,* 524.

Warfarin

Causal relationship o

Symptomatic cases of hepatic injury have been reported only very rarely.
Rehnquist reported 2 cases (1). One patient developed elevation of liver
enzyme concentrations after starting treatment with warfarin and hepar-

114

in, which returned to normal almost completely despite continuation of warfarin. The other patient developed jaundice and fever after the intake of an overdose (50 mg) but had pre–existing liver function disturbances. Jones et al (2) reported a case of intrahepatic cholestasis appearing 6 months after starting warfarin treatment. Histology showed moderate cholestasis and mild portal inflammation with bile duct proliferation.

Three fatal cases of a Reye–like syndrome were ascribed to the ingestion of a warfarin–containing rodenticide by children (3). However, this report has remained incidental.

Warfarin has occasionally been associated with hepatic rupture (4).

(1) Rehnqvist (1978) *Acta Med. Scand., 204,* 335. (2) Jones et al (1980) *Postgrad. Med. J., 56,* 671. (3) Mogilner (1974) *Isr. J. Med. Sci., 10,* 1117. (4) Roberts et al (1975) *Arch. Surg., 110,* 1152.

B.2. INDANEDIONES

Phenindione

Causal relationship +

During the period when phenindione was widely used, it was probably the anticoagulant most frequently implicated in causing hepatic injury. Fever, rash, eosinophilia and leukocytosis with atypical lymphocytes occurred in up to 3% of treated patients (1). Some 10% of this group showed signs of hepatic injury, i.e. liver enzyme elevations and/or jaundice (2). A rechallenge has been positive in several cases (4, 5); the hypersensitivity symptoms usually reappeared within 1–3 days. Both cholestasis and hepatocellular injury have been suggested by biochemical alterations and histology. The onset was mostly within 4 weeks with a variation of 10 days to 9 weeks after starting treatment (3). In fatal cases, death seems primarily to have been caused by severe generalized hypersensitivity, e.g. Lyell or Stevens–Johnson syndrome, renal failure or blood disorders (2). This anticoagulant has been largely abandoned in favor of the coumarin derivatives.

(1) Zimmerman (1978) *Hepatotoxicity,* p 510. Appleton–Century–Crofts, New York. (2) Perkins (1962) *Lancet, 1,* 127. (3) Klatskin (1975) In: Schiff (Ed), *Diseases of the Liver, 4th ed,* p 604. Lippincott, Philadelphia. (4) Brooks et al (1960) *Ann. Intern. Med., 52,* 706. (5) Makous et al (1954) *J. Am. Med. Assoc., 155,* 739.

C. PLATELET AGGREGATION INHIBITORS

Ticlopidine

Causal relationship o

Ticlopidine is a thrombocyte aggregation inhibitor which has led to several reports of blood dyscrasias, especially in France and The Netherlands (1–3). In the latter country, it was withdrawn from the market.

Hepatic injury has been reported less frequently. Deschamps et al (4) described 2 patients who developed a mixed cholestatic–hepatocellular pattern of injury in the first 6 weeks of treatment. No immunoallergic signs were associated with this reaction. Histology showed centrilobular cholestasis and acidophilic necrosis and mild portal mononuclear infiltration. Cholestatic jaundice was reported in a patient who had been treated for 3 months with this agent (5). Seven months after discontinuation, laboratory data had returned to normal. Concomitant syphilis in this patient (or its treatment?) was not held responsible by the authors. Indeed, cholestasis is unusual in syphilis (6), although the high APh levels as observed in this patient are often seen in syphilis.

(1) De Fraiture et al (1982) *Ned. Tijdschr. Geneeskd.*, *126*, 1051. (2) Chomienne et al (1983) *Rev. Méd. Thér.*, *13*, 589. (3) Meyer et al (1982) *Lyon Méd.*, *248*, 407. (4) Deschamps et al (1982) *Gastroentérol. Clin. Biol.*, *6*, 595. (5) Biour et al (1982) *Thérapie*, *37*, 217. (6) Sherlock (1982) *Diseases of the Liver and Biliary System, 6th ed*, p 437. Blackwell, London.

D. FIBRINOLYTICS

Streptokinase

Co–enzyme obtained from cultures of various
strains of *Streptococcus haemolyticus*   *Causal relationship* +

Liver enzyme abnormalities may occur (1). Sallen (2) described a patient who developed ASAT and APh elevations on the 4th day of streptokinase treatment. Fever accompanied the abnormalities. After normalization a rechallenge was immediately followed by fever and relapse. Urdahl (5) observed acute hepatitis, accompanied by fever, in a 30–year–old man. Discontinuation preceded recovery.

In 3 patients treated with streptokinase for deep venous thrombosis, spontaneous liver rupture developed. Two of them died. In none of the cases was underlying liver disease demonstrated (3). Analogous cases have been observed by others (4).

(1) Brogden et al (1973) *Drugs*, *5*, 375. (2) Sallen et al (1983) *Am. J. Gastroenterol.*, *78*, 523. (3) Eklöf et al (1978) *Läkartidningen*, *75*, 777. (4) Kriessmann et al (1977) *Fortschr. Med.*, *95*, 858. (5) Urdahl (1983) *Tidsskr. N. Laegeforen.*, *103*, 763.

11. Thyroid/antithyroid agents

A. 1. Thiouracils
   2. Thioimidazoles
B. Iodides

Introduction

Hyperthyroidism is associated with a high incidence of mild hepatic dysfunction, i.e. elevation of APh and ASAT and BSP retention (1). Occasionally, jaundice may be caused by congestive heart failure or aggravation of underlying Gilbert's disease. In the latter, histology is normal, while in the former, pericentral congestion and fibrosis may be seen. Rarely, cholestatic jaundice is encountered without a clear cause. Although it may be difficult to distinguish thyrostatic–induced hepatic injury from hyperthyroidism–induced injury (2), differentiation is mostly possible since the onset occurs when thyroid function has been normalized by adequate treatment. If hypothyroidism is induced, treatment may be followed by hepatic congestion and elevation of liver enzyme concentrations in the serum.

The antithyroid thiouracils (e.g. thiouracil, propylthiouracil) and thioimidazoles (e.g. methimazole, carbimazole) occasionally cause hepatic injury. Most cases have been ascribed to the use of propylthiouracil, but this is probably related to its more frequent use. Also some infrequently used drugs (e.g. methylthiouracil, aminothiazole) have only rarely been associated with jaundice (4). While the thiouracil derivatives are mostly associated with a hepatocellular pattern of injury, thioimidazoles seem to produce a mainly cholestatic type.

Most unwanted effects of these agents are immunoallergic rather than toxic (3). However, the mechanism of hepatic injury is unknown. Although the reaction is idiosyncratic because there is no dose–dependence and it is not reproducible in animals, it is not entirely clear whether the reaction is immunoallergic or metabolic. On the one hand, concurrent immunoallergic symptoms are infrequent and the latent period between starting therapy and appearance of injury is several months in a number of cases, which is not consistent with the immunoallergic 'sensitization period' of approximately 6 weeks. On the other hand, some cases show an accelerated reaction to rechallenge and in–vitro tests (lymphocyte stimulation test) have been positive. Cross–sensitivity between individual agents has only rarely been reported.

Iodides may cause hepatic injury when administered in high doses. In animal toxicity tests, these agents caused centrizonal necrosis. Therapeutic doses in man, however, are rarely a problem as regards hepatic injury.

(1) Anderson et al (1982) In: Schiff et al (Eds), *Diseases of the Liver, 5th ed*, p 167. Lippincott, Philadelphia. (2) Jansen et al (1982) *Neth. J. Med., 25*, 318. (3) Von Eickstedt (1980) In: Dukes (Ed), *Meyler's Side Effects of Drugs, 9th ed*, p 695. Excerpta Medica, Amsterdam. (4) Vanderlaan et al (1955) *Pharmacol. Rev., 7*, 301.

A.1. THIOURACILS

Propylthiouracil

Causal relationship +

Cases of acute (1–5, 7–14, 16, 18) and chronic (6, 14) hepatic injury have been reported in the medical literature, mainly of the hepatocellular type. It usually occurred within the first 2 months of therapy but in several cases only after 3–6 months (6, 10, 13, 16, 18). Concurrent fever and/or rash occurred in some cases (1, 2, 8); granulocytopenia/agranulocytosis was relatively frequent (1, 4, 8, 10). In 1 case hepatic injury was accompanied by a systemic lupus erythematosus–like syndrome (1). In some cases re–administration was performed and followed by recurrence of signs (10, 13). In 3 cases a lymphocyte stimulation test was performed which was positive in 2 cases (9, 16) but negative in 1 case (11). Apparent cross–sensitivity with methimazole was present in 1 case (16) but absent in 2 other cases (13, 16). Histology showed varying degrees of necrosis, ranging from mild to severe (9, 14, 15, 10) with or without bridging. A pattern resembling chronic active hepatitis (6, 13) has been observed with mild cirrhosis (13). These reactions are probably idiosyncratic since propylthiouracil shows little intrinsic hepatotoxic potential.

Preliminary results suggest that propylthiouracil protects animals against CCl_4–induced liver injury (17) and recent reports suggest that this agent may be beneficial in the short–term treatment of active alcoholic hepatitis (16).

(1) Amrhein et al (1970) *J. Pediatr., 76*, 54. (2) Anonymous (1969) *Med. Trib. Rep., 10*, 8. (3) Brody et al (1974) *Med. Ann. DC, 43*, 72. (4) Colwell et al (1952) *J. Am. Med. Assoc., 148*, 639. (5) Eisen (1953) *N. Engl. J. Med., 249*, 814. (6) Fedotin et al (1975) *Arch. Intern. Med., 135*, 319. (7) Ishizuli (1974) *Clin. Endocrinol., 22*, 1083. (8) Livingston et al (1947) *J. Am. Med. Assoc., 135*, 422. (9) Mihas et al (1976) *Gastroenterology, 70*, 770. (10) Nielsen et al (1980) *Ugeskr. Laeg., 142*, 3189. (11) Parker (1975) *Ann. Intern. Med., 82*, 228. (12) Reddy (1979) *J. Ntl. Med. Assoc., 71*, 1185. (13) Weiss et al (1980) *Arch. Intern. Med., 140*, 1184. (14) Safani et al (1982) *Arch. Intern. Med., 142*, 838. (15) Maddrey et al (1977) *Gastroenterology, 72*, 1348. (16)

Parker (1982) *Clin. Pharm., 1,* 471. (17) Orrego et al (1976) *Gastroenterology, 71,* 821. (18) Hanson (1984) *Arch. Intern. Med., 144,* 994.

Thiouracil

Causal relationship +

Incidental cases of hepatic injury have been reported in the medical literature, of a mainly cholestatic (1, 2) and a predominantly hepatocellular (3) pattern. The onset of these cases was within the first month of therapy (1–3). In 1 patient the reaction was accompanied by a maculopapular rash, fever and arthralgia (2). Rechallenge with a lower dose was followed by prompt recurrence of signs (2). One patient died (3). Histology showed centrilobular necrosis and cholestasis. In another case there was cholestasis without parenchymal damage (1).

Gargill (1) noted 2 cases of cholestatic jaundice in a group of 43 thiouracil–treated patients (1).

(1) Gargill et al (1945) *J. Am. Med. Assoc., 127,* 890. (2) Paschkis et al (1944) *J. Clin. Endocrinol., 4,* 179. (3) Holoubek et al (1948) *Am. J. Med., 5,* 138.

Thiourea

Causal relationship o

Jaundice, fever and rash secondary to periarteritis nodosa started after 1 month of therapy (1). Histology showed periarteritis in the portal areas as well as in other organs. This drug is no longer in use.

(1) Gibson et al (1945) *Lancet, 2,* 108.

A.2. THIOIMIDAZOLES

Carbimazole

Causal relationship +

Since carbimazole is metabolized to methimazole, one may expect that these agents will have the same potential to cause hepatic injury and will produce the same pattern. This indeed seems to be the case, although concurrent blood cell disorders have been reported less frequently so far in cases of carbimazole–associated hepatic injury.

There is mainly a cholestatic to mixed pattern of hepatic injury (1–4) with jaundice. Concurrent fever is reported (2, 3, 5). Symptoms appeared within the first 3 weeks (2, 3, 5) or after 3–4 months (1, 4). In 2 cases a rechallenge was performed and it was positive (2, 4) within 24 hours. A lymphocyte stimulation test was negative (2) but weakly positive in another case (1). Histology showed centrilobular cholestasis (3, 4), diffuse mild necrosis (3), bile duct multiplication (2, 3) and mild portal infiltration. In 1 case, bile duct damage and granulomas resembled early primary biliary cirrhosis, according to the authors (5). Electron microscopy showed non–specific hyperplasia and membrane alterations of endoplasmic reticulum and mitochondria (2). However, analogous changes may be seen in hyperthyroidism (6).

(1) Prost et al (1973) *Nouv. Presse Méd., 2,* 2479. (2) Lunzer et al (1975) *Gut, 16,* 913. (3) Efstratiadis et al (1982) *Dtsch. Med. Wochenschr., 107,* 1531. (4) Dinsmore et al (1983) *N. Engl. J. Med., 309,* 438. (5) Jenkins et al (1982) *Br. J. Clin. Pract., 36,* 415. (6) Anderson et al (1982) In: Schiff et al (Eds), *Diseases of the Liver, 5th ed,* p 167. Lippincott, Philadelphia.

Methimazole

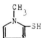
Causal relationship o/ +

Methimazole is a metabolite of carbimazole. As regards methimazole–associated hepatic injury, mainly cases of cholestatic jaundice have been described (1–6, 9), but occasionally the pattern is hepatocellular (8). Whereas rash/eosinophilia was not mentioned, concurrent agranulocytosis/bone marrow depression was frequently present (3, 4, 7). Onset was usually within 2 months after starting treatment. There were 2 fatal cases, although not secondary to a hepatic cause (3, 8). Biopsy showed centrilobular cholestasis often with (peri)portal infiltrate but without liver cell necrosis in most cases. There was focal necrosis in 1 case (8). The difficulty of proving a causal relationship to methimazole intake is demonstrated by 1 report of 3 hyperthyroid patients with cholestatic jaundice, 2 of whom already had signs of cholestasis before taking the drug (1).

(1) Jansen et al (1982) *Neth. J. Med., 25,* 318. (2) Efstratiadis et al (1982) *Dtsch. Med. Wochenschr., 107,* 1531. (3) Specht et al (1952) *J. Am. Med. Assoc., 149,* 1010. (4) Shipp (1955) *Ann. Intern. Med., 42,* 701. (5) Martinez–Lopez et al (1962) *Gastroenterology, 43,* 84. (6) Reinwein (1971) *Dtsch. Med. Wochenschr., 42,* 1640. (7) Rosenbaum et al (1953) *J. Am. Med. Assoc., 152,* 27. (8) Becker et al (1968) *J. Am. Med. Assoc., 206,* 1787. (9) Fischer et al (1973) *J. Am. Med. Assoc., 223,* 1028.

B. IODIDES

Iodides

KI, NaI   *Causal relationship* o

Iodides may rarely cause jaundice in man (1). When administered in high doses to animals, dose–dependent (2) necrosis has been noted, varying from mild focal necrosis and steatosis (3) of hepatocytes to marked centrizonal necrosis (2).

(1) Von Eickstedt (1980) In: Dukes (Ed), *Meyler's Side Effects of Drugs, 9th ed,* p 695. Excerpta Medica, Amsterdam. (2) Lavelle et al (1975) *Toxicol. Appl. Pharmacol., 33,* 52. (3) Webster et al (1957) *J. Pharmacol. Exp. Ther., 120,* 171.

12. Antidiabetic agents

A. Sulfonylureas
B. Biguanides

Introduction

Diabetes mellitus may be associated with hepatomegaly and fatty infiltration of liver cells. Moreover, patients on sulfonylureas and biguanides (mostly maturity–onset diabetes) are often obese, which is a known cause of fatty change. The incidence of fatty liver in diabetics over 60 years is estimated at 45% and is not correlated with the degree of control or with the duration of diabetes (1). In cases with mildly abnormal liver function tests or elevated liver enzyme levels during intake of antidiabetic agents, the possible responsibility of the underlying disease (either alone or in combination with the suspected drug) should always be borne in mind.

However, diabetes mellitus is not a cause of symptomatic hepatic injury and several of these cases in patients with diabetes can be attributed definitely to the use of sulfonylureas. Biguanides have only rarely been reported as a cause and with the exception of synthalin (2), they do not seem to be injurious to the liver, although biguanide–induced lactic acidosis is partly explained by inhibition of hepatic gluconeogenesis.

Most sulfonylureas have been associated occasionally with liver enzyme elevations – as have less frequently mentioned drugs, e.g. glisoxepide (3), chlorpentazide (4) gliclazide (5) – and/or symptomatic hepatic injury, but the incidence shows a wide range. Some of them have been associated with a hepatocellular pattern of injury in a relatively large percentage of recipients (e.g. glybuthiazol, carbutamide), suggesting an intrinsic toxic effect on the liver. Other sulfonylureas produce a mainly cholestatic pattern in a small percentage of patients (e.g. tolbutamide, chlorpropamide in therapeutic doses). The latter, however, may also cause hepatic injury if taken in overdose.

According to Zimmerman (2), the nitrophenyl structure is important for the hepatotoxic effect of carbutamide and glybuthiazol. Less convincing is an analogous effect of chlorophenyl compounds (chlorpropamide, azepinamide). Sulfonylureas are structurally related to sulfonamides and may be expected to have a similar tendency to cause immunoallergic reactions. Indeed, many cases of cholestatic hepatitis induced by chlorpropamide are accompanied by extrahepatic hypersensitivity signs, but not all related drugs seem to exhibit this pattern.

Sulfonylureas may inhibit the metabolism of alcohol and have a disulfiram–like action. This is especially the case with chlorpropamide.

An unusual report is that of marked ALAT/ASAT elevation in 2 patients, ascribed to use of insulin (6). One of them had HBsAg–negative chronic active hepatitis. A relation with insulin seems doubtful, but since insulin may occasionally cause allergic reactions, the possibility of immunoallergic hepatic injury should not be completely discounted.

(1) Alpers et al (1982) In: Schiff et al (Eds), *Diseases of the Liver, 5th ed*, p 813. Lippincott, Philadelphia. (2) Zimmerman (1978) *Hepatotoxicity*, p 436. Appleton–Century–Crofts, New York. (3) Kiesselbach et al (1974) *Arzneim.–Forsch.*, *24*, 447. (4) Jørgensen (1967) *Med. Monatsschr.*, *21*, 278. (5) Holmes et al (1984) *Drugs*, *27*, 301. (6) Hiramatsu et al (1982) *J. Jpn. Diabet. Soc.*, *25*, 1221.

A. SULFONYLUREAS

Acetohexamide

Causal relationship o

Although several (unspecified) cases of cholestatic jaundice have occurred (1), few have been described in detail. The incidence is believed to be lower with acetohexamide than with carbutamide and metahexamide (2), although such claims are difficult to (dis)prove. The pattern seems mainly hepatocellular (2, 3). In 1 case, postnecrotic cirrhosis was ascribed to this agent (3).

(1) AMA Council on Drugs (1965) *J. Am. Med. Assoc.*, *191*, 127. (2) Zimmerman (1978) *Hepatotoxicity*, p 436. Appleton–Century–Crofts, New York. (3) Goldstein et al (1966) *N. Engl. J. Med.*, *275*, 97.

Azepinamide

Causal relationship o

Cholestatic hepatitis appeared after 5 weeks of therapy with increasing doses to 600 mg/d (1). There was no recurrence after a challenge period of 2 months (500 mg/d).

(1) Weinstein et al (1963) *Am. J. Med. Sci.*, *84*, 432.

Carbutamide

Causal relationship o/ +

Carbutamide has been abandoned in many countries because of its frequent side effects. One of these – hepatic injury, which is sometimes fatal

(2, 3) – was estimated to occur in 0.5–1.5% (1) of recipients. Hepatic injury is mostly hepatocellular (1). In 2 studies, jaundice was reported in 1.4% (2) and 0.08% (3), respectively. Two cases, reported in more detail (2), showed onset within 4 weeks of therapy. Rash and fever were present in 1 case.

Carbutamide proved hepatotoxic in dogs (4, 5) and caused a high incidence of liver function disturbances in man (6). Nitrophenyl–containing sulfonylureas were supposed to produce a higher incidence of hepatic injury (1, 7). See also 'Glybuthiazol' and 'Metahexamide'.

(1) Zimmerman (1978) *Hepatotoxicity*, p 436. Appleton–Century–Crofts, New York. (2) Camerini–Davalos et al (1957) *Diabetes, 6,* 74. (3) Kirtley (1957) *Diabetes, 6,* 72. (4) Anderson et al (1957) *Diabetes, 6,* 2. (5) Sirek et al (1957) *Diabetes, 6,* 151. (6) Marble et al (1957) *Ann. NY Acad. Sci., 71,* 239. (7) Mach et al (1959) *N. Engl. J. Med., 261,* 438.

Chlorpropamide

C_3H_7 — NH — CO — NH — SO_2 —⟨benzene ring⟩— Cl   *Causal relationship* +

Mostly a cholestatic/mixed pattern is found (1–3, 6, 7, 14, 15). Granulomatous hepatitis (5) and a serum–sickness pattern with nephrotic syndrome, circulating immunocomplexes and hepatocellular injury have also been described (4). Onset is usually within 2 months (1–8, 14, 15). Rash/eosinophilia (1, 2, 4, 15) and exfoliative dermatitis (5) may appear concurrently. Rechallenge has been positive (3), but was negative in 3 cases (1). In 1 report the reaction was accompanied by pure red cell aplasia (15). In a study of 17 jaundiced patients, 8 had rash, 6 fever and 3 eosinophilia (17). Biopsy showed cholestasis (1–3, 7, 9) and minor necrosis or degeneration of hepatocytes (1–3, 5, 9). In 1 case, granulomas were found in liver and bone marrow, heavily infiltrated with eosinophils (5).

The incidence was estimated at 0.5% (3). No cross–sensitivity to tolbutamide was demonstrated in 2 cases (1, 3), but in 1 patient with chlorpropamide–associated jaundice, tolbutamide was held responsible for a relapse (14). Because of irreproducibility in animals (10, 11), a latent period of mostly 2 months and signs of hypersensitivity, the mechanism seems immunoallergic. Lower doses, however, seem to lead to a lower incidence (12) and some intrinsic toxicity is suggested by elevated APh levels in 25% of recipients in 1 study (13). Moreover, intrinsic toxicity has been suggested by the appearance of cholestatic jaundice in a patient who had taken an overdose (16).

(1) Hamff et al (1958) *Ann. NY Acad. Sci., 74,* 820. (2) Brown et al (1959) *J. Am. Med. Assoc., 170,* 2058. (3) Reichel et al (1960) *Am. J. Med., 28,* 654. (4) Appel et al (1983) *Am. J. Med., 74,* 337. (5) Rigberg et al (1976) *J. Am. Med. Assoc., 235,* 409. (6) Stewart et al (1959) *N. Engl. J. Med., 261,* 427. (7) Stocchi et al (1962) *Clin. Ter., 22,* 925. (8) Bloodworth (1963) *Metabolism, 12,* 287. (9) Hopper et al (1965) *Arch. Intern. Med., 115,* 128. (10) Knick (1958) *Ann. NY Acad. Sci., 74,* 858. (11) Schneider et al (1959) *Ann. NY Acad. Sci., 74,* 427. (12) Zimmerman (1978) *Hepato-*

toxicity, p 436. Appleton–Century–Crofts, New York. (13) Unger et al (1959) *Ann. NY Acad. Sci., 82*, 570. (14) Collens et al (1965) *NY State J. Med., 65*, 907. (15) Gill et al (1980) *Arch. Intern. Med., 140*, 714. (16) Frier et al (1977) *Clin. Toxicol., 11*, 13. (17) Pannekoek (1968) In: Meyler et al (Eds), *Side Effects of Drugs, 6th ed*, p 422. Excerpta Medica, Amsterdam.

Glibenclamide

Causal relationship o/+

Only a few cases of clinically overt hepatic injury have been reported (1–3), with cholestatic hepatitis (1, 2) and a hepatocellular pattern (3). Onset varied from within 4 weeks (2, 3) to 17 months (1). There were generalized hypersensitivity symptoms (2) with rash, fever, eosinophilia, renal failure and arteritis; this patient died secondary to bronchopneumonia. The concurrent use of a pyrazole derivative could also have been responsible in this patient. In 1 report readministration caused a relapse (3). Ingelmo (4) ascribed vasculitis and granulomatous hepatitis to the use of glibenclamide.

(1) Wongpaitoon et al (1981) *Postgrad. Med. J., 57*, 244. (2) Clarke et al (1974) *Diabetes, 23*, 739. (3) De Rosa et al (1980) *Epatologia, 26*, 73. (4) Ingelmo et al (1980) *Med. Clin. (Barcelona), 75*, 306.

Glybuthiazol

Causal relationship o/+

Seventeen of 31 patients (mostly treated with 1 g/d) developed hepatic dysfunction, 6 of them with jaundice. Eosinophilia was seen in 6 patients with hepatic dysfunction, 4 of them with jaundice. Biopsy showed varying degrees of diffuse parenchymal degeneration, scattered focal necrosis, and portal and periportal inflammation, in 3 cases with many eosinophils (1).

Occurrence of hepatic dysfunction was unrelated to age or to dose/duration of use or diabetic state (1). See also 'Carbutamide' and 'Metahexamide'.

(1) Davis et al (1959) *Can. Med. Assoc. J., 81*, 101.

Glyparamide

Causal relationship o

Glyparamide was mentioned by Zimmerman as a rare cause of hepatic injury, but no details were given (1).

(1) Zimmerman (1978) *Hepatotoxicity*, p 456. Appleton–Century–Crofts, New York.

125

Metahexamide

CH₃ — [structure: benzene ring with NH₂, S(=O)(=O)-NH-C(=O)-NH-cyclohexyl]

Causal relationship +

Both hepatocellular (1, 2, 5, 6) and cholestatic/mixed (6, 7, 9) patterns of injury have been reported. A causal relationship was proven in some cases by a prompt reaction to rechallenge (1, 4). Popper et al (2) mention massive and submassive necrosis in 7 patients on this drug. Cirrhosis has also been observed (5). Some cases of pericholangitis have been reported (4), whereas others exhibited focal necrosis with significant cholestasis (6, 7).

In 1 survey the incidence was 0.5% with a dose lower than 200 mg/d and 4.4% with a dose higher than 200 mg/d (3). In 1 study 4 of 6 patients on metahexamide had abnormal liver function compared to none of 7 on tolbutamide and 1 of 7 on chlorpropamide (4). One study noted transient APh elevations in 24% of recipients (5), but others found a lower percentage of up to 6% (7). Bradley (10) treated 85 diabetics with metahexamide. Two of them developed jaundice and 1 asymptomatic liver function disturbances. One of the patients had previously developed jaundice to carbutamide. A hepatotoxic effect of metahexamide is suggested by studies in animals, where high doses (≥ 100 mg/kg) caused fatty degeneration and necrosis of hepatocytes in rats (8), whereas in dogs these changes were already present at 10 mg/kg. See also 'Carbutamide'.

(1) Mach et al (1959) *N. Engl. J. Med., 261,* 438. (2) Popper et al (1965) *Arch. Intern. Med., 115,* 128. (3) Pollen et al (1960) *Diabetes, 9,* 25. (4) Drey et al (1959) *Metabolism, 8,* 676. (5) Unger et al (1959) *Ann. NY Acad. Sci., 82,* 570. (6) Dolger (1959) *Ann. NY Acad. Sci., 82,* 531. (7) Hamwi et al (1959) *Ann. NY Acad. Sci., 82,* 547. (8) Bänder (1959) *Ann. NY Acad. Sci., 82,* 508. (9) Granville–Grossman et al (1959) *Br. Med. J., 2,* 841. (10) Bradley (1959) *Ann. NY Acad. Sci., 82,* 513.

Tolazamide

[structure] N—NH—CO—NH—SO₂—[benzene ring]—CH₃

Causal relationship o

Insidious onset of jaundice was reported 1 month after starting therapy in a patient who recovered in 2.5 months after discontinuation. Biochemically a mixed pattern was observed. Biopsy showed marked centrilobular necrosis and cholestasis with mononuclear infiltrate (1). The patient was treated concurrently with clofibrate.

(1) Van Thiel et al (1974) *Gastroenterology, 67,* 506.

Tolbutamide

C₄H₉—NH—CO—NH—SO₂—[benzene ring]—CH₃

Causal relationship +

Mainly a cholestatic to mixed pattern was observed (1–5, 7), in 1 case resembling primary biliary cirrhosis (5). Onset occurred from 1 month (3, 4) to 1 year or more (1, 5, 7) after starting therapy. Rechallenge was positive in 2 reports (3, 7). Concurrent thrombocytopenia was observed (6, 7). Biopsy showed centrilobular (2, 3) or midzonal (1) cholestasis, (peri)portal lymphocytic infiltration (2, 3) and some fibrosis (3). Destructive cholangitis/cholangiolitis and disappearance of interlobular ducts have also been seen (5).

Balodimos et al (6) in a study of over 3300 patients noted 4 cases of liver involvement of which 3 were possibly unrelated to the drug (6). However, regular liver enzyme assessment is not mentioned in their study and they probably missed asymptomatic elevations.

(1) McMahon (1963) *Med. Ann., 32,* 509. (2) Popper et al (1965) *Arch. Intern. Med., 115,* 128. (3) Baird et al (1960) *Ann. Intern. Med., 53,* 194. (4) Collens et al (1965) *NY State J. Med., 65,* 907. (5) Gregory et al (1967) *Arch. Pathol., 84,* 194. (6) Balodimos et al (1966) *Metabolism, 15,* 957. (7) Ananth et al (1970) *Can. Med. Assoc. J., 103,* 1194.

B. BIGUANIDES

Buformin

$$NH_2-\underset{\underset{NH}{\|}}{C}-NH-\underset{\underset{NH}{\|}}{C}-NH-C_4H_9$$

Causal relationship o

One unspecified case of hepatic injury has been reported (1). The lymphocyte stimulation test was positive.

(1) Namihisa (1975) *Leber Magen Darm, 5,* 73.

Phenformin

$$NH_2-\underset{\underset{NH}{\|}}{C}-NH-\underset{\underset{NH}{\|}}{C}-NH-CH_2-CH_2-\text{C}_6\text{H}_5$$

Causal relationship o

A case of cholestatic jaundice after 1 week of usage was reported. Biopsy showed midzonal bile stasis (1).

Biguanides interfere with lactate metabolism in the liver and may cause lactic acidosis (2) of which secondary hepatic injury is not a usual feature.

(1) Smetana (1963) *Ann. NY Acad. Sci., 104,* 821. (2) Von Eickstedt (1980) In: Dukes (Ed), *Meyler's Side Effect of Drugs, 9th ed,* p 714. Excerpta Medica, Amsterdam.

13. Antiarrhythmics/Cardiac agents

A. Antiarrhythmic agents
B. Other cardiac agents

Introduction

Like other cardiovascular drugs, antiarrhythmics are often employed in a complicated clinical setting, e.g. after cardiac surgery in patients on multiple drugs. The assessment of a causal relationship between the drug and the suspected adverse reaction is always difficult under such circumstances.

Many antiarrhythmic drugs may occasionally cause hepatic injury. Both cholestatic and hepatocellular patterns of injury have been observed. Also, antiarrhythmics with beta–blocking properties (e.g. propafenone) (1, 4) have been associated with hepatic injury. With the exception of amiodarone, which causes elevation of ASAT/ALAT levels in a large proportion of patients (albeit often transient), these reactions are idiosyncratic. With some drugs the reactions are accompanied by extrahepatic signs of immunoallergy (e.g. quinidine, ajmaline) while these are absent with other drugs (e.g. disopyramide).

Since all antiarrhythmic agents have a negative inotropic effect, they may aggravate congestive heart failure and induce a rise in the concentration of liver enzymes or even jaundice, secondary to hepatic venous congestion (e.g. tocainide, disopyramide).

Mild liver enzyme elevations after starting treatment are common, but these values usually normalize despite continuation of therapy. The explanation for this observation is uncertain, but it has been considered as an adaptive response to the drug by enzyme induction. In a study comparing the antiarrhythmic agents prajmaline, disopyramide, propafenone and sparteine and the vasodilator nitroglycerin, all agents caused liver enzyme elevations in a number of patients 10–16 days after starting treatment (2).

Scillaren, a cardiac glycoside, inhibits $(Na^+ + K^+)$–ATPase and decreases blood flow; whereas the former is responsible for inhibition of the bile–salt–independent bile flow, according to Miyai et al (3) the latter may potentiate the decrease in bile flow and the appearance of morphological abnormalities. However, their study was performed in a perfused rat liver system.

(1) Schuff–Werner et al (1982) *Internist Prax.*, *22*, 475. (2) Engels et al (1984) *Fortschr. Med.*, *102*, 53. (3) Miyai et al (1982) *Exp. Mol. Pathol.*, *36*, 333. (4) Konz et al (1984) *Dtsch. Med. Wochenschr.*, *109*, 1525.

A. ANTIARRHYTHMIC AGENTS

Ajmaline (see also 'Prajmaline')

Causal relationship + +

Several symptomatic cases of hepatic injury have been associated with the intake of ajmaline. Most frequently reported was a cholestatic pattern of injury with or without mild to moderate ASAT/ALAT elevations (4, 5, 7–9, 10, 12–15). In some cases a hepatocellular pattern predominated (12). The onset was mostly within the first 6 weeks of therapy, but a latent period of 120 days has also been reported (12). In a Japanese study of 69 cases, the mean latent period was 8 days (11). Fever accompanied the hepatic injury in most cases (1–10, 14, 15). Eosinophilia (1, 2, 8, 9, 13, 14), thrombocytopenia (6, 7), agranulocytosis (6), pancytopenia (12) and renal dysfunction (6, 7) were less frequent. One case of prolonged cholestasis (> 1 year) with xanthoma formation started 11 days after a short course of ajmaline and sex hormones (3); unfortunately, there was no follow–up. Another case of prolonged cholestasis ended in biliary cirrhosis (5). In some cases, readministration was followed by relapse (3, 7, 9, 13). In a number of cases a lymphocyte stimulation test was performed and found to be positive (6–8, 10, 13, 14).

Histology showed mostly centrilobular cholestasis, either with (2, 3, 9, 14) or without (1, 3, 8, 14, 15) mild/moderate necrosis. Portal inflammation is usually present and is mainly mononuclear, although the presence of eosinophils (without quantification) has been mentioned in most biopsy reports. Electron microscopy showed dilatation of the endoplasmic reticulum. The microfilamentous network of the hepatocytes was reduced and disorganized. Biliary canaliculi were enlarged with blunted microvilli. According to the authors, this pattern resembled that seen with cytochalasin B (15).

The above–mentioned signs and symptoms seem compatible with an immunoallergic mechanism. It is striking that rash is infrequent and that some cases (2), including one reported to us, have a very short latent period (< 1 week) between first intake and onset, despite first use. This has also been reported for prajmaline.

(1) Dölle (1962) *Med. Klin.*, *57*, 1648. (2) Möckel (1965) *Med. Klin.*, *60*, 294. (3) Beermann et al (1971) *Acta Med. Scand.*, *190*, 241. (4) Andersson et al (1973) *Läkartidningen, 70*, 2134. (5) Einarsson et al (1973) *Läkartidningen, 70*, 1288. (6) Offenstadt et al (1976) *Ann. Méd. Interne, 127*, 622. (7) Guyon et al (1978) *Nouv. Presse Méd.*,

7, 1558. (8) Hecht et al (1978) *Méd. Chir. Dig.*, *7*, 473. (9) Pariente et al (1980) *Gastroentérol. Clin. Biol.*, *4*, 240. (10) Mizoguchi et al (1979) *Gastroenterol. Jpn.*, *14*, 19. (11) Sameshima et al (1974) *Jpn. J. Gastroenterol.*, *71*, 799. (12) Rubinstein et al (1981) *Ugeskr. Laeg.*, *143*, 3304. (13) Kato et al (1979) *Gastroenterol. Jpn.*, *14*, 216. (14) Labadie et al (1983) *Méd. Chir. Dig.*, *12*, 181. (15) Monges et al (1983) *Gastroentérol. Clin. Biol.*, *7*, 540.

Amiodarone

Causal relationship +

Amiodarone is used for a variety of arrhythmias, preferably when other antiarrhythmic agents have failed and when a negative inotropic effect should be avoided. A mild (up to 4–fold the normal value) increase in serum aminotransferase levels in the first few months after starting treatment is common. An incidence of 40–55% (1, 2), but also a lower incidence of 10–20% (3, 4), has been mentioned in the literature, often transient despite continuation of use. Occasionally, liver enzyme elevations are marked and recur on readministration (2). According to Harris et al (3), these elevations correlate with the plasma concentration of amiodarone and its metabolite, desethylamiodarone (3).

More serious, and not completely unexpected, cases of phospholipidosis and cirrhosis have been described (8, 9). The diethylaminoethoxy–3,5–diiodophenyl side–chain of amiodarone resembles Coralgil (4,4′–diethylaminoethoxyhexestrol), a vasodilator, which in Japan has caused over 100 cases of hepatosplenomegaly with phospholipidosis in all hepatic cell types as well as in lymphatic tissues, bone marrow, kidney, lung and myocardium (5). Cirrhosis developed in some of these cases. Like all drugs that may cause phospholipidosis, amiodarone has an apolar ring structure with a polar side–chain. Indeed, amiodarone has caused phospholipidosis in animal toxicity testing (6). The problem with amiodarone is that it has a half–life of up to 2.5 months (7) and that the drug and its metabolite may reach liver tissue levels of several g/kg.

Lim et al (8) described a patient who developed neuropathy and liver dysfunction after 19 months of treatment. Histology showed periportal and centrilobular fibrosis, later progressing to fatal micronodular cirrhosis despite discontinuation of the drug 5 months before his death. Electron microscopy showed lamellar inclusion bodies in the liver cells. Significant amounts of amiodarone and desethylamiodarone were still present in liver tissue. Poucell et al (9) found roughly the same features in 3 of their patients. Hepatomegaly and liver enzyme elevations were discovered after 1–2 years of therapy (600 mg/wk). Fibrosis, cholangitis, a mixed inflammatory infiltrate and cytoplasmic granules were found in all cases. Mallory bodies and cirrhosis were present in 2 of them. Electron microscopy showed numerous pericanalicular lysosomal inclusion bodies with a laminated structure, resembling fingerprints, in hepatocytes and in endothelial, biliary epithelial and Kupffer cells. This pattern

130

also resembles perhexiline–induced damage and, indeed, this drug also has a relatively long half–life (up to 2 weeks) and the above–mentioned structural properties. Additional cases can be expected to be reported in the near future.

(1) Heger et al (1981) *N. Engl. J. Med., 305*, 539. (2) McGovern et al (1983) *Br. Med. J., 287*, 175. (3) Harris et al (1983) *Circulation, 67*, 45. (4) Plomteaux et al (1969) *Eur. J. Pharmacol., 8*, 369. (5) Lüllmann et al (1975) *C.R.C. Crit. Rev. Toxicol., 4*, 185. (6) Bockhardt (1979) *Inaugural Dissertation*, University of Kiel. (7) Stäubli et al (1983) *Eur. J. Clin. Pharmacol., 24*, 485. (8) Lim et al (1984) *Br. Med. J., 288*, 1638. (9) Poucell et al (1984) *Gastroenterology, 86*, 926.

Aprindine

Causal relationship +

Cholestatic (3), mixed (1) and hepatocellular (2) patterns of hepatitis have been observed; immunoallergic signs were absent. There was no hypotension. Onset was within 3 weeks, resolving in 2 months. Biopsy showed diffuse hepatitis, with mild necrosis and mononuclear infiltration (1, 2), centrilobular bile staining and thrombi, and portal infiltration (3).

Rechallenge was positive within 1–4 days (1–3), however with spontaneous normalization despite continuation of aprindine (2) in 1 of these cases.

(1) Brandes et al (1976) *Dtsch. Med. Wochenschr., 101*, 111. (2) Herlong et al (1978) *Ann. Intern. Med., 89*, 359. (3) Elewaut et al (1977) *Acta Gastroenterol. Belg., 40*, 236.

Detajmium bitartrate (see also 'Ajmaline' and 'Prajmaline')

Causal relationship o/ +

One case of cholestatic jaundice starting 12 days after initial intake was reported (1). Normalization occurred within $3^1/_2$ weeks after discontinuation. Fever and mild eosinophilia were present. Biopsy showed bile stasis with a few thrombi and small necrotic foci. There was a rich periportal eosinophilic infiltrate.

(1) Mölleken et al (1980) *Z. Ges. Inn. Med., 7*, 296.

Disopyramide

Causal relationship o/+

Several cases have been reported of hepatic injury with biochemically a cholestatic (1, 3, 4, 6–8), mixed (2) or mainly hepatocellular (5, 6, 9) pattern. In 1 case, disseminated intravascular coagulation accompanied hepatic injury (9). In another case, hepatic dysfunction was probably secondary to disopyramide–induced cardiac failure (10). The appearance of symptoms was mostly within the first 2 weeks of therapy (1, 4–7). Normalization of liver enzymes took several months (1–4, 8). With the exception of peripheral eosinophilia in 1 patient (2), immunoallergic signs were absent. A lymphocyte stimulation test, however, has been positive (6). When biopsy was performed in a few cases, histology showed fatty droplets in the cytoplasm (1) and non–specific inflammatory changes (5).

The causal relationship between disopyramide intake and the reported cases of hepatic injury is difficult to evaluate. Concurrent use of ajmaline (1), hypotension (5, 9), preceding operation (7, 8), underlying illness and scanty documentation complicate the evaluation of these cases. However, hepatic dysfunction secondary to cardiac failure, which occurred twice in the same patient (10), seems probable in vulnerable patients. The Japanese Health Authorities estimated the occurrence of hepatic injury at 0.35% with jaundice in 0.09% (6). These data were based on 6294 patients using disopyramide; no details on the design of the study were provided.

(1) Meinertz et al (1977) *Lancet, 2,* 829. (2) Riccioni et al (1977) *Lancet, 2,* 1363. (3) Anonymous (1979) *Jpn. Med. Gaz., 20 Sept,* 10. (4) Craxi et al (1980) *Ann. Intern. Med., 93,* 150. (5) Tonkin et al (1980) *Chest, 77,* 125. (6) Anonymous (1981) *Jpn. Med. Gaz., 20 June,* 11. (7) Edmonds et al (1980) *Eur. J. Clin. Pharmacol., 18,* 285. (8) Bakris et al (1983) *Mayo Clin. Proc., 58,* 265. (9) Doody (1982) *South. Med. J., 75,* 496. (10) Scheinman et al (1980) *Yale J. Biol. Med., 53,* 361.

Mexiletine

Causal relationship o

Pernot et al (1, 2) described 6 cases of a predominantly hepatocellular type of injury. In these cases, liver enzyme elevations were discovered within 1 month of starting treatment. Although several patients had complicated cardiovascular histories and/or preceding operation, mexiletine was considered to be the most likely causative factor. A biopsy performed in 1 patient showed minimal necrosis and centrilobular bile staining. There was a mixed portal infiltrate of mononuclear cells and polymorphs.

The authors found liver enzyme elevations in 10 of 25 patients on mexi-letine, whereas in a comparable group of patients not on mexiletine, only 9 of 116 had liver enzyme elevations (2). Although these figures may give some indication, they should be carefully interpreted since they do not originate from a prospective controlled study.

(1) Pernot et al (1983) *Presse Méd., 12,* 1938. (2) Pernot et al (1983) *Thérapie, 38,* 695.

Prajmaline (see also 'Ajmaline')

Causal relationship + +

One study of 61 cases (6) showed a mainly cholestatic pattern. This was confirmed by other cases (1, 2, 4, 5, 7, 9, 10, 12), although cases with a hepatocellular pattern may occur (3). Onset is mostly in the first few months of treatment (1, 3–5, 7, 8, 12), as was seen in 93% in a study of 61 cases (6), almost invariably starting with fever (1–9, 12). Eosinophilia (1, 4, 7, 8, 12) is frequent (65%) (6), rash less so (6.5%) (6). Biopsy in the study (33 biopsied patients) showed cholestasis as being most frequent (32 pts). There was minimal necrosis (6 pts), steatosis (15 pts), infiltration with lymphocytes (14 pts)/eosinophils (7 pts) and fibrosis (11 pts). Other authors have observed granulomas (3, 7, 8), 'reactive hepatitis' (5), peri-portal necrosis with collapse (2) and chronic hepatitis (3).

According to Engels (6), women and younger users are more vulnera-ble. Rechallenge was positive within 1–3 days (1–3, 5–7); macrophage in-hibition factor was positive in 2 cases (7). In 2 cases granular deposits of IgG and IgA were observed on bile canaliculi (7). The lymphocyte stim-ulation test was negative (7). Engels estimated the frequency at 0.012% (6) but did not correct for under–reporting. A very short latent period ($\leqslant 7$ days) during first use in several cases (6, 8) is odd, although concur-rent drug therapy may have been responsible. There may be large indi-vidual differences in metabolism of prajmaline and the plasma level after intake of 60 mg may show a 33–fold variation. A relationship to sparteine oxidation capacity has been demonstrated (11) and it would be interest-ing to discover whether patients with hepatic injury belong to the slow or fast metabolizers of prajmaline.

(1) Rotmensch et al (1980) *Postgr. Med. J., 56,* 738. (2) Weiss et al (1978) *Méd. Chir. Dig., 7,* 527. (3) Henning et al (1975) *Z. Gastroenterol., 13,* 501. (4) Pantlen (1976) *Dtsch. Med. Wochenschr., 101,* 1855. (6) Engels (1977) *Inaugural Dissertation.* Uni-versity of Tübingen. (7) Rotmensch et al (1981) *Z. Gastroenterol., 19,* 691. (8) Nas-chitz et al (1981) *Leber Magen Darm, 11,* 264. (9) Berlinger (1981) *Med. Welt, 43,* 1621. (10) Ritterman et al (1983) *Gastroenterohepatol. Arh., 2,* 100. (11) Reetz et al (1984) Paper presented at: 90. Tagung der Deutschen Gesellschaft für innere Medizin, Wiesbaden, 1984. (12) Kleinman et al (1983) *Ital. J. Gastroenterol., 15,* 33.

Procainamide

Causal relationship +

It is well known that procainamide is a frequent cause of drug–induced systemic lupus erythematosus (SLE). Although the rare reports of symptomatic hepatic injury in the literature seem to bear no relation to this syndrome, we know of 1 case in which liver enzyme elevations accompanied a procainamide–associated SLE syndrome.

The literature consists of cases with a mild to moderate, mixed to hepatocellular pattern of injury (1, 2, 5), whereas granulomas predominate in other cases (3, 4). Some cases exhibited fever as a concurrent symptom (1, 5). One patient had previously developed a rash to quinidine but did not show this reaction to procainamide (1). The onset was mostly in the early weeks of treatment. A rechallenge was followed by a relapse (1, 4). Histology performed in some cases showed granulomas (3, 4), epithelioid without caseation or giant cells (4), and accompanied by chronic–active–hepatitis–like features (3).

Berg et al (3) found antimitochondrial antibodies of the M3 type, which differ from those seen with primary biliary cirrhosis, and suggested that these might be characteristic of drug–induced disease (3). Rotmensch (4) looked for lymphocyte stimulation and macrophage migration inhibition but obtained negative results. However, mast cell degranulation was positive and, according to the author, humoral immunogenic mechanisms may have played a role.

(1) King et al (1963) *J. Am. Med. Assoc., 186,* 603. (2) Zimmerman (1978) *Hepatotoxicity,* p 510. Appleton–Century–Crofts, New York. (3) Berg et al (1981) In: Davis et al (Eds), *Drug Reactions and the Liver,* p 105. Pitman Medical, London. (4) Rotmensch et al (1978) *Ann. Intern. Med., 89,* 646. (5) Farber (1974) *Postgrad. Med. J., 56,* 155.

Quinidine

Causal relationship +

Several cases have been observed (1–13), mostly of a mild, mixed cholestatic–hepatocellular pattern without jaundice. Only some reports mentioned jaundice (16) or scleral icterus (17). Fever was mostly present (1–5, 7–9, 12–15, 17), less frequently accompanied by rash (11, 14), lymphadenopathy (4, 7), hemolytic anemia (14), eosinophilia (15) or thrombocytopenia (11, 14). All patients recovered quickly after discontinuation. With some exceptions (6, 14), most cases started within 1 month after initial

134

treatment (1, 2, 4, 5, 7–9, 15, 17, 18). Biopsy showed non–caseating granulomas (4, 5, 11, 14, 15, 17) consisting of epithelioid cells (4, 11), focal (6) and centrilobular necrosis with an infiltrate of round cells, eosinophils and plasma cells (9). Marked centrilobular cholestasis was noted in 1 report (16).

There was a prompt reaction to rechallenge (1–7, 9, 14, 17). In a series of 487 quinidine users, 32 cases (6.5%) of a hypersensitivity reaction included 10 cases (2%) of hepatic injury (14). Four of them had granulomatous hepatitis. In 4 of 9 patients the direct and indirect Coombs tests were positive in the presence of quinidine. Rotmensch (15) noted a positive macrophage migration inhibition factor but a negative lymphocyte stimulation and mast cell degranulation test.

(1) Colding (1969) Ugeskr. Laeg., 131, 1657. (2) Deisseroth et al (1972) Ann. Intern. Med., 77, 595. (3) Murphy et al (1973) Ann. Intern. Med., 78, 785. (4) Chajek et al (1974) Ann. Intern. Med., 81, 774. (5) Chajek (1975) Ann. Intern. Med., 82, 282. (6) Handler et al (1975) Arch. Intern. Med., 135, 871. (7) Herman et al (1975) J. Am. Med. Assoc., 234, 310. (8) Roque (1976) RI Med. J., 59, 407. (9) Koch et al (1976) Gastroenterology, 70, 1136. (10) Dzur (1976) J. Am. Med. Assoc., 235, 908. (11) Bramlet et al (1980) Arch. Intern. Med., 140, 395. (12) Deglin et al (1980) Drug Intell. Clin. Pharm., 14, 216. (13) Slezak (1981) Med. J. Aust., 1, 139. (14) Geltner et al (1976) Gastroenterology, 70, 650. (15) Rotmensch et al (1981) Z. Gastroenterol., 19, 691. (16) Hogan et al (1984) Can. Med. Assoc. J., 130, 973. (17) Urdahl et al (1983) Tidsskr. Nor. Laegefor., 103, 760. (18) Chagnon et al (1983) Méd. Armées, 11, 577.

Tocainide

Causal relationship o

Some unspecified cases of hepatitis have been reported and were attributed to intake of this agent (1, 2) which has only recently come into general use. ALAT/ASAT elevation was observed 6 weeks after initial treatment (2). Histology, 20 months after discontinuation of the drug, showed chronic active hepatitis. Nauta et al (3) reported heart failure and jaundice with very high ASAT/ALAT values in a 61–year–old man who had been treated with tocainide for 2 months (1200 mg/d). Recovery occurred in 6 weeks after discontinuation (3). Histology showed liver cell dropout in the centrilobular area.

(1) Horn et al (1980) Am. Heart J., 100, 1037. (2) Levin et al (1982) Clin. Res., 30, 200a. (3) Nauta et al (1984) Int. J. Cardiol., 5, 89.

Verapamil

Causal relationship +

See also 'Papaverine' which shows some structural resemblance. Some cases of hepatic injury have been described with biochemical signs of mild (2, 4) to marked (1, 3) hepatocellular injury. In 1 of these cases, jaundice followed a prodromal stage of abdominal pain, low–grade fever, arthralgia and vomiting, and was accompanied by eosinophilia (4). In the other cases, immunoallergic signs were absent. The onset/discovery was 2–3 weeks after starting treatment (1–4). A rechallenge in 1 of the cases was followed by an accelerated reaction with a higher ALAT peak, which suggests that an immunoallergic mechanism played a role (1). Histology in 1 case showed moderate cholestasis and a mixed infiltrate with many eosinophils in the portal area (4).

(1) Brodsky et al (1981) *Ann. Intern. Med., 94,* 490. (2) Stern et al (1982) *N. Engl. J. Med., 306,* 612. (3) Nash et al (1983) *J. Am. Med. Assoc., 249,* 395. (4) Guarascio et al (1984) *Br. Med. J., 288,* 362.

B. OTHER CARDIAC AGENTS

Amrinone

Causal relationship o/ +

Liver enzymes were elevated despite increased hemodynamics in 2 patients with cardiac failure (1). One case was reported of cholestatic jaundice (no further details given) 10 days after starting amrinone, with rash, generalized vasculitis, pulmonary infiltration and thrombocytopenia (2). The latter occurs frequently with this agent (2). Rechallenge was positive in 1 case (1).

(1) Dunkman et al (1983) *Am. Heart J., 105,* 816. (2) Wilmshurst et al (1983) *Br. Heart J., 49,* 447.

136

14. Antimicrobial agents

Introduction

Topically administered antimicrobial agents are not discussed in this Chapter.

Antimicrobial agents comprise a wide range of products which may interfere with the growth of micro–organisms in several ways but which may also be the cause of a wide variety of adverse effects, including hepatic injury.

These agents are systemically administered in, sometimes severely debilitated, patients in complicated clinical situations. Under these cir-

137

cumstances, it may be difficult to determine a causal relationship between hepatic injury and the suspected drug.

Micro–organisms may involve the liver primarily (e.g. viral hepatitis) or secondarily (e.g. sepsis) and any drug which is administered during the period of active disease may be falsely incriminated of causing hepatic injury. Moreover, patients with chronic liver disease may suffer relapse coinciding with administration of the suspected agent. On the other hand, one should never ascribe too readily signs or aggravation of hepatic injury to underlying hepatic disease.

Antimicrobial agents can cause hepatic injury through a toxic effect (e.g. high intravenous doses of tetracyclines), metabolic idiosyncrasy (e.g. isoniazid) or immunoallergy (e.g. quinine, sulfonamides). Moreover, they may cause or aggravate hepatic damage indirectly, e.g. secondary to a Jarisch–Herxheimer reaction, anaphylactic shock or porphyric attack.

Mild to moderate elevation of ASAT concentrations may occur after intramuscular administration, especially of irritating agents (e.g. gentamicin, carbenicillin) (1). For this reason it is advisable to measure ALAT levels simultaneously since this enzyme is more specific to the liver and is as sensitive as ASAT. Unfortunately, there are still many studies which assess ASAT in the serum as the only aminotransferase.

(1) Knirsch et al (1970) *N. Engl. J. Med., 282,* 1081.

A. ANTHELMINTICS/SCHISTOSOMICIDES

Important helmintic infections such as schistosomiasis, hydatidosis, ascariasis, trichiniasis, toxocariasis and fascioliasis may cause liver damage varying from mild elevations of liver enzyme concentrations to complete biliary obstruction. Usually the diagnosis can be made by non–invasive diagnostic procedures and liver biopsy (which may be contraindicated, e.g. hydatid cysts). In non–specific cases, when the infection is suspected and treated, it may be difficult to decide whether mild liver enzyme elevations are drug–induced or related to the underlying illness.

Fever and peripheral eosinophilia are relatively frequent and should not be confused with drug–induced immunoallergic liver injury. The same applies to liver granulomas, but ova, larvae and/or cysts usually facilitate differentiation.

Many anthelmintics are absorbed poorly or not at all from the gastrointestinal tract (e.g. mebendazole) and are unlikely candidates for liver injury unless in high doses or when erosions facilitate absorption. Others are well–absorbed (e.g. levamisole, piperazine) or reach the liver after parenteral administration.

Tetrachloroethylene may cause the same pattern of centrizonal necrosis and steatosis as CCl_4. Most cases of liver damage are accidental. Used as an anthelmintic in low doses, it is hardly absorbed and is non–toxic to the liver. Occasional serum aminotransferase elevations have been ascribed to niridazole (1), oxamniquine (2), pyrantel (3, 8), albendazole (4) and praziquantel (5), but a relation to the drug is sometimes uncertain. Flavaspidic acid, a constituent of the male fern, may cause hyperbilirubinemia by interfering with the uptake of bilirubin from sinusoidal blood (6). Dichlorophen in overdose may cause hepatic necrosis (7).

(1) Kanani et al (1970) *J. Trop. Med. Hyg., 73,* 162. (2) Lambertucci et al (1982) *Trans. R. Soc. Trop. Med. Hyg., 76,* 751. (3) Dukes (1980) In: Dukes (Ed), *Meyler's Side Effects of Drugs, 9th ed,* p 536. Excerpta Medica, Amsterdam. (4) Cortes et al (1982) *Compend. Invest. Clin. Latinoam., 2,* 63. (5) Chen et al (1982) *J. Formosan Med. Assoc., 81,* 1434. (6) Kenwright et al (1974) *Gut, 15,* 220. (7) *The Extra Pharmacopoeia, 28th ed,* p 90. Pharmaceutical Press, London, 1982. (8) Coutinho et al (1984) *Rev. Inst. Med. Trop. Sao Paulo, 26,* 38.

Hycanthone

Causal relationship +

Hycanthone is a metabolite and the 4–hydroxymethyl analog of lucanthone, one of the first antischistosomal drugs. It is structurally related to the thioxanthene derivatives (see 'Neuroleptics'). Besides schistosomiasis, for which it is administered in single doses of 3 mg/kg i.m., its use as an antitumor drug is experimental (1). Although both cholestasis and hepatocellular injury may occur (10), the latter is far more frequent. The drug is considered to be contraindicated in patients with underlying liver disease, febrile bacterial infections or patients treated with potentially cholestatic agents, in the latter because inhibition of biliary excretion of hycanthone and metabolites may produce toxic concentrations (3). Several cases of fatal hepatic necrosis have been reported (1, 2, 4–11, 14), often preceded by persistent vomiting, which may start 3 hours after injection and is followed by hepatic injury after 1 to several days. Its appearance after the 5th day is uncommon (3). The incidence is unknown, but has been estimated at $1:10$–20×10^3 (12). In 2723 patients, treated with 1–3 mg/kg for schistosomiasis no liver toxicity was reported (12). On the other hand, 15 of 17 courses in 7 patients with advanced refractory breast cancer, treated with 70 mg/m^2/d for 5 days, were followed by hepatic injury, which strongly suggests a toxic effect, especially since ASAT/ALAT elevation followed the first injections by a few days (1). This high incidence was confirmed by others (13). Histology has showed varying degrees of hepatocellular necrosis with bridging, steatosis, moderate cholestasis (11), and cirrhosis (10). One case of chronic persistent hepatitis, 1 year after injection (11), seems speculative since hycanthone is rapidly excreted. Animal toxicity tests in dogs and monkeys confirmed the hepatotoxic effect of hycanthone (1). In mice, hycanthone was associated with hepatic tumors (15), but this was not confirmed by others.

(1) Haq et al (1980) *Cancer Treat. Rep., 64,* 929. (2) Buchanan et al (1978) *S. Afr. Med. J., 53,* 257. (3) Dennis (1978) *S. Afr. Med. J., 54,* 137. (4) Farid et al (1972) *Br. Med. J., 2,* 88. (5) Andrade et al (1974) *Rev. Inst. Med. Trop. Sao Paulo, 16,* 160. (6) Marinho et al (1974) *Trop Dis. Bull., 71,* 1038. (7) Marinho et al (1975) *Trop. Dis. Bull., 72,* 821. (8) Tshiani et al (1979) *Trop. Dis. Bull., 76,* 365. (9) Legha et al (1978) *Cancer Treat. Rep., 62,* 1173. (10) Goncalves et al (1978) *Trop. Dis. Bull., 75,* 371. (11) Cohen (1978) *Gastroenterology, 75,* 103. (12) Cook et al (1976) *Ann. Trop. Med. Parasitol., 70,* 109. (13) Kovach et al (1979) *Cancer Treat. Rep., 63,* 1965. (14) Mengistu (1982) *Ethiop. Med. J., 20,* 145. (15) Haese et al (1973) *J. Pharmacol. Exp. Ther., 186,* 430.

Levamisole

Causal relationship o/+

As an anthelmintic, levamisole is usually given in a single dose or for 2–3 days. The drug has immunomodulating properties. Elevated ASAT levels in the serum necessitated discontinuation of therapy in 2 of 11 patients on 100–200 mg/d for 2 consecutive days/week for recurrent pyoderma (1). Onset occurred after 2 and 6 months respectively and levels returned to normal after discontinuation. Readministration was followed by relapse within a week.

Levamisole has been used in the treatment of chronic viral hepatitis but with little or no success.

(1) Papageorgiu et al (1982) *J. Clin. Lab. Immunol., 8,* 121.

Mebendazole

Causal relationship +

Mebendazole is hardly absorbed from the gastrointestinal tract and therefore hepatic injury may seem unexpected. However, erosions may facilitate increased absorption and relatively small amounts may be sufficient for an immunoallergic type of reaction.

ASAT/ALAT elevations are occasionally noted during short–term treatment (1). Seitz et al (2) noted hepatic injury in a 76–year–old man who was treated with 2 g/d for echinococcosis cysts in the liver. Forty–nine days after starting treatment rash and elevation of aminotransferase levels occurred which improved after discontinuation. After a low–dose challenge (100–300 mg/d, climbing dose) aminotransferase concentrations rose markedly and to a higher level (2). Junge et al (3) described a patient who developed hepatitis after 2 months of treatment for echinococcosis (3.5 g/d). After dechallenge liver enzyme levels normalized almost completely in 1 month. A challenge dose (1.5 g) was followed by marked ASAT/ALAT elevation. Histology showed minimal lobular necrosis and an increase in Kupffer cells.

140

(1) Beard et al (1978) *Med. J. Aust., 1,* 633. (2) Seitz et al (1983) *Z. Gastroenterol., 21,* 324. (3) Junge et al (1983) *Z. Gastroenterol., 21,* 736.

Niclofolan

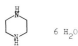

Causal relationship o

Cholestatic jaundice was reported in a patient with fascioliasis. Rash and eosinophilia were present. Onset occurred in 1 week after starting treatment, with subsidence in 3 weeks. Biopsy showed pronounced centrilobular cholestasis and mild portal infiltration with many eosinophils (1).

Since fascioliasis may produce the same clinical picture, this case remains speculative.

(1) Reshef et al (1982) *Br. Med. J., 285,* 1243.

Piperazine

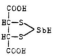

6 H_2O

Causal relationship o/+

One case was reported of acute hepatocellular injury with deep jaundice, starting 3–4 weeks after the intake of 1 dose (unspecified). Biopsy showed slight confluent necrosis and cholestasis in the centrilobular area (1).

Rechallenge was positive within a week, producing a more serious pattern with confluent necrosis and bridging.

(1) Hamlyn et al (1976) *Gastroenterology, 70,* 1144.

Stibocaptate

COOH
|
HC—S
| >SbE
HC—S
|
COOH

Causal relationship +

Inorganic antimony compounds cause liver injury in animals when administered in high doses (1). In patients treated for leishmaniasis with organic compounds, fatty degeneration of liver, heart and kidneys occurred (2). Although leishmaniasis itself may be a cause of steatosis, the presence of Leishman–Donovan bodies with Kupffer cell hyperplasia and portal infiltration/fibrosis facilitates differentiation. The same holds true for schistosomiasis, another indication for these drugs, which can be easily differentiated from drug–induced hepatic injury by the presence of ova in the majority of cases. Trivalent antimony derivatives (e.g.

stibophen, stibocaptate and antimony potassium tartrate), are considered more toxic than pentavalent derivatives (e.g. sodium stibgluconate). These agents are now less frequently used. ASAT elevations caused by stibocaptate are frequent (up to 65%) and probably dose–dependent (2, 4). These elevations may appear as early as the 2nd day of therapy (200 mg/d i.m. for 10 days) and as late as the 4th day after completion of therapy (4). In a small study, 82% of patients had ornithine carbamyl transferase elevations in serum (3). Occasionally, a case of severe hepatic injury occurs, as seen in a series of some 1200 patients treated for half a year (5). Histology showed microvesicular steatosis but also ova deposits and fibrosis; nevertheless, the reaction was ascribed to stibocaptate.

(1) Klatskin (1975) In: Schiff (Ed), *Diseases of the Liver, 4th ed*, p 610. Lippincott, Philadelphia. (2) Spingarn et al (1963) *Am. J. Med., 34,* 477. (3) Manson–Bahr (1972) In: Meyler et al (Eds), *Side Effects of Drugs, 7th ed*, p 433. Excerpta Medica, Amsterdam. (4) Waye et al (1962) *Am. J. Cardiol., 10,* 829. (5) Rugemalila (1980) *East Afr. Med. J., 57,* 720.

Tiabendazole

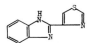

Causal relationship o/ +

A cholestatic (1, 4, 6) or mixed (2) pattern has been observed starting mostly in 2 weeks (1, 4–6). There was concomitant low–grade fever (1, 4–6), rash (1, 4) and eosinophilia (1, 6); these signs may however sometimes be related to underlying helmintic diseases. In 3 cases keratoconjunctivitis sicca was present (1, 5) without signs of primary–biliary–cirrhosis–like disease. Another case, however, resembled primary biliary cirrhosis (4). Normalization was prolonged in several cases (1, 5, 6), varying from 4 to 6.5 months. There was a prompt reaction to rechallenge in 2 cases (1, 3). Biopsy showed bile staining of hepatocytes with occasional necrosis and bile plugs.

One author reported abnormal liver tests in 5 of 14 patients (36%) (3), another a much lower incidence of 3% (7). The mechanism is unknown but may be related to immunomodulating properties or by hapten–protein formation and a subsequent immunological reaction (1).

(1) Rex et al (1983) *Gastroenterology, 85,* 718. (2) Hennekeuser et al (1969) *Tex. Rep. Biol. Med., 27, Suppl 2,* 581. (3) Bayles (1971) *Arch. Dermatol., 104,* 476. (4) Jalota et al (1974) *Am. J. Trop. Med. Hyg., 23,* 676. (5) Fink et al (1979) *Ophthalmology, 86,* 1892. (6) Feregrino et al (1976) *Prensa Med. Mex., 41,* 167. (7) Zimmerman (1978) *Hepatotoxicity,* p 498. Appleton–Century–Crofts, New York.

B. ANTIBIOTICS

The underlying illness for which antibiotics are administered may be associated with significant hepatic injury. In a patient with high fever who develops jaundice during treatment with an antibiotic, sepsis induced by an insensitive organism will be a more likely explanation for hepatic injury than the administered drug.

The use of antibiotics may be associated with complicated clinical circumstances, which often make it difficult to assess their eventual responsibility for hepatic injury.

Some antibiotic groups (e.g. high–dose i.v. tetracyclines, macrolides (except oleandomycin)), definitely cause hepatic injury in man, but for several other groups (e.g. aminoglycosides) a causal relationship is less certain.

B.1. PENICILLINS

Semisynthetic penicillins Although not yet proven, it is generally assumed that the semisynthetic penicillins (e.g. oxacillin) are a more frequent cause of hepatic injury than the natural penicillins (e.g. benzylpenicillin).

Several studies mention mild elevation of ASAT concentrations, but these may be ascribed partly to intramuscular administration. In particular, concentrated solutions of penicillins with irritating properties (e.g. carbenicillin) may injure skeletal muscle with subsequent ASAT release (1). This may also result from extravasation during intravenous administration but is probably less marked.

Besides the agents listed below, occasional liver enzyme elevations have been ascribed to most penicillins (e.g. mezlocillin (2), bacampicillin (3), dicloxacillin (5)), usually without much significance. One study mentioned cases of hepatic injury by sulbenicillin and pyrimidine penicillin in which a causal relationship was suggested by a positive lymphocyte stimulation test to drug–containing serum (4).

(1) Knirsch et al (1970) *N. Engl. J. Med., 282*, 1081. (2) Parry et al (1982) *J. Antimicrob. Chemother., 9, Suppl a*, 273. (3) Scheife et al (1982) *Pharmacotherapy, 2*, 313. (4) Namihisa et al (1975) *Leber Magen Darm, 5*, 73. (5) *The Extra Pharmacopoeia, 28th ed*, p 1154. Pharmaceutical Press, London, 1982.

Natural penicillins Natural penicillins are a very rare cause of hepatic injury. In the cases reported, the onset was usually within 2 weeks and was secondary to or accompanied by shock (1, 4), rash (3, 6–8) or exfoliative dermatitis (1, 5), fever and/or eosinophilia (1–3, 5, 7, 8). A serum–sickness–like pattern may be present (2, 8). A positive lymphocyte stimulation test was found in 5 cases (11). Including cases of shock and ischemic necrosis, both hepatocellular injury and a predominantly cholestatic pattern (2, 3, 6, 7, 9) have been observed. In 1 case recovery took almost a year and showed signs of chronicity (3). Skin tests with penicillin and complement–dependent cytotoxicity assays were positive (3). Another case of prolonged (> 1 year) cholestatic hepatitis was reported but no details were given (12). The mechanism in the observed cases seems to be immunoallergic; hepatic lesions have not been reproduced in animals

(13), although a toxic effect of high doses on protein metabolism of rat hepatocytes has been observed (10).

(1) Valdivia–Barriga et al (1963) *Gastroenterology, 45,* 114. (2) Goldstein et al (1974) *Arch. Pathol. Lab. Med., 98,* 114. (3) Girard et al (1967) *Helv. Med. Acta, 34,* 23. (4) Murphy et al (1962) *Arch. Pathol. Lab. Med., 73,* 13. (5) Rabinovitch et al (1948) *J. Am. Med. Assoc., 138,* 496. (6) Beeley et al (1976) *Lancet, 2,* 1297. (7) Möckel (1965) *Med. Klin., 60,* 294. (8) Felder et al (1950) *J. Am. Med. Assoc., 143,* 361. (9) Williams et al (1981) *Dig. Dis. Sci., 26,* 470. (10) Vonen et al (1982) *Acta Pharmacol. Toxicol., 51,* 81. (11) Namihisa et al (1975) *Leber Magen Darm, 5,* 73. (12) Dubin et al (1960) *Am. J. Med., 29,* 55. (13) Klatskin (1975) In: Schiff (Ed), *Diseases of the Liver,* 4th ed, p 604. Lippincott, Philadelphia.

Ampicillin

Causal relationship o

Acute hepatic necrosis was reported in 1 case, ultimately fatal, starting after 15 days of treatment; there was rash and eosinophilia (1). Liver injury and Stevens–Johnson syndrome were observed in a patient on ampicillin and cephalexin (2).

The leukocyte migration inhibition test (3) and the lymphocyte stimulation test (4) were positive in some unspecified cases.

(1) Caravati et al (1971) *Dig. Dis. Sci., 16,* 803. (2) McArthur et al (1975) *NZ Med. J., 81,* 390. (3) Morizane (1978) *Gastroenterol. Jpn., 13,* 281. (4) Namihisa et al (1975) *Leber Magen Darm, 5,* 73.

Carbenicillin

Causal relationship +

Several cases of hepatic injury, mostly mild (2–5) have been ascribed to the intravenous use of carbenicillin. Rechallenge was positive in 5 cases (2, 3); there was rash (2, 3) and eosinophilia (2). Biopsy showed spotty necrosis and minimal portal mononuclear infiltration (2). A higher incidence of ALAT/ASAT elevations was reported with carbenicillin than with piperacillin (4) or ticarcilline (5) in some studies. Knirsch et al (1) noted ASAT elevations only after intramuscular, but not after intravenous, administration in the same individuals. Creatinine phosphokinase accompanied ASAT elevation, whereas ALAT remained normal. They suggested that muscle damage was responsible.

(1) Knirsch et al (1970) *N. Engl. J. Med., 282,* 1081. (2) Wilson et al (1975) *J. Am.*

Med. Assoc., 232, 818. (3) Graft et al (1982) J. Pediatr., 100, 497. (4) Shariffi et al (1982) J. Urol. (Baltimore), 128, 755. (5) Parry et al (1978) Am. J. Med., 64, 961.

Cloxacillin

Causal relationship +

Cases of cloxacillin–associated hepatic injury have so far been reported only infrequently (1, 2). In 1 case, icteric cholestatic hepatitis with severe intrahepatic cholestasis and a few scattered foci of necrosis appeared after 2–3 weeks of therapy; no immunoallergic signs were observed (2).

Rechallenge was positive within 4 days (1, 2). There was a positive macrophage inhibition factor test (2).

(1) Berger et al (1977) Lancet, 2, 95. (2) Enat et al (1980) Br. Med. J., 1, 982.

Flucloxacillin

Causal relationship o/ +

Non–symptomatic hepatic injury has been suggested by moderate ASAT/ ALAT elevations in a hemodialysis patient with infections treated with oral flucloxacillin. There was a temporal relationship to intake and a rechallenge was positive (1).

(1) Lobatto et al (1982) Neth. J. Med., 25, 47.

Methicillin

Causal relationship o

Elevated liver enzyme levels were reported in 21.3% of 75 pediatric patients receiving 200 mg/kg/d i.v. for 3–39 days (1), but no abnormalities were observed in 28 patients (62.5–200 mg/kg/d) treated for 2–23 days (2).

(1) Kitzing et al (1981) Am. J. Dis. Child., 135, 52. (2) Nahata et al (1982) Dev. Pharmacol. Ther., 4, 117.

Nafcillin

Causal relationship o

Elevated liver enzymes were reported in several studies (1–3). In one study comparing methicillin (200 mg/kg/d i.v.) with nafcillin (150 mg/kg/d i.v.), mild ASAT/ALAT elevations were noted in up to 25% of patients on nafcillin for 21–39 days. Eosinophilia was ascribed to this agent in 24% (2). Nahata et al (1) found a much lower incidence despite a comparable regimen. Another study showed minimal ASAT elevation in a few patients but eosinophilia in up to 20% (3). In a patient with ASAT/ALAT elevation in response to oxacillin, use of nafcillin was followed by a relapse (4). Subsequent cefalotin, 5 months later, was again followed by liver enzyme elevation.

(1) Nahata et al (1982) *Dev. Pharmacol. Ther., 4,* 117. (2) Kitzing et al (1981) *Am. J. Dis. Child., 135,* 52. (3) Feldman et al (1978) *J. Pediatr., 93,* 1029. (4) Miller et al (1983) *Clin. Pharmacol., 2,* 465.

Oxacillin

Causal relationship o/+

Several cases have been reported, biochemically of a hepatocellular pattern (1, 3–17) varying from mild ALAT/ASAT elevations to high values (5, 8, 11, 17). Cholestatic hepatitis has also been described (2). Onset is within 1 month in almost every case and often within 10 days (5–7, 9, 11, 13) after starting therapy (often high i.v. doses). Confounding factors are, of course, sepsis and in many cases parenteral drug abuse. Concurrent eosinophilia (5, 6, 12–14) and rash (6, 12) may occur; rechallenge was positive in 1 case (6). Immunological testing was positive in 1 case (lymphocyte stimulation test etc.) (16). One study showed a higher incidence of penicillin allergy in a group of patients with oxacillin–induced hepatic injury (6).

(1) Huang et al (1963) *Antimicrob. Agents Chemother.,* 237. (2) Ten Pas et al (1965) *J. Am. Med. Assoc., 191,* 674. (3) Walker et al (1967) *Am. J. Dis. Child., 114,* 64. (4) Dismukes (1973) *J. Am. Med. Assoc., 226,* 861. (5) Olans et al (1976) *J. Pediatr., 89,* 835. (6) Onorato et al (1978) *Ann. Intern. Med., 89,* 497. (7) Klein et al (1976) *Am. J. Gastroenterol., 65,* 546. (8) Bruckstein et al (1978) *Am. J. Med., 64,* 519. (9) Pollock et al (1978) *Arch. Intern. Med., 138,* 915. (10) Halloran et al (1979) *Arch. Intern. Med., 139,* 376. (11) Denny et al (1979) *Ann. Intern. Med., 90,* 277. (12) Taylor et al (1979) *Ann. Intern. Med., 90,* 857. (13) McKelvie et al (1982) *Hosp. Pharm.,*

17, 562. (14) Goldstein et al (1978) *Am. J. Gastroenterol., 70,* 171. (15) Nahata et al (1982) *Dev. Pharm. Ther., 4,* 117. (16) Mizoguchi et al (1980) *Gastroenterol. Jpn., 15,* 14. (17) Michelson (1981) *Can. J. Hosp. Pharm., 34,* 83.

Piperacillin

Causal relationship o

In a comparative study of patients with complicated urinary tract infections ASAT/ALAT/APh elevations were noted in 1/1/1 of 29 patients on piperacillin (mean: 181 mg/kg/d i.v.) as against 6/7/4 of 27 patients on carbenicillin (mean: 270 mg/kg/d i.v.) (1). Elevated liver enzyme levels (ASAT/APh) were also reported in 3% of 758 patients (2).

(1) Sharifi (1982) *J. Urol. (Baltimore), 128,* 755. (2) Fortner et al (1982) *Pharmacotherapy, 2,* 287.

Ticarcillin

Causal relationship o/+

Mild elevations of ASAT concentrations have been noted in 1–4% (1–3) but may be partly ascribed to intramuscular administration. However, concurrent APh elevations (3) suggest mild liver injury in some patients. Clinical trials in 1433 patients of all age groups showed ALAT elevations in 1% (4). In 3 patients with carbenicillin–induced hepatic injury no reaction followed ticarcillin (4). In a patient with ticarcillin–associated granulocytopenia, concurrent ASAT elevation, fever and eosinophilia had also been present during a preceding course with the same drug (6). Parry et al (5) studied ticarcillin and tobramycin versus carbenicillin and gentamycin: ASAT elevations were encountered in 23% on the latter regimen as against 3% on the former.

(1) Nelson et al (1978) *Pediatrics, 61,* 858. (2) Wise (1978) In: *Ticarcillin. Proceedings, International Symposium, Switzerland, 1977.* Excerpta Medica, Amsterdam. (3) Pines et al (1974) *Chemotherapy, 20,* 39. (4) Graft et al (1982) *J. Pediatr., 100,* 497. (5) Parry et al (1978) *Am. J. Med., 64,* 961. (6) Ohning et al (1982) *Am. J. Dis. Child., 136,* 645.

B.2. CEPHALOSPORINS

Hepatic enzyme elevations in serum may occur during use of cephalo-sporins. They are often transient and may disappear despite continua-tion of therapy; these drugs seem to give rise only rarely to clinical signs of hepatic injury. There are some important points: Firstly, intramuscu-lar administration (of any drug) may cause ASAT elevation, in which case the drug may be falsely incriminated of producing hepatic injury. Secondly, bacterial infections for which the drug has been administered may be responsible for mild liver enzyme elevations as well as cholestatic jaundice (1). Since it is very unusual to perform a clinical trial of anti-infectious drugs with placebo as control, many studies are open or dou-ble–blind with another cephalosporin as control. Hence the causal rela-tionship between enzyme elevations and drug intake may be difficult to establish. Nevertheless, the (sometimes high) incidence of ASAT/ALAT elevations in some studies and even after intravenous administration suggests that cephalosporins may indeed cause liver enzyme release un-der certain, largely unknown, circumstances. It is unclear whether this is directly related to the high biliary concentration of some of these agents. Eosinophilia is also fairly frequent but accompanies in only some cases liver enzyme elevations; probably it is not related and does not give much insight into an eventual mechanism of hepatic injury. Although the ability to produce clinically significant hepatic injury is less certain, mild liver enzyme elevations have been noted during the use of most agents, e.g. cefotaxime (13), cefuroxime (4), cefamandole (5), ceftizoxime (6), cefotiam (7), cefsulodin (8), cefoxitin (9) and cefadroxil (10). Also, studies of new agents, e.g. cefotetan (11) and cefpiramide (12), have shown that liver enzyme elevations are not uncommon, albeit often diffi-cult to ascribe directly to drug use.

Bleeding complications, such as seen in debilitated patients with some cephalosporins (e.g. moxalactam), are probably not of hepatic origin but related to interference with vitamin–K–producing gut flora and suppres-sion of platelet function (2). Several cephalosporins (e.g. cefoperazone, cefamandole and moxalactam) may cause disulfiram–like reactions (3).

Zimmerman et al (1979) *Gastroenterology, 77,* 363. (2) Carmine et al (1983) *Drugs, 26,* 279. (3) Van Klingeren (1982) In: Dukes (Ed), *Side Effects of Drugs, Annual 6,* p 240. Excerpta Medica, Amsterdam. (4) Brogden et al (1979) *Drugs, 17,* 233. (5) Several authors (1979) *Chemotherapy (Tokyo), 27,* S–5. (6) Yoshida et al (1982) *Jpn. J. Antibiot., 34,* 112. (7) Several authors (1979) *Chemotherapy (Tokyo), 27,* S–3. (8) Miki et al (1983) *Chemotherapy (Tokyo), 31,* 254. (9) Van Winzum (1978) *J. Antimicrob. Chemother., 4, Suppl B,* 91. (10) Motohiro et al (1983) *Jpn. J. Anti-biot., 36,* 93. (11) Nagamatsu et al (1983) *Jpn. J. Antibiot., 36,* 1199. (12) Suzuki et al (1983) *Chemotherapy (Tokyo), 31, Suppl 1,* 542. (13) Carmine (1983) *Drugs, 25,* 223.

Cefacetrile

N≡C-CH₂-CONH—[structure: β-lactam/cephem ring with COOH and —CH₂OCOCH₃ substituents]

Causal relationship o

Mildly elevated liver enzyme levels have been reported (1). In a study of 27 patients with cellulitis, pneumonia or pyelonephritis, 8 developed mild to moderate ALAT elevation. Eosinophilia was noted in 4 cases. Treatment was with 6–9 g/d i.v. or i.m. (1).

(1) Hodges et al (1973) *Antimicrob. Agents Chemother.*, *3*, 228.

Cefaclor

[structure: phenyl—CH(NH₂)—CO—NH—cephem ring with COOH and Cl substituents]

Causal relationship o

Transient liver enzyme elevation was reported in 0.5% of 1851 patients (1). A case of mild cholestatic jaundice, accompanied by rash, was noted in a child with pneumonia treated with 120 mg/kg/d. Jaundice appeared after 10 days of treatment; there was complete recovery after discontinuation (2).

(1) Fujii (1979) *Postgrad. Med. J.*, *55, Suppl 4*, 88. (2) Bosio (1983) *J. Toxicol. Clin. Toxicol.*, *20*, 79.

Cefalexin

[structure: phenyl—CH(NH₂)—CO—NH—cephem ring with COOH and CH₃ substituents]

Causal relationship o/+

Hepatic necrosis (1, 2), fatal in 1 case (2) as well as a cholestatic (3) and mixed (4) pattern of injury have been observed, but few details were given. A rechallenge was positive in 1 case (2). The lymphocyte stimulation test was positive (2–4). In 1 case a lymphokine was isolated which produced cholestasis when injected into the mesenteric vein of dogs (3).

(1) Kanetaka et al (1973) *Acta Pathol. Jpn.*, *23*, 617. (2) Namihisa et al (1975) *Leber Magen Darm*, *5*, 73. (3) Mizoguchi et al (1979) *Gastroenterol. Jpn.*, *14*, 19. (4) Mizoguchi et al (1980) *Gastroenterol. Jpn.*, *15*, 14.

Cefalotin

[structure: thiophene—CH₂-CO-NH—cephem ring with COOH and —CH₂-O-C(=O)-CH₃ substituents]

Causal relationship o

Hepatic injury has been reported in some cases (1, 2); cholestatic jaundice has been ascribed to cefalotin. Fever, eosinophilia and jaundice appeared after 17 days of treatment which subsided after discontinuation. In another (unspecified) case a lymphocyte stimulation test was positive in the presence of drug–containing serum (2). In 1 case of liver enzyme elevation to oxacillin, treatment with nafcillin and later cefalotin was followed by a relapse (3).

(1) Schaefer et al (1975) *Münch. Med. Wochenschr., 117,* 251. (2) Namihisa et al (1975) *Leber Magen Darm, 5,* 73. (3) Miller et al (1983) *Clin. Pharm., 2,* 465.

Cefoperazone

Causal relationship o

Elevated ALAT/ASAT and APh levels were reported in 2.7% of 756 patients (2–4 g/d) (1), also in 4.8% of 466 patients (2 g/d) (2). ALAT/ASAT elevation was seen in 7 of 35 patients (2–4 g/d i.v.) with normal pre–treatment values. There was no deterioration in abnormal pre–treatment values (3).

(1) Shibata (1980) *Clin. Ther., 3,* 173. (2) Mashimo (1980) *Clin. Ther., 3,* 159. (3) Carlberg et al (1982) *J. Antimicrob. Chemother., 10,* 483.

Cefazolin

Causal relationship o

Mild ALAT/ASAT elevations have been reported (1, 2). One case has been reported of prolonged cholestatic jaundice starting after 5 days of treatment with cefazolin (1 g/d i.m.), cefadroxil (1 g/d p.o.) and mefenamic acid (500 mg/d p.o.). A positive lymphocyte stimulation test was seen with cefazolin (3). Biopsy showed cholestasis without necrosis.

(1) *J. Infect. Dis.,* 1973, *128, Suppl.* (2) *Infection,* 1974, *2, Suppl 1.* (3) Ammann et al (1982) *Lancet, 2,* 337.

Ceforanide

Causal relationship o

Mild and transient elevations of ALAT/ASAT levels have been reported

150

in several studies (1–3). An occasional case of hepatitis was seen (4), possibly related to high doses taken for 2–4 weeks.

(1) Smyth et al (1979) *Antimicrob. Agents Chemother.*, *16*, 615. (2) Musher et al (1980) *Antimicrob. Agents Chemother.*, *17*, 254. (3) Burch et al (1979) *Antimicrob. Agents Chemother.*, *16*, 386. (4) Cooper et al (1981) *Antimicrob. Agents Chemother.*, *19*, 256.

Ceftazidime

Causal relationship o

Elevated liver enzymes, especially ALAT/ASAT, have been reported in several studies in frequencies ranging from 3% (1) and 6–9% (2–4) to 20% (5, 6). Dose and administration were similar in most studies (1–6 g/d i.m. or i.v.).

(1) Daikos et al (1981) *J. Antimicrob. Chemother.*, *8, Suppl B*, 331. (2) Petterson et al (1981) *J. Antimicrob. Chemother.*, *8, Suppl B*, 303. (3) Gozzard et al (1982) *Lancet, 1,* 1152. (4) Clumeck et al (1983) *Antimicrob. Agents Chemother.*, *24*, 176. (5) De Sandre et al (1981) *J. Antimicrob. Chemother.*, *8, Suppl B*, 307. (6) Rusconi et al (1984) *Antimicrob. Agents Chemother.*, *25*, 395.

Ceftriaxone

Causal relationship o

In a study of 55 patients with infections of urinary tract, respiratory tract or soft tissue treated with 2 g/d for at least 5 days, 16% developed ASAT and/or APh elevations. Eosinophilia was noted in 8% (1).

(1) Gnann et al (1982) *Antimicrob. Agents Chemother.*, *22,* 1.

Moxalactam

Causal relationship o

Mildly elevated aminotransferase and APh levels have been reported in approximately 3% of patients (1, 2). Other studies give much higher figures (3, 4). A comparison of moxalactam (1 g/d; 41 patients) and cefazolin (2 g/d; 41 patients) in patients with urinary tract infections showed a significantly higher incidence of liver enzyme elevations (37% vs 15%) (4), but this was not confirmed by others (5). Cholestatic hepatitis was seen in 1 case (6). Moxalactam has been associated with bleeding disorders, probably due to interference with vitamin–K–producing gut flora and to suppression of platelet function (1). Hypoprothrombinemia with a hematoma in the right liver lobe developed in a woman after 8 days of therapy (7). Thomas et al (8) reported a patient with liver abscess associated with the use of moxalactam. It was suggested that superinfection with insensitive enterococci was directly related to the use of moxalactam.

(1) Carmine et al (1983) *Drugs, 26,* 279. (2) Iwai et al (1981) *Jpn. J. Antibiot., 34,* 799. (3) Varghese et al (1982) *Chemotherapy (Basel), 28,* 417. (4) Lea et al (1982) *Antimicrob. Agents Chemother., 22,* 32. (5) Konno et al (1982) *Chemotherapy (Tokyo), 30,* 62. (6) Lagast et al (1982) *Antimicrob. Agents Chemother., 22,* 604. (7) Sylvester et al (1984) *Minn. Med. J., 67,* 141. (8) Thomas et al (1983) *Arch. Intern. Med., 143,* 1780.

B.3. LINCOMYCINS

Hepatic injury by lincomycin has been reported mainly after high doses. Too little is known for a clear picture to emerge.

Clindamycin

$H_3C-H_2C-H_2C-$ [chemical structure: pyrrolidine N-CH$_3$ ring, CO-NH-CH, Cl-CH-CH$_3$, sugar ring with OH, OH, SCH$_3$]

Causal relationship o

There are rare reports of overt hepatocellular injury (1, 2); the causal relationship is difficult to assess because of preceding/concurrent use of methotrexate and fusidic acid (1) and sepsis (2). Indications of a hepatotoxic effect were found in dogs on 600 mg/kg (3) and some studies of parenteral administration in man showed ALAT/ASAT elevations in 20–50% (4).

(1) Craig (1974) *Br. Med. J., 3,* 43. (2) Elmore et al (1974) *Am. J. Med., 57,* 627. (3) Gray et al (1971) *Toxicol. Appl. Pharmacol., 19,* 217. (4) Zimmerman (1978) *Hepatotoxicity,* p 480. Appleton–Century–Crofts, New York.

B.4. MACROLIDES

The ability of macrolides to produce hepatic injury is unequivocal. The esters of oleandomycin and erythromycin (esterification facilitates gastrointestinal absorption), troleandomycin and erythromycin estolate have been incriminated in the causation of many cases of cholestatic jaundice.

An increasing number of reports on the other erythromycin esters

152

probably reflects changing prescribing habits and demonstrates that the hepatic injury is not exclusively caused by the estolate, as was formerly thought. A recent study even suggested a higher incidence for the stearate than for the estolate, but needs further confirmation (1).

Midecamycin has been associated occasionally with mild liver enzyme elevations (2), but, as far as we know, not with clinical cases.

(1) Inman et al (1983) *Br. Med. J.*, *286*, 1954. (2) Fujii et al (1983) *Chemotherapy (Tokyo)*, *31*, 54.

Erythromycin

L-cladinose

Causal relationship + +

Because of its instability in gastric acid, erythromycin is mostly administered as salt or ester. The latter is a known and unequivocal cause of hepatic injury, although in a minority of patients. Most reported cases concern the estolate ester, but previous claims that this was the only injurious form have been contradicted by analogous cases ascribed to the ethylsuccinate (1–9, 23, 30), the propionate (10–12) and the stearate ester (13). Moreover, 1 case was ascribed to the use of non–esterified erythromycin (14).

It is widely accepted – but not proven – that the estolate produces hepatic injury more frequently than the other forms. This assessment is based largely on extensive reporting in the literature (up to 55 cases in 1983) (15). Moreover, 93% of 418 cases reported to the Food and Drug Administration between 1969 and 1978 comprised the estolate form (16). The role of more extensive use of the latter and of selective reporting of known (and thus easily recognized) reactions is uncertain. Nevertheless, the incidence of reports of hepatic injury due to the estolate was more than 20–fold that due to other forms. Moreover, these findings were consistent over several years and were widely confirmed in several other countries; several health commissions advised cautious use. On the other hand, a recent study with prescription event monitoring in 12,208 patients showed no cases of jaundice ascribed to the estolate as against 3 ascribed to the stearate (17). The incidence was estimated at less than 0.1% (17), which is much lower than that previously mentioned (2–4%) (18).

Serum aminotransferase elevations ascribed to the use of the estolate have been noted in up to 38% (13). In a controlled study 9.9% had ASAT elevations as against 1.8% in the control group (19).

Less frequent is symptomatic hepatic injury. Most reports concern a

153

mixed to cholestatic pattern of injury. Funck–Brentano et al (15) compared the clinical features of cases of hepatic injury to the estolate as reported in the medical literature with ethylsuccinate and propionate. There were no significant differences. Most cases presented with abdominal pain, nausea and jaundice. Approximately half the patients had fever and/or hepatomegaly. The latter was especially frequent in children. First symptoms appeared in most cases within the first 5–15 days after starting therapy. In the majority of cases there was rapid recovery after discontinuation. The incidence of eosinophilia was higher with the ethylsuccinate and the propionate (80–100%) than with the estolate (45%), but the small numbers in the first two groups make it difficult to assess the significance. Rash was rarely reported. In the cases of estolate–associated injury in which a rechallenge was performed, there was an accelerated reaction, mostly within 2 days (15). This was also observed with single cases of ethylsuccinate–induced (2, 5) and propionate–induced (11) injury. Cross–sensitivity was observed in 2 cases (8, 10) of estolate hepatitis with ethylsuccinate and propionate, respectively. Antinuclear factor was negative while mitochondrial and microsomal antibodies were not present (15). Lymphocyte stimulation tests (only performed in cases with estolate–associated injury) have been both positive (20, 29) and negative (10, 21, 22). Histology mostly showed centrilobular cholestasis with mononuclear and eosinophilic infiltration, both portal and lobular. Necrosis was less frequent and mostly mild to moderate (15). There was no significant difference in histology between the esters. Although controlled studies have not so far been reported, hepatic injury is generally believed to be less frequent in children (16, 24).

The mechanism is unknown. Mild intrinsic toxicity is suggested by the high incidence of aminotransferase elevations in some studies (13, 19). In clinically overt cases an immunoallergic reaction may be superimposed on this mild intrinsic toxicity by a change in the antigenic structure. Several suggestions have been made to explain a higher incidence of estolate–induced hepatic injury: higher blood levels due to better absorption (25), toxicity of the propionate and lauryl sulfate moiety of the molecule (26) or a strong antigenic capacity of the estolate (27). Erythromycin estolate was more toxic than the erythromycin base in cell cultures and in the perfused rat liver (28), but the difference from the propionate was not significant.

(1) Klatskin (1975) In: Schiff (Ed), *Diseases of the Liver, 4th ed*, p 604. Lippincott, Philadelphia. (2) Bena (1979) *J. Kansas Med. Soc., 80,* 418. (3) Greenlaw et al (1979) *Drug Intell. Clin. Pharm., 13,* 236. (4) Stein (1979) *Drug Intell. Clin. Pharm., 13,* 612. (5) Viteri et al (1979) *Gastroenterology, 76,* 1007. (6) Zafrani et al (1979) *Dig. Dis. Sci., 24,* 385. (7) Sullivan (1980) *J. Am. Med. Assoc., 243,* 1074. (8) Keeffe et al (1982) *Dig. Dis. Sci., 27,* 701. (9) Funck–Brentano et al (1982) *Gastroentérol. Clin. Biol., 6,* 1044. (10) Tolman et al (1974) *Ann. Intern. Med., 81,* 58. (11) Pessayre et al (1976) *Arch. Fr. Mal. Appar. Dig., 65,* 405. (12) Ponsot et al (1982) *Gastroentérol. Clin. Biol., 6,* 594. (13) Ticktin et al (1963) *Ann. NY Acad. Sci., 104,* 1080. (14) Hosker et al (1983) *Postgrad. Med. J., 59,* 514. (15) Funck–Brentano et al (1983) *Gastroentérol. Clin. Biol., 7,* 362. (16) Anonymous (1979) *FDA Drug Bull.,*

9, 26. (17) Inman et al (1983) *Br. Med. J., 286*, 1954. (18) Australian Drug Evalua-tion Committee (1971) *Med. J. Aust., 1*, 1203. (19) McCormack et al (1977) *Anti-microb. Agents Chemother., 12*, 630. (20) Cooksley et al (1977) *Aust. NZ J. Med., 7*, 291. (21) Gafter et al (1979) *NY State J. Med., 79*, 87. (22) Lunzer et al (1975) *Gastroenterology, 68*, 1284. (23) Phillips (1983) *Can. Med. Assoc. J., 129*, 411. (24) Ginsburg et al (1976) *J. Pediatr., 89*, 872. (25) Keller et al (1980) In: Dukes (Ed), *Meyler's Side Effects of Drugs, 9th ed*, p 452. Excerpta Medica, Amsterdam. (26) Dujovne et al (1972) *J. Lab. Clin. Med., 79*, 832. (27) Gilbert (1962) *J. Am. Med. Assoc., 182*, 1048. (28) Zimmerman (1978) *Hepatotoxicity*, p 468. Appleton–Centu-ry–Crofts, New York. (29) Namihisa et al (1975) *Leber Magen Darm, 5*, 73. (30) Diehl et al (1984) *Am. J. Med., 76*, 931.

Josamycin

Causal relationship o

In a study in 30 neonates treated for a variety of infections with josamy-cin (50 mg/kg/d) for up to 10 days, 6 showed a moderate and 2 a marked increase in APh concentration in the serum. In one of them, serum aminotransferase levels were moderately elevated. Premature infants de-veloped the reaction more frequently (1). Morizane (2) mentioned 3 un-specified cases of hepatic injury; in 2 of these leukocyte migration inhibi-tion was demonstrated.

(1) Masser et al (1982) *Drugs Exp. Clin. Res., 8*, 313. (2) Morizane (1978) *Gastroen-terol. Jpn., 13*, 281.

Troleandomycin

Causal relationship + +

The formula represents oleandomycin; troleandomycin is the triacetyl ester. Whereas oleandomycin has not been reported as a cause of hepatic injury, troleandomycin has. Jaundice was reported as early as 1962 to oc-cur in up to 4% of recipients of this drug (1). Hepatic dysfunction was demonstrated in over 50% of patients taking 1 g/d for 2 weeks (1), but lower doses may also cause mild liver enzyme elevations which respond to dose reduction or resolve despite continuation (2). A dose of 250 mg/d is usually safe (2). In the former study (1) histology showed moderate cholestasis and cellular abnormalities and portal mononuclear infiltration. A challenge in 3 patients was positive (1). Since 1978 many reports have appeared of cholestatic jaundice caused by the combination of this drug with oral contraceptives (3–16). Miguet et al (3) saw 24 cases of cholestatic jaundice on this combination as against 1 on each drug separately. These 24 patients had safely used contraceptives for several months or years; within 1 month after starting treatment with this drug (mean dose 1.9 g/d) jaundice appeared, preceded by pruritus. Biochemistry suggested a cholestatic to mixed pattern of injury; biopsy showed pure cholestasis only (3). The other reports (4–16) are practically identical. Although occasional rash and eosinophilia (3) and a positive lymphocyte stimulation test (15) suggest an immunoallergic mechanism in some patients, a toxic cause seems more likely, since most cases occur in the first 10 days of therapy and present a picture of pure cholestasis. A different mechanism may possibly involve cholestatic jaundice caused by the use of troleandomycin without oral contraceptives, which seems to imply an additional necrotic component. It has been suggested that this drug causes a steroid cholestasis through inhibition of contraceptive metabolism (3). The demonstration that clearance of other steroids is also inhibited by troleandomycin is compatible with this theory (2).

(1) Ticktin et al (1962) *N. Engl. J. Med., 267,* 964. (2) Zeiger et al (1980) *J. Allergy Clin. Immunol., 66,* 438. (3) Miguet et al (1980) *Gastroentérol. Clin. Biol., 4,* 420. (4) Perol et al (1978) *Nouv. Presse Méd., 7,* 4302. (5) Goldfain et al (1979) *Nouv. Presse Méd., 8,* 1099. (6) Rollux et al (1979) *Nouv. Presse Méd., 8,* 1694. (7) Treille et al (1979) *Rev. Méd. Alpes Fr., 8,* 317. (8) Buffet et al (1979) *Concours Méd.,* 7215. (9) Girard et al (1980) *Lyon Méditerr. Méd., 16,* 2335. (10) Mauerhoff et al (1980) *Louvain Méd., 99,* 153. (11) Le Verger (1980) *Ouest Méd., 33,* 1087. (12) Haber et al (1980) *Acta Gastroenterol. Belg., 43,* 475. (13) Fevery (1981) *Tijdschr. Geneeskd., 37,* 201. (15) Namihisa et al (1975) *Leber Magen Darm, 5,* 73.

B.5. TETRACYCLINES

Tetracyclines cause steatosis, both in animals and man, mainly after intravenous administration in subjects with decreased renal function. Most cases have been reported after the use of tetracycline but chlortetracycline (7), demechlortetracycline (13), oxytetracycline (15) and rolitetracycline (19) have also been incriminated. These agents are discussed together. The use of lower doses and the avoidance of intravenous administration have made this problem less frequent. Minocycline (21) and doxycycline have rarely or not at all been associated with hepatic injury, probably because they are effective at relatively low oral doses and because these agents do not depend entirely on the kidney for their excretion.

Studies comparing doxycycline and tetracycline in rats demonstrated a significant increase in hepatic triglyceride content in tetracycline–treated rats but not in doxycycline–treated rats at comparable blood levels of both drugs (20).

156

Tetracycline

Causal relationship +

Most cases of hepatic injury were reported 15–30 years ago. Characteristically, within 10 days after starting intravenous administration of a high daily dose (> 1.5 g/d), nausea and abdominal pain were followed by lethargy, hemorrhage, hypotension, hypoglycemia and ultimately coma (1). With some exceptions (2) most of these cases ran a fatal course. Serum aminotransferase and bilirubin levels showed mostly only a moderate increase. Histology demonstrated centrilobular (3, 4) but also panlobular (3, 4) microvesicular steatosis with little or no necrosis/cholestasis or infiltration with inflammatory cells. Proximal renal tubules may also show fine fatty infiltration (4). Clinically and morphologically this pattern resembles Reye syndrome (5) and Jamaican vomiting disease (6).

Most cases have been reported in pregnant women, often treated for urinary tract disease (1–4), and these cases were indistinguishable from fatty liver of pregnancy. Several other cases, however, in non–pregnant women without renal disease (8), in children with renal disease (10) and in men (9, 11) demonstrated that every human may be afflicted. Occasionally, lower intravenous doses (12) and oral overdosage in a man with impaired renal function (13) caused hepatic damage. Recently 2 cases were ascribed to topical administration (14).

The mechanism is toxic. Human experiments in pregnant women (!) demonstrated a dose–dependent degree of steatosis (15). Testing in animals and with isolated perfused rat liver demonstrated that decreased fat egress from the hepatocyte, through a decrease in lipoprotein synthesis, was partly responsible for the steatosis (16, 17). Possibly, increased uptake of fatty acids, increased formation of triglycerides or decreased oxidation of fatty acids plays an additional role (17). Increased susceptibility in mature females was observed in mice (18) but not in rats (17). Estrogen administration seemed to aggravate hepatic injury (19), possibly also in males (11).

Moreover, the antianabolic action of tetracyclines may further impair a decreased renal function and enhance its own toxicity since the main route of excretion is via the urinary tract.

(1) Zimmerman (1978) *Hepatotoxicity,* p 468. Appleton–Century–Crofts, New York. (2) Meihoff et al (1967) *Obstet. Gynecol., 29,* 260. (3) Whalley et al (1964) *J. Am. Med. Assoc., 189,* 357. (4) Kunelis et al (1965) *Am. J. Med., 38,* 359. (5) Reye et al (1963) *Lancet, 2,* 749. (6) Tanaka (1979) In: Vinken et al (Eds), *Handbook of Clinical Neurology, Vol 37,* p 511. North Holland Publishing Company, Amsterdam. (7) Schwindt et al (1967) *Am. J. Surg., 113,* 387. (8) Peters et al (1967) *Am. J. Surg., 113,* 622. (9) Robinson et al (1970) *Am. J. Dig. Dis., 15,* 857. (10) Lloyd–Still et al (1974) *J. Pediatr., 84,* 366. (11) Winterling et al (1965) *Calif. Med., 102,* 314. (12) Rutenberg et al (1952) *N. Engl. J. Med., 247,* 797. (13) Mandel (1966) *Ohio*

State Med. J., 62, 333. (14) Wenk et al (1981) J. Reprod. Med., 26, 135. (15) Allen et al (1966) Am. J. Obstet. Gynecol., 95, 12. (16) Hansen et al (1968) Proc. Soc. Exp. Biol. Med., 128, 143. (17) Breen et al (1975) Gastroenterology, 69, 714. (18) Estler et al (1981) Dev. Pharmacol. Ther., 3, 189. (19) Böcker et al (1981) Arch. Pharmacol., 316, R22. (20) Böcker et al (1981) Arzneim.–Forsch., 31, 2118. (21) Namihisa et al (1975) Leber Magen Darm, 5, 73.

Minocycline

Causal relationship o

See 'Tetracyclines'. Clinically overt hepatic injury has been reported only rarely; 1 unspecified case showed a positive lymphocyte stimulation test (1). A case of jaundice and liver enzyme elevation was associated with minocycline (400 mg/d i.v.) (2). Histology showed diffuse steatosis.

(1) Namihisa et al (1975) Leber Magen Darm, 5, 73. (2) Burette et al (1984) Arch. Intern. Med., 144, 1491.

B.6. CHLORAMPHENICOLS

The clinical significance of chloramphenicol–induced hepatic injury has always been trivial compared with aplastic anemia. With decreasing use, hepatic injury due to these agents has become extremely rare.

Chloramphenicol

Causal relationship o/ +

Many cases have been reported as part of the chloramphenicol–hepatitis–aplastic anemia syndrome described by Hodgkinson (1). Characteristically, cholestatic jaundice preceded the symptoms (1–7) and in several cases the onset of aplasia (1, 4, 6, 7). The data, however, are scanty because many older cases are less well documented. Except in 1 case (8) with a rash, immunoallergic signs were absent. The onset was usually in 1–2 months, when the drug was already discontinued, followed directly or after some months by aplasia. With an occasional exception (8), all patients died, usually secondary to aplasia. Differentiation from viral hepatitis as the cause of aplasia may be difficult. Hodgkinson suggested modified detoxification by hepatic injury as a possible cause of aplastic anemia, but this does not explain cases of aplasia without overt hepatic injury (4, 6).

(1) Hodgkinson (1973) Med. J. Aust., 1, 939. (2) Hawkins et al (1952) Br. Med. J.,

2, 423. (3) Wolman (1952) *Br. Med. J., 2*, 426. (4) Hargraves et al (1952) *J. Am. Med. Assoc., 149*, 1293. (5) Foot et al (1963) *Br. Med. J., 1*, 403. (6) Hodgkinson (1954) *Lancet, 1*, 285. (7) Hodgkinson (1971) *Lancet, 1*, 1014. (8) Casale et al (1982) *J. Pediatr., 101*, 1025.

Thiamphenicol

Causal relationship o

One unspecified case of hepatic injury with a positive lymphocyte stimulation test has been reported (1).

(1) Namihisa et al (1975) *Leber Magen Darm, 5,* 73.

B.7. AMINOGLYCOSIDES

Hepatic injury associated with the use of aminoglycosides is incidental and scantily documented. Apparently it is not very significant in view of their widespread use for years. Their intramuscular administration may cause elevation of ASAT concentrations due to muscle damage.

Some newer aminoglycosides which have been associated with occasional liver enzyme elevations are amikacin (1), sisomicin and netilmicin (2).

(1) Keller (1984) In: Dukes (Ed), *Meyler's Side Effects of Drugs, 10th ed*, p 492. Elsevier, Amsterdam. (2) Noone et al (1984) *Drugs, 27,* 548.

Gentamicin

Causal relationship o

Liver enzyme levels and bilirubin in the serum are occasionally elevated (1). Some 33 cases of hepatic effects ascribed to the use of this drug had been reported to the U.S. Food and Drug Administration up to 1981 (2).

(1) *The Extra Pharmacopoeia, 28th ed*, Pharmaceutical Press, London, 1982. (2) *ADR Highlights, Feb. 17,* 1981.

Kanamycin

Causal relationship o

There is 1 report of 9 cases of severe bridging necrosis, 1 of which was caused by kanamycin. Recovery was uneventful. Eight cases were confirmed by rechallenge, 1 by in–vitro testing. No further details were given (1).

(1) Imoto et al (1979) *Ann. Intern. Med., 91,* 129.

Streptomycin

Causal relationship o

One unspecified case of hepatic injury has been reported in which leukocyte migration inhibition was demonstrated (1).

(1) Morizane (1978) *Gastroenterol. Jpn., 13,* 281.

Tobramycin

Causal relationship o

Hepatotoxicity (no specification) was reported in 12 of 3506 patients (1). Up to 1981, 116 suspected cases of hepatic injury by tobramycin, starting after 1–20 days of therapy, had been reported to the U.S. Food and Drug Administration (2). Some of these 'possible' cases have been described (2).

(1) Bendush et al (1977) *Med. J. Aust., 2, Suppl 3,* 22. (2) *ADR Highlights, Feb. 17,* 1981.

B.8. POLYPEPTIDES

Liver damage by polypeptides has been only rarely reported, with the exception of saramycetin.

Colistin

Causal relationship o

A case was reported of combined renal and hepatic injury starting within several days after first administration (6.5 mg/kg/d i.m.). ASAT and urea nitrogen levels returned to normal 1 week after discontinuation of the drug. Histology showed vacuolic degeneration of the epithelium of the proximal convoluted tubules in the kidney and centrilobular areas of focal necrosis in the liver (1). Kidney damage may occur in up to 20% of treated patients and is dose–dependent (2).

(1) Katz (1963) *Med. Ann. DC, 32,* 408. (2) Keller et al (1980) In: Dukes (Ed), *Meyler's Side Effects of Drugs, 9th ed,* p 452. Excerpta Medica, Amsterdam.

Saramycetin   *Causal relationship* +

Saramycetin is a parenterally administered polypeptide antibiotic which has been used in the treatment of histoplasmosis and blastomycosis. Almost every patient treated with therapeutic doses showed impairment of BSP excretion and the majority developed hyperbilirubinemia, whereas 20–40% had increased levels of ASAT and APh (1).

(1) Witorsch et al (1966) *Am. Rev. Tuberc., 93,* 876.

B.9. RIFAMYCINS

Rifamycins are excreted into the bile. These agents may cause hyperbilirubinemia, both conjugated and unconjugated, although the latter is more marked. The most important representative is rifampicin which is used mainly in tuberculosis. This agent may potentiate the hepatotoxic effect of isoniazid, probably through enzyme induction.

Rifampicin

Causal relationship +

Rifampicin may cause hyperbilirubinemia by interfering with the uptake of the unconjugated form and excretion of the conjugated (2) form, which may produce total bilirubin levels of up to 3 mg/100 ml, 3 hours after ingestion (2). BSP elimination is decreased (2).

The ability to induce cellular damage is more equivocal. Since rifampicin is used mostly in combination with isoniazid, an agent with a proven hepatotoxic potential, little is known about an injurious effect on the liver of rifampicin alone. Combination with ethambutol, however, may also cause (mostly mild and transient) signs of injury (5, 9), sometimes with allergic signs (10). Rare cases have been ascribed to rifampicin alone (4, 6, 9); challenge with rifampicin alone was positive in some cases (6, 7) but in the cases of Scheuer et al (7) isoniazid was used throughout. One of us treated a patient, who had fever, chills and liver enzyme elevations with a combined regimen of rifampicin, isoniazid and ethambutol. After normalization, treatment with rifampicin alone was followed within hours by a recurrence of all signs. Because this drug, through enzyme induction (8), seems to shorten the latent period between intake of isoniazid and onset of hepatitis (3), cases were at first ascribed to rifampicin (7). Today it is generally assumed that rifampicin enhances the risk of isoniazid–induced hepatic injury by enzyme induction with subsequently increased formation of toxic intermediate (see 'Isoniazid').

Rifampicin may precipitate porphyria cutanea tarda (1).

(1) Millar (1980) *Br. J. Dis. Chest*, *74*, 405. (2) Capelle et al (1972) *Gut*, *13*, 366. (3) Pessayre et al (1977) *Gastroenterology*, *72*, 284. (4) Rothwell et al (1974) *Br. Med. J.*, *2*, 481. (5) Blanchon et al (1973) *Poumon Coeur*, *29*, 739. (6) Nebout et al (1974) *Nouv. Presse Méd.*, *3*, 733. (7) Scheuer et al (1974) *Lancet*, *1*, 421. (8) Miguet et al (1977) *Gastroenterology*, *72*, 924. (9) Lees et al (1971) *Tubercle*, *52*, 182. (10) Grennan et al (1976) *Tubercle*, *57*, 259.

Rifamycin SV

Causal relationship +

See 'Rifampicin'. Rifamycin SV interferes with bilirubin clearance, mainly by inhibition of its excretion (1). Elevated serum transaminase levels were seen in up to 30% of patients who were treated with a combination of rifamycin SV and isoniazid (2).

(1) Acocella et al (1965) *Gastroenterology*, *49*, 526. (2) Baronti et al (1966) *Ann. Med. Sondalo*, *14*, 55.

B.10. MISCELLANEOUS ANTIBIOTICS

Some members of this group have been mentioned as a cause of hepatic injury. In addition to the drugs discussed below, others have been associated occasionally with elevation of liver enzyme concentrations, e.g. fosfomycin (1), spectinomycin and cycloserine (2). Tyrothricin, a mixture of tyrocidine and gramicidine, may cause hemolysis and renal and liver damage after parenteral administration (2). It is still in use in throat tablets, in which form it is harmless to the liver.

Aztreonam, which shows some structural resemblance to penicillins and cephalosporins and is effective against penicillinase–producing gonococci, has been associated with mild liver enzyme and bilirubin elevations in up to 20% of recipients in 1 study (3).

(1) *Chemotherapy (Tokyo)*, 1975, *23*, 1649. (2) *The Extra Pharmacopoeia, 28th ed*, p 1076. Pharmaceutical Press, London, 1982. (3) Sattler et al (1984) *Lancet, 1*, 1315.

Fusidic acid/Sodium fusidate

R = -O-CO-CH₃

Causal relationship o/ +

Jaundice occurred in 38 of 112 patients on fusidic acid compared to 2 of 101 patients on other antimicrobial agents; both groups had staphylococcal bacteremia (1). Intravenous administration was associated with a higher incidence of jaundice than oral treatment (48% and 13%, respectively). In 93%, jaundice appeared within 48 hours after first administration (1). Although hemolysis could not be excluded, at least in some cases jaundice was cholestatic. Humble (1) pointed to the structural resemblance to steroids and this is compatible with a recent case of biochemically pure, steroid–like cholestasis (4). Some additional cases of cholestatic jaundice have been reported (2, 3).

(1) Humble et al (1980) *Br. Med. J., 1*, 1495. (2) Manten (1980) In: Dukes (Ed), *Meyler's Side Effects of Drugs, Annual 4*, p 198. Excerpta Medica, Amsterdam. (3) Talbot et al (1980) *Br. Med. J., 2*, 308. (4) McAreavey et al (1983) *Scott. Med. J., 28*, 179.

Novobiocin

Causal relationship +

Novobiocin increases the serum level of unconjugated bilirubin (1), which sometimes leads to jaundice (2), particularly in neonates (3, 4). Novobiocin reduces bilirubin conjugation by inhibition of glucuronyl transferase (1), but may possibly also reduce excretion of conjugated bilirubin (5) or uptake of the unconjugated form (1). Hypersensitivity reactions

163

were reported in 12.7% of patients (6), occasionally with severe hepatic necrosis (6, 7).

Novobiocin may be used as a test in Gilbert's syndrome (8).

(1) Hargreaves et al (1963) *Nature (London), 200,* 1172. (2) Cox et al (1959) *N. Engl. J. Med., 261,* 139. (3) Sutherland et al (1961) *Am. J. Dis. Child., 101,* 447. (4) Hargreaves et al (1962) *Lancet, 1,* 839. (5) Billing et al (1965) In: *The Biliary System,* p 215. Davis, Philadelphia. (6) Bridges et al (1957) *J. Pediatr., 50,* 579. (7) Persico (1966) *Policlinico, 73,* 1607. (8) Demeulenaere et al (1982) In: *Ziekten van Lever en Galwegen.* Story–Scientia, Ghent.

C. ANTIMYCOTICS

Fungal infections are a rare cause of hepatic injury. In immunocompromised patients these infections are more frequent, especially among patients with hematological malignancies (1). Cases of hepatic involvement have been reported, caused by Candida (1) and Trichosporon (2) infections. Usually these infections cause granulomatous hepatitis and this, combined with the clinical picture and demonstration of the organism, makes it possible to differentiate from drug–induced hepatic injury. Largely the same considerations apply to coccidioidomycosis and blastomycosis.

Antimycotics may cause hepatic injury but probably not very often. Although agents like ketoconazole and flucytosine cause elevations of liver enzyme concentrations in a significant number of patients, serious hepatic injury appears to be relatively infrequent. Although the mechanism is unknown, the absence of immunoallergic signs and the frequent liver enzyme elevations suggest an intrinsic toxic effect but apparently with a wide range of susceptibility. It has been speculated that the mild liver enzyme elevations may be partly explained by a sort of Jarisch–Herxheimer reaction, secondary to the release of mycotoxins, some of which appear to be toxic (4).

An antifungal agent which has only rarely been associated with hepatic injury is amphotericin. As far as we know, only 1 case of fatal liver failure has been ascribed to this otherwise toxic agent (3).

(1) Bodey et al (1978) *Cancer, 41,* 1610. (2) Korinek et al (1983) *Gastroenterology, 85,* 732. (3) Carnecchia et al (1960) *Ann. Intern. Med., 53,* 1027. (4) Janssen et al (1983) *Am. J. Med., 74,* 80.

C.1. ANTIBIOTICS

Griseofulvin

Causal relationship o/ +

Griseofulvin–induced hepatic injury has 3 aspects. Firstly, the drug interferes with porphyrin metabolism, possibly through increased formation of δ–aminolevulinic acid synthetase (1). In some cases, griseofulvin was held responsible for a flare–up in patients with acute intermittent porphyria (2, 3), accompanied by ALAT elevation. Hepatic injury is usually absent in this disease, although BSP excretion is disturbed and non–specific changes in aminotransferase levels were reported in up to 13% of patients (4). Disturbed BSP excretion has also been ascribed to griseofulvin in cases of porphyria cutanea tarda (5), but no significant influence on porphyrin excretion was noted. Secondly, some cases/studies have been reported of griseofulvin–suspected hepatic injury (6–9). Besides disturbed BSP excretion there was transient ASAT elevation in over 50% of patients, which normalized after 4 weeks of therapy (6). Another report of 73 cases of possible griseofulvin–induced hepatitis, resulting from a German questionnaire, is difficult to interpret because of a lack of essential data (9). Two cases of cholestatic jaundice have been ascribed to the use of griseofulvin, both appearing after 1 to several months of therapy (7, 8). In one of these cases, jaundice was prolonged; normalization took 7 months (7). In the other case, facial edema caused discontinuation; however, when jaundice developed for the first time, during the second course, immunoallergic signs were absent (8). Biopsy in the latter case showed cholestasis and scattered foci of lymphocytic infiltration. Thirdly, high doses of griseofulvin can produce focal necrosis, a disturbance in porphyrin metabolism, and hepatocellular carcinoma in mice (10). In another study, oral intake of 250 mg/d in mice for 12–14 weeks caused hepatomegaly (x 2.5–8.5 increase in size compared with control mice), nodular hyperplasia, precancerous changes in hepatocytes, and 'hepatomas' (11). Although the relevance to use in man, at a much lower dose, is uncertain, prolonged use should be discouraged.

(1) Doeglas (1975) In: Dukes (Ed), *Meyler's Side Effects of Drugs, 8th ed*, p 648. Excerpta Medica, Amsterdam. (2) Redeker et al (1964) *J. Am. Med. Assoc., 188*, 466. (3) Berman et al (1968) *J. Am. Med. Assoc., 192*, 1005. (4) Demeulenaere et al (1982) *Ziekten van Lever en Galwegen*. Story–Scientia, Ghent. (5) Schlenzka et al (1971) *Dermatol. Monatsschr., 157*, 88. (6) Simon et al (1971) *Arch. Dermatol. Forsch., 241*, 148. (7) Breinstrup et al (1966) *Ugeskr. Laeg., 128*, 145. (8) Chiprut et al (1976) *Gastroenterology, 70*, 1141. (9) Götz et al (1972) *Hautarzt, 11*, 485. (10) Hurst et al (1963) *Br. J. Dermatol., 75*, 105. (11) Astahova (1983) In: Dukes (Ed), *Side Effects of Drugs, Annual 7*, p 287. Excerpta Medica, Amsterdam.

C.2. IMIDAZOLES

Econazole

Causal relationship o

An unspecified case of hepatitis after 4 months of treatment was reported during a trial in 6 persons (1).

(1) Drouhet et al (1978) *Mykosen, Suppl 1*, 192.

Clotrimazole

Causal relationship o/ +

An increase in serum bilirubin, APh and/or aminotransferase levels occurred in 5–15% of 314 patients with deep–seated mycoses and in 13 volunteers who received 60 mg/kg per day (oral) for 1 month (1).

(1) Doeglas (1975) In: Dukes (Ed), *Meyler's Side Effects of Drugs, 8th ed*, p 651. Excerpta Medica, Amsterdam.

Ketoconazole

Causal relationship +

Ketoconazole has recently been introduced as an effective oral antifungal agent. It is an imidazole derivative related to miconazole. In some trials, mostly mild liver enzyme elevations were noted sometimes in more than 10% of cases (1, 2, 13), but these were often transient despite continuation. However, several cases of moderate to very high liver enzyme elevations have been reported with symptoms consistent with hepatitis such as malaise, nausea and jaundice (3–16, 18–20). In these cases the onset was within 1–6 months after starting therapy with 200–400 mg/d. Biochemically the pattern was mainly hepatocellular (3–16, 18–20) but occasionally cholestatic (11, 16). In 1 of these cases readministration after normalization caused a relapse after 14 days (4). Also, in another case a rechallenge was positive (18). Jaundice was frequent but immunoallergic signs were absent. In some cases normalization took place despite continuation of ketoconazole (8, 13). Histology confirmed the mainly hepatocellular pattern in most patients, with necrotic areas of varying severity and mononuclear infiltration. In some cases, signs of chronic hepatitis were present (9, 10, 15), but in 1 these could be attributed to alcohol abuse (15). In a study of 33 cases from 54 reports to the U.S. Food and Drug Administration, Lewis et al (16) categorized the clinical data. There was a female preponderance. After a latent period varying from 11 to 168 days, after starting treatment with an average daily dose of 200 mg, 82% developed jaundice. This was preceded and/or accompanied by

166

gastrointestinal symptoms in up to 40%. Fever occurred in 12%, but rash or eosinophilia was absent. A hepatocellular pattern was noted in 55% and a cholestatic pattern in 15%, whereas 27% showed evidence of a mixed pattern of injury. A biopsy performed in only 3 patients showed abnormalities varying from cellular unrest to massive necrosis (16). An additional case of fatal hepatic necrosis was reported by Duarte et al (19). The manufacturer received 31 reports on 300,000 users (17), but such figures are difficult to interpret because of potential underreporting. The suggestion made by the manufacturer that preceding use of griseofulvin increases the risk of hepatotoxicity seems speculative (17). Although the mechanism is unknown, the above–mentioned data suggest metabolic idiosyncrasy. Apparently there is no dose–dependence although very high doses have induced hepatic injury in animals (16). The mild and transient liver enzyme elevations shortly after starting therapy may be explained either as an adaptive response to a mildly intrinsic hepatotoxin or as secondary to a sort of Herxheimer reaction to released mycotoxins, reflecting successful therapy (17, 21). The latter, however, is somewhat speculative.

(1) Brass et al (1980) *Rev. Infect. Dis.*, *2*, 656. (2) Hawkins et al (1981) *Ann. Intern. Med.*, *95*, 446. (3) Petersen et al (1980) *Ann. Intern. Med.*, *93*, 791. (4) Heiberg et al (1981) *Br. Med. J.*, *283*, 825. (5) Horsburgh et al (1982) *Lancet*, *1*, 860. (6) Tkach (1982) *Cutis*, *29*, 482. (7) Svejgaard et al (1982) *Ann. Intern. Med.*, *96*, 788. (8) Firebrace (1981) *Br. Med. J.*, *283*, 1058. (9) Van Dijke (1983) *Ned. Tijdschr. Geneeskd.*, *127*, 339. (10) Kramer et al (1983) *Ned. Tijdschr. Geneeskd.*, *127*, 343. (11) Boëtius et al (1983) *Ned. Tijdschr. Geneeskd.*, *127*, 341. (12) Bekkers (1983) *Ned. Tijdschr. Geneeskd.*, *127*, 1114. (13) Rollman et al (1983) *Br. J. Dermatol.*, *108*, 376. (14) Okumura et al (1983) *Gastroenterol. Jpn.*, *18*, 142. (15) Pegram et al (1983) *Arch. Intern. Med.*, *143*, 1802. (16) Lewis et al (1984) *Gastroenterology*, *86*, 503. (17) Janssen et al (1982) *Janssen Res. News*, *33*, 18. (18) Henning et al (1983) *Z. Gastroenterol.*, *21*, 709. (19) Duarte et al (1984) *Arch. Intern. Med.*, *144*, 1069. (20) Svedhem (1984) *Scand. J. Inf. Dis.*, *16*, 123. (21) Janssen et al (1983) *Am. J. Med.*, *74*, 80.

C.3. MISCELLANEOUS ANTIMYCOTICS

Flucytosine

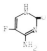

Causal relationship o/ +

As an antimetabolite (see also 'Cytostatics'), flucytosine may be a suspected hepatotoxin. Indeed, liver enzyme elevations are reported to occur in 5–10% of recipients (1, 2) and are claimed to be dose–related and reversible (2). Mostly these elevations are not accompanied by symptoms (1). Occasionally, patchy necrosis of hepatocytes was seen on biopsy (3). Two fatal cases were ascribed to the use of this drug (4). Besides a complicated clinical course which started 6–8 weeks after starting treatment with flucytosine (8 g/d) for candida endocarditis, autopsy revealed marrow aplasia and periportal and midzonal liver cell necrosis with collapse of the reticular framework.

(1) Doeglas (1978) In: Dukes (Ed), *Side Effects of Drugs, Annual 2*, p 242. Excerpta Medica, Amsterdam. (2) *The Extra Pharmacopoeia, 28th ed*, p 723. Pharmaceutical Press, London, 1982. (3) Bennett (1977) *Ann. Intern. Med., 86*, 319. (4) Record et al (1971) *Br. Med. J., 1*, 262.

D. ANTIPROTOZOAL AGENTS

Hepatic damage occurs during malaria but is minimal. Rupture of individual liver cells, liberating merozoites into the peripheral blood, does not give rise to significant functional alteration (1). One may, however, expect mild and short–lasting elevations of serum aminotransferase levels in some cases.

Antimalarials have only rarely been associated with hepatic injury. Quinine and mepacrine have caused hepatic injury as part of a hypersensitivity reaction.

Of the important protozoal infections, i.e. amebiasis, trypanosomiasis and trichomoniasis, the first two (may) cause hepatic involvement. Differentiation from drug–induced hepatic injury is usually simple unless mild to moderate liver enzyme elevations are the only sign. Drugs which have most often been incriminated of causing hepatic injury are the inorganic and organic arsenicals.

Emetine in high doses or after prolonged exposure may cause damage to the heart, liver, kidneys and skeletal muscle (2).

Of several drugs, liver enzyme elevations have occasionally been reported but, as far as we know, without severe liver damage, e.g. dehydroemetine (3), ornidazole (4), tinidazole (4), niridazole (8), melarsoprol (5) and difetarsone. In a study of the latter drug, a pentavalent arsenical, transient ASAT and/or APh elevations were noted in up to 6% of recipients (6). Suramin, an intravenously administered drug used in the early stages of *Trypanosoma rhodesiense* infections, caused a storage disease in rats treated with high doses (250–500 mg/kg). Large amounts of glycosaminoglycans accumulate in the liver, kidneys, spleen and other organs. Histology suggests lysosomal storage disease, resembling mucopolysaccharidosis (7). Although an interesting model, the problem is however of little clinical significance.

Several antiprotozoal agents may cause hyperbilirubinemia secondary to hemolysis.

(1) Marcial–Rojas et al (1982) In: Schiff et al (Eds), *Diseases of the Liver, 5th ed*, p 1165. Lippincott, Philadelphia. (2) *The Extra Pharmacopoeia, 28th ed*, p 980. Pharmaceutical Press, London, 1982. (3) Clark (1977) *Adv. Drug React. Bull. Oct.*, 232. (4) Sabchareon et al (1980) *Southeast Asian J. Trop. Med. Publ. Hlth, 11*, 282. (5) *The Extra Pharmacopoeia, 28th ed*, p 980. Pharmaceutical Press, London, 1982. (6) Keystone et al (1983) *Trans. R. Soc. Trop. Med. Hyg., 77*, 84. (7) Constantopoulos et al (1983) *Am. J. Pathol., 113*, 266. (8) Kanani et al (1970) *J. Trop. Med. Hyg., 73*, 162.

D.1. ANTIMALARIALS

Amodiaquine

Causal relationship o

Cases of hepatic injury have been described during treatment of rheumatoid arthritis (1) and systemic lupus erythematosus (2). Jaundice appeared after 10 days (2) and 4 and 16 weeks (1) in these cases, ending in hepatic failure in 1 of them (1). Reversible agranulocytosis was present in 1 patient (2). Biopsy showed zones of necrosis and lymphocytic proliferation (1) and biliary cirrhosis in the fatal case.

(1) Pomeroy et al (1959) *Arthr. Rheum., 2,* 396. (2) Perry et al (1962) *J. Am. Med. Assoc., 179,* 598.

Chloroquine

Causal relationship o

Chloroquine is not a hepatotoxin. Even in overdose it does not cause significant liver damage. It increases the urinary excretion of porphyrins. When used in high doses (0.5–1 g/d) in the treatment of porphyria cutanea tarda (PCT), it may precipitate an acute reaction with elevation of serum aminotransferases (1–3) and even centrilobular necrosis (1). But lower doses (1 g/week) were also associated with ASAT elevations in these patients (1). Some concern about a possible hepatotoxic effect during such treatment was expressed by some authors (2, 3, 5). However, a study by Chlumska et al (4) with a low dose (250 mg/wk) suggested a decrease in the incidence of aminotransferase elevations without morphological changes during treatment. Cainelli et al (5) compared hydroxychloroquine (400 mg/wk) with phlebotomy for PCT. Although clinical and biochemical signs improved, 40% on the drug and 23% after phlebotomy showed an increase in the extent of necrosis, inflammation and fibrosis. The authors expressed their concern about a possible aggravation of underlying liver disease by the drug.

(1) Taljaard et al (1972) *Br. J. Dermatol., 87,* 261. (2) Cripps et al (1962) *Arch. Dermatol., 5,* 575. (3) Sweeney et al (1965) *Br. Med. J., 1,* 1281. (4) Chlumska et al (1980) *Br. J. Dermatol., 102,* 261. (5) Cainelli et al (1983) *Br. J. Dermatol., 108,* 593.

169

Mepacrine

Causal relationship +

Agress (1) described 5 cases of combined toxic epidermal necrolysis and hepatic injury. Onset was within 1 month after starting treatment, with jaundice, fever, lymphadenopathy, rash, leukocytosis and eosinophilia. In 2 of them a rechallenge was positive. Patch tests were positive in most cases. Histology showed mainly hepatocellular necrosis. Unspecified cases of hepatitis and skin disorders with a 100% fatality rate were mentioned by another author (2).

(1) Agress (1946) *J. Am. Med. Assoc., 131,* 14. (2) Livingood et al (1945) *J. Am. Med. Assoc., 129,* 1091.

Pyrimethamine

Causal relationship o

Some cases of hepatic injury were associated with the antimalarial combination pyrimethamine + sulfadoxine (see 'Sulfonamides'). These reactions are usually ascribed to the sulfa–component. Pyrimethamine, which is largely without side effects, was suspected of causing liver dysfunction in 2 of 7 psoriatic patients treated with a high dose (1).

(1) Dibella et al (1977) *Arch. Dermatol., 113,* 172.

Quinine

Causal relationship +

Granulomatous hepatitis of moderate severity was reported in 1 case, with fever, polyarthralgia and gastrointestinal symptoms. There were several episodes due to irregular use. Biopsy showed diffuse fatty change and scattered intralobular microgranulomas composed of histiocytes and some eosinophils (1). The diagnosis of granulomatous hepatitis was however questioned in this case (2).

Rechallenge was positive within 48 hours (1). Quinine may be expected to cause the same pattern of injury, with the same frequency as its isomer, quinidine; the reaction is probably immunoallergic.

(1) Katz et al (1983) *Br. Med. J., 286,* 264. (2) Nirodi (1983) *Br. Med. J., 286,* 647.

170

D.2. MISCELLANEOUS ANTIPROTOZOAL AGENTS

Arsphenamine

Causal relationship +

Formerly used in the treatment of syphylis, arsphenamine is now mainly of historical interest. However, it is worth noting because the pattern of drug–induced intrahepatic cholestasis through an immunoallergic mechanism was first postulated by Hanger and Gutman on the basis of arsphenamine–induced jaundice (1). Characteristically, gastrointestinal symptoms and/or immunoallergic symptoms (rash, fever, Quincke's edema) developed after the 2nd or 3rd injection, followed after several days by jaundice of the 'obstructive type' without extrahepatic obstruction. Parenchymal degeneration was absent or mild (1). A mainly hepatocellular pattern, however, may also be produced by this agent (1).

(1) Hanger et al (1940) *J. Am. Med. Assoc., 115, 263.*

Carbarsone

Causal relationship o/ +

Cases with a predominantly hepatocellular (1, 2) and a cholestatic (2–4) pattern of injury within 1 month after starting therapy have been described. There was concurrent exfoliative dermatitis (1) and central nervous system involvement (3, 4), the latter suggesting too high a dose. Biopsy showed hepatocellular steatosis and necrosis (1) and cholestasis (2–4) resembling immunoallergic arsphenamine cholestasis. Contamination with arsanilic acid, was possibly the causative factor (3). According to Epstein et al (1), cases of jaundice and exfoliative dermatitis had also been reported during use of acetarsol, a structurally related organic arsenical.

(1) Epstein (1936) *J. Am. Med. Assoc., 106,* 769. (2) Nelson (1956) *J. Am. Med. Assoc., 160,* 764. (3) Radke et al (1957) *Ann. Intern. Med., 47,* 418. (4) Schwartz et al (1965) *J. Am. Med. Assoc., 191,* 678.

Furazolidone

Causal relationship +

Furazolidone structurally resembles nitrofurantoin. The drug has been

171

used in several types of intestinal infection. It has a disulfiram–like effect in alcohol users and may precipitate (hemolytic) jaundice in patients with glucose–6–phosphate dehydrogenase deficiency. Occasionally, hepatic injury follows the use of the drug. In 1 such case with mild cholestatic hepatitis, fever and eosinophilia, a prompt reaction to rechallenge suggested an immunoallergic mechanism (1). On the other hand, possible conversion to hydrazines in rats (2) may favor a mechanism analogous to that of iproniazid hepatotoxicity.

A peculiar case concerns a patient with nitrofurantoin–associated rash and cholestatic hepatitis who experienced an exacerbation of the symptoms after intravaginal administration of furazolidone (3), which suggests cross–reactivity in some cases. Although the drug is hardly absorbed from the gastrointestinal tract, even a small percentage is apparently sufficient to produce hepatic injury; erosions probably enhance absorption.

(1) Löwenberg (1970) *Ned. Tijdschr. Geneeskd., 114,* 1404. (2) Stern et al (1967) *J. Pharmacol. Exp. Ther., 156,* 492. (3) Engel et al (1975) *Arch. Intern. Med., 135,* 733.

Hydroxystilbamidine

Causal relationship o

Hydroxystilbamidine has both antifungal and antiprotozoal properties. It has been claimed to be less toxic than stilbamidine (1). It is used mainly in blastomycosis and leishmaniasis. Cases of hepatic injury have been described (1, 2). One of these concerned a child showing features of Reye's syndrome with apathy, convulsions and subsequent death after 1 month of therapy. Autopsy showed microvesicular steatosis of liver cells and proximal tubules and cerebral edema (1).

(1) Oberman et al (1958) *Ann. Intern. Med., 48,* 1401. (2) Bennett (1974) *N. Engl. J. Med., 290,* 320.

Metronidazole

Causal relationship o

Animal toxicity tests revealed histological liver changes in monkeys treated with 45–240 mg/kg/d (1). Human use at therapeutic doses seems largely free of hepatic involvement, but a few cases have been reported. In 1 case severe ASAT/ALAT elevations occurred within several days after treatment with metronidazole (2 g/24 h i.v.). This patient, however, had been treated with several drugs and had been operated upon shortly before (2). In another case the intake of 1 tablet daily was followed by fever and chills after 4 days with subsequent jaundice after 9 days. Laboratory data suggested cholestatic hepatitis (3).

In vulnerable persons metronidazole causes a disulfiram–like effect if taken in combination with alcohol.

(1) Nir (1980) In: Dukes (Ed), *Side Effects of Drugs, Annual 4*, p 204. Excerpta Medica, Amsterdam. (2) Appleby et al (1983) *Clin. Pharmacol. Ther.*, *2*, 373. (3) Fagin (1965) *J. Am. Med. Assoc.*, *193*, 1128.

Pentamidine

H_2N-C ⟨⟩ $-O-(CH_2)_5-O-$ ⟨⟩ $-C-NH_2$
 HN   NH

Causal relationship o/ +

ASAT elevations have been seen in some studies in up to 7% of cases, but may have been caused partly by intramuscular administration (1, 2). In 1 patient with leishmaniasis, liver enzyme elevations disappeared after discontinuation and reappeared on rechallenge (3). In a study of 38 patients with acquired immunodeficiency syndrome (AIDS), pentamidine was associated with a higher incidence (30%) of liver enzyme elevations than cotrimoxazole, both administered for pneumocystosis. However, with cotrimoxazole, these were more severe. The high incidence in both groups is probably partly explained by underlying viral infections (4); it has been suggested that AIDS patients have a higher incidence of adverse effects than other patient populations.

(1) Waalkes et al (1970) *Clin. Pharmacol. Ther.*, *11*, 505. (2) Western et al (1970) *Ann. Intern. Med.*, *73*, 695. (3) Lichey et al (1979) *Münch. Med. Wochenschr.*, *121*, 665. (4) Gordin et al (1984) *Ann. Intern. Med.*, *100*, 495.

Stilbamidine

H_2N-C ⟨⟩ $-HC=CH-$ ⟨⟩ $-C-NH_2$
 HN   NH

Causal relationship o

Stilbamidine has been used in trypanosomiasis and kala azar (leishmaniasis) but has largely been abandoned because of its neurotoxicity. Some cases of liver cell necrosis with hepatic failure, appearing 1–3 months after completion of therapy, were attributed to the drug (1). In these cases the reaction was ascribed partly to the use of older preparations which contained large amounts of toxic degradation products. Steatosis was seen after administration to animals (1).

(1) Kirk et al (1944) *Ann. Trop. Med.*, *38*, 99.

Tryparsamide

$$HO-\overset{\overset{\displaystyle O}{\|}}{As}-ONa$$

NH-CH$_2$-CO-NH$_2$

Causal relationship o/ +

Tryparsamide is an organic arsenical used in trypanosomiasis with central nervous system involvement. Because of its oculotoxicity it has largely been abandoned in favor of melarsoprol. It is still used, however, in combination with suramin for late *Trypanosoma gambiense* infection (1). Cases of liver damage, varying from mild injury to severe fatal hepatic necrosis, have been observed with therapeutic doses; in some cases the pattern is mainly cholestatic (2). In animal toxicity tests, massive doses of both organic and inorganic arsenicals produce acute liver necrosis (3) which suggests dose–dependent and intrinsic toxicity. On the other hand, low intermittent doses of these agents may cause an immunoallergic type of hepatic injury (see 'Arsphenamide').

(1) *The Extra Pharmacopoeia, 28th ed.* Pharmaceutical Press, London, 1982. (2) Harvey (1975) *The Pharmacological Basis of Therapeutics, 5th ed,* p 924. Macmillan, New York. (3) Klatskin (1975) In: Schiff (Ed), *Diseases of the Liver, 4th ed,* p 604. Lippincott, Philadelphia.

E. ANTIVIRAL AGENTS

Hepatic injury may be caused by several of the viruses for which these drugs are administered. This complicates the assessment of a causal relationship in cases of suspected drug–induced hepatic injury.

Some of these agents have been used in the treatment of acute or chronic viral hepatitis but without much success.

Since several antiviral agents have cytostatic properties, also for human cells, hepatic injury is not completely unexpected. Nevertheless, most agents seem remarkably free from hepatotoxicity and hepatic injury has mostly been limited to mild liver enzyme elevations.

Interferon may induce fever, shivering, malaise and pain and erythema at the site of injection. Serum aminotransferase levels may be mildly elevated but occasionally necessitate discontinuation of therapy (1). It is not clear whether these reactions are caused by interferon or by contaminating proteins (2).

Intravenous administration of aciclovir (3) and vidarabine (4) have been associated with elevation of serum aminotransferase levels, with the latter in up to 17%.

Ribavirin (1 g/d for 5 days) has caused hyperbilirubinemia in almost one–third of recipients (5).

174

(1) Sherwin et al (1982) *J. Am. Med. Assoc., 248*, 2461. (2) *The Extra Pharmaco-poeia, 28th ed*, p 822. Pharmaceutical Press, London, 1982. (3) Richards et al (1983) *Drugs, 26*, 378. (4) Whitley et al (1981) *N. Engl. J. Med., 304*, 313. (5) Magnusson et al (1977) *Antimicrob. Agents Chemother., 12*, 493.

Idoxuridine

Causal relationship o

Pure cholestasis was found in a man treated with 30 g for 8 days (1). In another case there was APh and bilirubin elevation 13 days after starting treatment (2). One study showed ALAT/ASAT or APh elevation in 5 of 8 patients treated with 100 mg/kg/d (3); however, all were being treated for systemic herpes simplex, a possible cause of hepatic injury. Bone marrow depression seems a far more serious consequence of this antiviral inhibitor of DNA synthesis.

(1) Dayan et al (1969) *Lancet, 2*, 1073. (2) Silk et al (1970) *Lancet, 1*, 411. (3) Boston Interhospital Virus Study Group and the NIAID–Sponsored Cooperative Antiviral Clinical Study (1975) *N. Engl. J. Med., 292*, 599.

Isothiazole thiosemicarbazone (see also thioacetazone)

Causal relationship o/ +

In a study of 147 patients with smallpox 18 became jaundiced (1). Only unconjugated bilirubin was elevated without signs of hemolysis or liver damage. The authors suggested that the drug interferes with the conjugation process in the hepatocyte. The drug is structurally related to thioacetazone.

(1) Rao et al (1965) *Ann. NY Acad. Sci., 130*, 118.

Xenazoic acid

Causal relationship o

Intrahepatic cholestasis has been observed during or subsequent to treatment with this antiviral agent (1, 2). Jaundice appeared after 5–16 days (1, 2), accompanied by fever (1, 2), rash (1) and eosinophilia (1); histology showed cholestatic hepatitis. However, in 1 case there was viral hepatitis in the neighborhood (2). Recovery took several months (1).

(1) Hecht et al (1965) *Arch. Mal. Appar. Dig., 54,* 615. (2) Herbeuval et al (1966) *Thérapie, 21,* 781.

F. ANTILEPROTIC AGENTS

Lepromatous leprosy may cause multiple small sinusoidal granulomas (1), but these can be easily differentiated from occasional dapsone–induced liver granulomas by their pattern and by the demonstration of acid–fast micro–organisms.

(1) Edmondson et al (1982) In: Schiff et al (Eds), *Diseases of the Liver, 5th ed,* p 303. Lippincott, Philadelphia.

Dapsone

$$H_2N-\langle\rangle-SO_2-\langle\rangle-NH_2$$

Causal relationship +

Dapsone is used against leprosy and herpetiform dermatitis. It is also used in combination regimens against malaria. As a sulfone, it is chemically related to the sulfonamides. Rarely dapsone may cause severe hypoalbuminemia with ascites and cardiac failure, after several years of treatment (3, 10). The drug may cause jaundice by hemolysis or secondary to hepatic injury. The latter occurs largely as part of the 'dapsone syndrome', a generalized hypersensitivity reaction with fever, exfoliative dermatitis, lymphadenopathy, methemoglobinemia, anemia and jaundice with hepatocellular damage (1, 2, 6–8). Although these signs are not invariably present, they often occur in combination and the reaction may resemble infectious mononucleosis. The blood picture may show atypical lymphocytes and eosinophilia. One patient had an allergic reaction to sulfapyridine (4). The pattern is not entirely hepatocellular; mostly cholestasis is also present and seems to predominate in some cases (5). The onset is usually in the first weeks of treatment. Histology, in a few cases, showed focal or more extensive necrosis (2) and granulomatous hepatitis (8). The syndrome is claimed to be less severe if therapy has been started with less than 100 mg/d, but it has appeared even with low doses given for a short period (6). However, according to Frey et al (7), the 'dapsone syndrome' became rare after a change to a dose regimen of 25 mg/wk, gradually increasing to 100 mg/d. Malnourished patients are more likely to develop the reaction (2). Despite the fact that a dose–dependent effect was suspected, the reaction is probably immunoallergic. Successful desensitization has been performed by Browne (9).

(1) Allday et al (1951) *Lancet, 2,* 205. (2) Jellife (1951) *Lancet, 1,* 1343. (3) Kingham

176

et al (1979) *Lancet, 2,* 662. (4) Millikan et al (1970) *Arch. Dermatol., 102,* 220. (5) Stone et al (1978) *Arch. Dermatol., 114,* 947. (6) Tomecki et al (1981) *Arch. Dermatol., 117,* 38. (7) Frey et al (1981) *Ann. Intern. Med., 94,* 777. (8) Kromann et al (1982) *Arch. Dermatol., 118,* 531. (9) Browne (1963) *Br. Med. J., 2,* 664. (10) Foster et al (1981) *Lancet, 2,* 806.

G. SULFONAMIDES

All sulfonamides are analogs of p–aminobenzoic acid. Formerly used for various infectious disorders, the employment of sulfonamides as mono-therapy is now mainly restricted to certain protozoal and urinary tract infections. However, they are often used in combination with trimetho-prim and pyrimethamine. Related generic drugs are the sulfonylureas, thiazides and carbonic anhydrase inhibitors. Sulfonamides consist of a large group of compounds with a wide range of absorption and excretion. Most of the older long–acting sulfonamides are now used infrequently.

Although animal toxicity tests have suggested that high doses have a hepatotoxic effect, the clinical features, low frequency and appearance in human subjects at a normal or even low–normal dose suggests an idio-syncratic reaction of the immunoallergic type. However, in cases with a serum–sickness–like pattern, one cannot completely discard the possi-bility of a dose–dependent effect.

Hepatic injury to combination products (e.g. co–trimoxazole) or com-pounds (e.g. sulfasalazine) are usually ascribed to the sulfa–moiety. How-ever, we know 1 case of a generalized hypersensitivity reaction with mo-derate ASAT/ALAT elevations to sulfasalazine, confirmed by a positive reaction to inadvertent readministration. Subsequent treatment with sulfapyridine and 5–aminosalicylic acid remained without a reaction, suggesting that the whole compound may have been responsible instead of the sulfa–moiety.

Sulfonamides may cause hyperbilirubinemia without hepatic injury by hemolysis in vulnerable persons (e.g. glucose–6–phosphate dehydrogen-ase deficiency).

G.1. INDIVIDUAL AGENTS

Causal relationship + +

Mainly a hepatocellular to mixed pattern of injury is observed (1), al-though a cholestatic pattern has been described several times recently (2–5, 15). In a review of 106 cases of sulfonamide–associated hepatic inju-ry from the literature, Dujovne et al (1) found fever in 25 cases; rash was found in 22 cases and eosinophilia in 7 of 29 patients in whom counts were done. In 36 of the 106 cases, hepatic injury developed within 4 weeks, especially after intraperitoneal administration (1). The case-fatality rate was estimated at more than 10% (1) but may be partly ascrib-ed to concurrent agranulocytosis (19), aplastic anemia (22) or other concurrent organ involvement. More recent cases were also reported to be accompanied by rash/Stevens–Johnson syndrome (4, 10, 12–14, 16, 26), eosinophilia (12, 16, 26) and fever (3–5, 10, 13, 16, 26), sometimes as part of a multisystem reaction (13, 16). The reaction may resemble serum sickness. Hepatic injury started within 6 weeks of therapy (2–5, 9–16, 26) except for 1 case (9). Rechallenge was positive in 2 days (1, 3, 6–8) or 1–2 weeks (9). Fries et al (6) demonstrated cross–sensitivity between sulfamethoxazole and sulfisoxazole in 1 case. A fatal course was observed in 3 cases (11, 13, 14). In 1 case of chronic active hepatitis, discontinuation resulted in recovery (8). Biopsy shows a picture varying from massive (1, 11, 14, 18) to diffuse focal (1, 9, 12) necrosis. There is bile accumulation with no (3, 4) or little (2, 5, 15) cellular degeneration/necrosis. Liver granulomas (10, 17, 18), chronic active hepatitis (8), mild fibrosis (9) and eosinophilic infiltration have been reported (1, 9, 10).

Some textbooks estimate the incidence of hepatic injury at 0.6% of recipients for sulfanilamide and less for other compounds (20, 21) but we do not believe that the available data from the medical literature permit such a conclusion about a different incidence for the individual agents since too many factors remain unknown. Although animal toxicity tests have demonstrated a hepatotoxic effect of sulfonamides (23, 24), the mechanism in the clinically overt cases seems to be immunoallergic. The lymphocyte stimulation test, reported in some cases, was positive (25).

See also individual compounds for references.

(1) Dujovne et al (1967) *N. Engl. J. Med.*, 277, 785. (2) Coto et al (1981) *South. Med. J.*, 74, 887. (3) Steinbrecher et al (1981) *Dig. Dis. Sci.*, 26, 756. (4) Ghishan (1983) *Clin. Pediatr.*, 22, 212. (5) Magee et al (1982) *Dig. Dis. Sci.*, 27, 1044. (6) Fries et al (1966) *N. Engl. J. Med.*, 274, 95. (7) Rammelkamp (1948) *Blood, 3*, 1411. (8) Tönder et al (1974) *Scand. J. Gastroenterol.*, 9, 93. (9) Iwarson et al (1979) *Acta Med. Scand.*, 206, 219. (10) Espiritu et al (1967) *J. Am. Med. Assoc.*, 202, 161. (11) Colucci et al (1975) *J. Am. Med. Assoc.*, 233, 952. (12) Shaw (1970) *Johns Hopkins Med. J.*, *126*, 130. (13) Brøckner et al (1978) *Lancet, 1*, 831. (14) Caravati et al (1971) *Dig. Dis. Sci.*, *16*, 803. (15) Nair et al (1980) *Ann. Intern. Med.*, *92*, 511. (16) Knudsen et al (1977) *Ugeskr. Laeg.*, *139*, 1007. (17) Hartroft (1944) *Can. Med. Assoc. J.*, *51*, 23. (18) More et al (1946) *Am. J. Pathol.*, *22*, 703. (19) Ziegler et al (1945) *N. Engl. J. Med.*, *233*, 59. (20) Klatskin (1975) In: Schiff (Ed), *Diseases of the Liver, 4th ed*, p 604. Lippincott, Philadelphia. (21) Zimmerman (1978) *Hepatotoxicity*, p 481. Appleton–Century–Crofts, New York. (22) Denny et al (1946) *Am. J. Med. Sci.*, *211*, 659. (23) Machella et al (1941) *Proc. Soc. Mayo Clin.*, *16*, 174. (24) Streicher (1945) *Am. J. Dig. Dis.*, *12*, 267. (25) Namihisa (1975) *Leber Magen Darm, 5*, 73. (26) Vestergaard Olsen et al (1982) *Lancet, 2*, 994.

Sulfadiazine

See 'Sulfonamides'.

(1) Herbut et al (1945) *Arch. Pathol.*, *40*, 94. (2) Ziegler et al (1945) *N. Engl. J.*

Med., *233*, 59. (3) Ducci et al (1946) *Rev. Med. Chile*, *74*, 55. (4) Hoffman (1955) *Gastroenterology*, *29*, 247.

Sulfadimethoxine

See 'Sulfonamides'.

(1) Esperitu et al (1967) *J. Am. Med. Assoc.*, *202*, 985.

Sulfadoxine

See 'Sulfonamides'. A drug–safety monitoring group analyzed 137 adverse reactions to the combination agent pyrimethamine/sulfadoxine, reported during 10 years (2); 24 cases concerned reactions of the liver and biliary system but remained unspecified.

Cases of Lyell (1) and Stevens–Johnson syndrome (3), accompanied by eosinophilia and jaundice (1, 4) or mildly elevated liver enzymes (3), have been reported, but 1 of these twice (1, 4). Usually sulfadoxine is held responsible for such reactions; a troublesome factor is the long half–life (blood, 4–8 days) which may be dangerous in patients with a severe hypersensitivity reaction.

(1) Vestergaard Olsen et al (1982) *Lancet*, *2*, 994. (2) Koch–Weser et al (1982) *Lancet*, *2*, 1459. (3) Ligthelm et al (1983) *Ned. T. Geneeskd.*, *127*, 1735. (4) Christensen et al (1983) *Ugeskr. Laeg.*, *145*, 245.

Sulfamethizole

See 'Sulfonamides'.

(1) Namihisa (1975) *Leber Magen Darm*, *5*, 73. (2) Iwarson et al (1979) *Acta Med. Scand.*, *206*, 219. (3) Tönder et al (1974) *Scand. J. Gastroenterol.*, *9*, 93.

Sulfamethoxazole

See 'Sulfonamides' and 'Cotrimoxazole'.

(1) Case records of the Massachusetts General Hospital (1965) *N. Engl. J. Med.*,

273, 440. (2) Fries et al (1966) *N. Engl. J. Med.*, *274*, 95. (3) Macoul (1966) *N. Engl. J. Med.*, *275*, 39. (4) Dujovne et al (1967) *N. Engl. J. Med.*, *277*, 785. (5) Caravati et al (1971) *Dig. Dis. Sci.*, *16*, 803. (6) Steinbrecher et al (1981) *Dig. Dis. Sci.*, *26*, 756. (7) Shaw et al (1970) *Johns Hopkins Med. J.*, *126*, 130. (8) Ghishan (1983) *Clin. Pediatr.*, *22*, 212. (9) Knudsen et al (1977) *Ugeskr. Laeg.*, *139*, 1007. (10) Namihisa (1975) *Leber Magen Darm*, *5*, 73.

Sulfamethoxypyridazine

See 'Sulfonamides'.

(1) Hershfield et al (1958) *NY State J. Med.*, *58*, 1508. (2) Stocchi et al (1962) *Clin. Ter.*, *22*, 925. (3) Tisdale (1958) *N. Engl. J. Med.*, *258*, 687. (4) Iwarson et al (1979) *Acta Med. Scand.*, *206*, 219. (5) Tönder et al (1974) *Scand. J. Gastroenterol.*, *9*, 93.

Sulfanilamide

See 'Sulfonamides'. One case of hepatic injury ascribed to sulfanilamide ointment has been reported (12).

(1) Hageman et al (1937) *J. Am. Med. Assoc.*, *109*, 642. (2) Saphirstein (1938) *Urol. Cutan. Rev.*, *42*, 101. (3) Bannick et al (1938) *J. Am. Med. Assoc.*, *111*, 770. (4) Garvin (1938) *J. Am. Med. Assoc.*, *111*, 2283. (5) Cline (1938) *J. Am. Med. Assoc.*, *111*, 2384. (6) Fitzgibbon et al (1939) *Calif. West. Med.*, *50*, 123. (7) Long (1938) *Ohio State Med. J.*, *34*, 977. (8) Watson et al (1940) *Arch. Intern. Med.*, *65*, 825. (9) Russell (1940) *Ann. Intern. Med.*, *14*, 168. (10) Berger et al (1941) *J. Lab. Clin. Med.*, *26*, 785. (11) Roche et al (1943) *J. Fl. Med. Assoc.*, *30*, 196. (12) Magee et al (1982) *Dig. Dis. Sci.*, *27*, 1044.

Sulfapyridine

See 'Sulfonamides' and 'Sulfasalazine'.

(1) More et al (1946) *Am. J. Pathol.*, *22*, 703. (2) Singh (1942) *Indian Med. Gaz.*, *77*, 96. (3) Han et al (1969) *N. Engl. J. Med.*, *280*, 547.

Sulfasuxidine

See 'Sulfonamides'.

(1) More et al (1946) *Am. J. Pathol.*, *22*, 703.

Sulfathalidine

See 'Sulfonamides'.

(1) Dykes et al (1965) *J. Am. Med. Assoc., 193,* 339.

Sulfathiazole

See 'Sulfonamides'.

(1) Simon et al (1943) *Can. Med. Assoc. J., 48,* 23. (2) Gotschalk (1945) *Hawai Med. J., 4,* 185. (3) Krusius (1947) *Ann. Med. Intern. Fenn., 36,* 83. (4) Rammelkamp (1948) *Blood, 3,* 1411. (5) More et al (1946) *Am. J. Pathol., 22,* 703.

Sulfisoxazole

See 'Sulfonamides'.

(1) Rodgers et al (1964) *Arch. Intern. Med., 114,* 637. (2) Case Records of the Massachusetts General Hospital (1965) *N. Engl. J. Med., 272,* 254. (3) Dykes et al (1965) *J. Am. Med. Assoc., 193,* 339. (4) Fries et al (1966) *N. Engl. J. Med., 274,* 95. (5) Shaw (1970) *Johns Hopkins Med. J., 126,* 130.

G.2. COMBINATION PRODUCTS

Cotrimoxazole

Combination product of sulfamethoxazole and trimethoprim (5:1)

See 'Sulfonamides' and 'Sulfamethoxazole'. Although unproven, most cases of cotrimoxazole–induced hepatitis (1–6) have been ascribed to the sulfa–compound instead of to trimethoprim. No conclusive cases of hepatic injury caused by the latter have so far been described. A high incidence of liver enzyme elevations, often severe, and of other adverse effects was noted in a study in AIDS patients who had received high doses for pneumocystosis (8). Although concurrent viral infections could alone have been responsible, the increased overall incidence of side effects suggested an additive effect.

(1) Coto et al (1981) *South. Med. J., 74,* 887. (2) Ghishan (1983) *Clin. Pediatr., 22,* 212. (3) Colucci et al (1975) *J. Am. Med. Assoc., 233,* 952. (4) Brøckner et al (1978) *Lancet, 1,* 831. (5) Knudsen et al (1977) *Ugeskr. Laeg., 139,* 1007. (6) Nair et al

(1980) *Ann. Intern. Med.*, *92*, 512. (7) Kossow (1981) *Mil. Med.*, *149*, 80. (8) Gordin et al (1984) *Ann. Intern. Med.*, *92*, 512.

Salazosulfapyridine (sulfasalazine)

Causal relationship +

Since the first description of sulfasalazine–associated hepatic injury in 1967, approximately 18 cases have been published (1–17). Most cases showed the same features of a generalized hypersensitivity reaction with rash, fever, lymphadenopathy, leukocytosis with atypical lymphocytes, and eosinophilia as the most common signs. Less frequent but more serious were a decrease in renal function (1, 5, 9), beginning pulmonary fibrosis (14) and thrombocytopenia (7). The onset was usually within 2 months after starting therapy with a dose varying from 2 to 6 g/d. In 3 patients the reaction was fatal (1, 2, 14). A rechallenge in 6 patients was positive with recurrence of all abnormalities within 1–3 days (7, 11, 12, 15, 16). Liver biopsies performed in some of these patients showed focal (5, 11) or moderate to massive (9, 14), predominantly centrilobular liver cell necrosis. Fibrotic changes were present in 2 cases (9, 15). Infiltration was mainly mononuclear, although eosinophils predominated in 1 case (5). A skin biopsy in some patients showed vasculitis (8, 12, 14). In some patients non–caseating granulomas were present (3, 4, 13, 17). Most of the above–mentioned cases demonstrated the same type of hypersensitivity reaction. A latent period of several weeks, the accelerated reaction to rechallenge, the hypersensitivity symptoms, the low incidence and the dose independence are consistent with an immunoallergic mechanism. Circulating immune complexes were demonstrated in 2 cases (8, 14) but were absent in 2 other patients (12, 15). A lymphocyte stimulation test to sulfasalazine was positive in 1 case (14) but negative in 2 other cases (8, 12). Testing of sulfasalazine alone is of limited value since this compound is split in the colon into 5–aminosalicylic acid and sulfapyridine. The latter moiety is held responsible for most of the adverse effects of sulfasalazine. One of our cases demonstrated the hypersensitivity reaction to sulfasalazine, which was proven by an immediate relapse after inadvertent re–administration. Treatment with sulfapyridine and 5–aminosalicylic acid per rectum was uneventful, which suggests that in some cases the whole molecule is responsible for the hypersensitivity reaction.

(1) Randall (1967) *Ann. Intern. Med.*, *66*, 1052. (2) Caravatti et al (1971) *Am. J. Dig. Dis.*, *16*, 803. (3) Rafoth (1974) *Dig. Dis.*, *19*, 465. (4) Callen et al (1978) *South. Med. J.*, *71*, 1159. (5) Chester et al (1978) *Arch. Intern. Med.*, *138*, 1138. (6) Jacobs et al (1978) *Gastroenterology*, *75*, 1193. (7) Kanner et al (1978) *Dig. Dis.*, *23*, 956. (8) Mihas et al (1978) *J. Am. Med. Assoc.*, *239*, 2590. (9) Sotolongo et al (1978) *Gastroenterology*, *75*, 95. (10) Zimmerman (1978) *Hepatotoxicity, 1st ed*, p 481. Appleton–Century–Crofts, New York. (11) Gulley et al (1979) *Am. J. Gastroenterol.*, *72*, 561. (12) Losek et al (1981) *Am. J. Dis. Child.*, *135*, 1070. (13) Namias et al (1981)

J. Clin. Gastroenterol., *3*, 193. (14) Larcan et al (1982) *Thérapie*, *37*, 315. (15) Smith et al (1982) *Aust. NZ J. Med.*, *12*, 76. (16) Lennard et al (1983) *Br. Med. J.*, *287*, 96. (17) Fich et al (1984) *Am. J. Gastroenterol.*, *79*, 401.

H. ANTITUBERCULOUS AGENTS

Tuberculosis may cause granulomas in the liver through miliary dissemination. These may be differentiated from drug–induced granulomas by the demonstration of caseating necrosis, acid–fast staining or culture of an unfixed portion of the biopsy. Tuberculosis, however, is seen relatively often in patients with other infectious diseases which may injure the liver or in severe immunocompromised patients. Of course, these causes should be excluded before a diagnosis of 'tuberculostatic–induced hepatic injury' is made.

There is convincing evidence from several clinical studies that antituberculous regimens are potentially harmful to the liver. Since they are often administered in combination regimens, it is usually difficult to incriminate one agent in particular.

It is impossible to compare the incidence of hepatic injury produced by the different individual agents. With the exception of isoniazid prophylactic studies, data on monotherapy with other agents are either lacking or are derived from uncontrolled studies during the early years of tuberculosis therapy. Nevertheless, it is beyond reasonable doubt that some drugs (e.g. isoniazid or pyrazinamide) are more hepatotoxic than others (e.g. ethambutol).

It appears from the literature that isoniazid, pyrazinamide, ethionamide and thioacetazone cause the highest incidence of hepatic injury which made several of these agents second–choice drugs in the treatment of tuberculosis. With the exception of the latter these agents are more or less related to nicotinamide and nicotinic acid.

Other agents have occasionally been associated with mild liver enzyme elevations (e.g. capreomycin and cycloserine) (1).

(1) *The Extra Pharmacopoeia, 28th ed*, p 1564. Pharmaceutical Press, London, 1982.

p–Aminosalicylic acid (PAS)

Causal relationship + +

Simpson et al (1) presented data of 277 recorded cases (including their own observations and literature cases) with a hypersensitivity reaction to PAS (1) (see Table 1). Hepatic involvement was reported in a significant number, with jaundice in 23%. Besides rash, fever and eosinophilia

TABLE 1 *Features of 277 cases of PAS-induced hypersensitivity (1)*

Total number	277
Fever	271
Skin rash	199
Lymphadenopathy	58
Jaundice	64
Hepatomegaly	72
Leukocytosis	94
Eosinophilia	84
Abnormal lymphocytes	57
Abnormal hepatic function	81
Sensitivity to streptomycin	30
Sensitivity to isoniazid	13
Desensitized	93
Death	11

which often accompanied hepatic injury, less common features were Löffler's syndrome, renal impairment and blood disorders (1). The onset was usually within 2–6 weeks after starting treatment, rarely later but occasionally earlier. This hypersensitivity reaction was reported in up to 5% of recipients (1) and, in cases accompanied by lymphadenopathy, hepatosplenomegaly and atypical lymphocytes, resembled a serum sickness syndrome (1, 6, 11).

The pattern of hepatic injury has been variably reported as hepatocellular, often fatal (2, 3, 10), or cholestatic (7, 8) but mixed patterns also occur (1). A rechallenge, often during desensitization, was positive in several cases (4, 5, 7). Both patch testing (1, 5) and a lymphocyte stimulation test have been positive (9).

In cases where a biopsy or autopsy was performed, histology showed varying degrees of necrosis, either mild or absent with bile stasis, or massive (2, 3, 10).

Obviously PAS produces a different clinical pattern from that of the other salicylates. Sodium–PAS causes identical reactions. A curious fact is that several patients were also reported to be hypersensitive to streptomycin or isoniazid. Since cross–sensitivity is unlikely, considering the lack of structural similarity, this suggests an immunoderegulation. On the other hand, successful desensitization in many cases (1) seems incompatible with such a theory.

(1) Simpson et al (1960) *Am. J. Med., 29,* 297. (2) Paine (1958) *J. Am. Med. Assoc., 167,* 285. (3) Bellamy et al (1956) *Ann. Intern. Med., 44,* 764. (4) McKendrick (1951) *Lancet, 2,* 668. (5) Cuthbert (1950) *Lancet, 2,* 209. (6) Lichtenstein et al (1953) *J. Am. Med. Assoc., 152,* 606. (7) Hensler et al (1957) *Am. Rev. Tuberc., 76,* 132. (8) Bower (1964) *Am. Rev. Resp. Dis., 89,* 440. (9) Morizane (1978) *Gastroenterol. Jpn.,*

13, 281. (10) Hansen et al (1955) *Dis. Chest, 28,* 577. (11) Zimmerman (1963) *Ann. NY Acad. Sci., 104,* 954.

Ethambutol

$$CH_3-CH_2-CH-NH-CH_2-CH_2-NH-CH-CH_2-CH_3$$
$$\underset{CH_2OH}{|} \qquad\qquad \underset{CH_2OH}{|}$$

Causal relationship o

Although liver function abnormalities may occur (1), they are mostly difficult to ascribe to ethambutol because of concurrent use of isoniazid, pyrazinamide or other hepatotoxic tuberculostatics in most studies. Occasionally, hepatic injury has possibly been caused, but these cases were usually poorly documented (2–4). In 1 case with drug fever and moderate liver enzyme elevations, only the drug fever was reproducible after readministration.

(1) Meyer et al (1980) In: Dukes (Ed), *Meyler's Side Effects of Drugs, 9th ed,* p 524. Excerpta Medica, Amsterdam. (2) Davey (1966) *Med. J. Aust., 1,* 789. (3) Haegi (1969) *Helv. Med. Acta, Suppl 49,* 81. (4) Tapalaga et al (1982) *Rev. Roum. Sér. Méd. Interne, 20,* 231.

Ethionamide

Causal relationship +

The incidence of hepatic injury, including mild liver enzyme elevations, has been variably reported in percentages of more than 20 in some studies, usually at a dose of 0.5–1 g/d (1). In 1 study abnormal ASAT values were observed in up to 37%, accompanied by gastrointestinal symptoms in two–thirds of these cases (3). Most studies, however, gave an estimation of up to 5% (1). In most cases reported, other tuberculostatics were used concomitantly. Pernod (2) noted 6 cases of jaundice in 222 treated patients. Most cases appeared after several months of treatment; fever was present in less than half the cases whereas rash or eosinophilia were infrequent (1). Rechallenge was positive in some cases (2, 4). A high incidence in patients with diabetes mellitus has been reported (1), but the significance of this remains uncertain.

The mechanism is unknown. Two studies noted a positive lymphocyte stimulation test in cases of ethionamide–associated hepatitis (5, 6), but with the exception of these results the evidence for an immunoallergic mechanism is not very convincing.

(1) Conn et al (1964) *Am. Rev. Resp. Dis., 90,* 542. (2) Pernod (1965) *Am. Rev. Resp. Dis., 92,* 39. (3) Simon et al (1969) *Scand. J. Resp. Dis., 50,* 314. (4) Moulding et al (1962) *Am. Rev. Resp. Dis., 86,* 252. (5) Namihisa et al (1975) *Leber Magen Darm, 5,* 73. (6) Kato et al (1979) *Gastroenterol. Jpn., 14,* 216.

Isoniazid (INH)

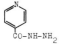

CO-NH-NH₂

Causal relationship + +

INH may cause hepatocellular damage, varying from mild and transient (1, 6) ALAT/ASAT elevations in 10–20% (1, 6, 7) to overt hepatic injury in 0.5–2% (2, 3, 6), the highest percentage being in the elderly. These figures are mostly derived from studies of the prophylactic use of INH alone (300 mg/d). Children/young adults are not affected unless high doses have been used (9), in which case a patient may sometimes be successfully treated with a lower dose and without recurrence (5, 26). Although mainly acute hepatocellular, mixed patterns and chronic forms have been reported, both in approximately 10% (4). Onset is mostly after 2 months or more (15% ≤ 1 month) (6), with gastrointestinal symptoms (55%), 'flu'–like symptoms (35%) or jaundice (10%) (4). Case–fatality rate varied between 3% (6) and 13% (4), but was sometimes higher (8); black women seemed most at risk (6), whereas the role of pre–existing liver damage or alcoholism is unclear. Both a bilirubin level above 20 mg/100 ml and onset after 2 months were associated with a high mortality (4). Immunoallergic signs were absent, with the exception of mild eosinophilia in some cases (4). Rash is rare but may occur (4, 10). By biopsy it was impossible to distinguish the lesions from severe viral hepatitis (11), with massive necrosis or less severe with focal necrosis, sinusoidal acidophilic bodies, ballooning degeneration and occasionally cholestasis (4, 6, 8). Patterns resembling chronic active hepatitis and/or cirrhosis may be seen (4).

The reaction is probably secondary to metabolic idiosyncrasy. Hepatotoxicity is probably due to acetylhydrazine (12, 13), a metabolite of INH. Rapid acetylators seemed more vulnerable (13), but this has been challenged by others (5, 21, 22, 29). In fact, there are at least 4 metabolic pathways responsible (12).

If combined with enzyme–inducing agents (rifampicin), the incidence of both asymptomatic and symptomatic hepatic injury may be enhanced to 20–21% and 5–6%, respectively (14). The incidences, however, vary per study and depend on the extent of liver enzyme assessments. Whereas a retrospective study in children suggested an incidence of moderate to severe liver enzyme elevations in 3.3% (27), a prospective study demonstrated moderate ASAT/ALAT elevation in 44% of children on rifampicin and INH (28). The latent period between first intake and onset of disease seems to be markedly shortened, often to 10 days or less (15). Fulminant hepatitis was partly ascribed to preceding general anesthesia (15, 16) and/or the use of enzyme inducers other than rifampicin (15–17, 23). The mechanism of the interaction is possibly by induction of enzymes involved in the activation of acetylhydrazine to toxic metabolites.

It has been suggested, however, that an immunological reaction may

186

also play a role. Although Dove et al (20) did not find lymphocyte stimulation in the presence of INH in 14 patients with hepatic injury, others have claimed positive results (18, 19, 24). In a recent study, Warrington (25) performed a lymphocyte stimulation test in 61 patients, shortly after starting with INH: 38% reacted positively to INH, isonicotinic acid or albumin conjugates of these haptens. In these 38%, subsequent liver dysfunction developed in over 58% as against 22.7% in the group of non–responders.

(1) Sharer et al (1969) *Ann. Intern. Med., 71*, 1113. (2) Garibaldi et al (1972) *Am. Rev. Resp. Dis., 106*, 357. (3) Thompson et al (1982) *Bull. Wld Health Org., 60*, 555. (4) Black et al (1975) *Gastroenterology, 69*, 289. (5) Mantero et al (1983) *G. Mal. Infett. Parassit., 35*, 1385. (6) Mitchell et al (1976) *Ann. Intern. Med., 84*, 18. (7) Bailey et al (1974) *Ann. Intern. Med., 81*, 200. (8) Maddrey et al (1973) *Ann. Intern. Med., 79*, 1. (9) Bassetti et al (1982) *Drugs Exp. Clin. Res., 8*, 255. (10) Zolov et al (1969) *Int. Arch. Allergy, 35*, 179. (11) Black et al (1976) *Gastroenterology, 70*, 978. (12) Timbrell (1981) In: *Drug Reactions and the Liver*, p 190. Pitman Medical, London. (13) Mitchell et al (1975) *Clin. Pharmacol. Ther., 18*, 70. (14) Powell Jackson et al (1981) In: *Drug Reactions and the Liver*, p 197. Pitman Medical, London. (15) Pessayre et al (1977) *Gastroenterology, 72*, 284. (16) Lenders et al (1983) *Ned. Tijdschr. Geneeskd., 127*, 420. (17) Dervaux et al (1980) *Ned. Tijdschr. Geneeskd., 124*, 1008. (18) Namihisa et al (1975) *Leber Magen Darm, 5*, 73. (19) Mathews et al (1971) *J. Allergy, 47*, 105. (20) Dove et al (1972) *Am. Rev. Resp. Dis., 106*, 485. (21) Musch et al (1982) *Klin. Wochenschr., 60*, 513. (22) Dickinson et al (1981) *J. Clin. Gastroenterol., 3*, 271. (23) Wright et al (1982) *N. Engl. J. Med., 307*, 1325. (24) Warrington et al (1978) *Clin. Exp. Immunol., 32*, 97. (25) Warrington et al (1982) *Clin. Allergy, 12*, 217. (26) Danielides et al (1983) *Am. J. Gastroenterol., 78*, 378. (27) O'Brien et al (1983) *Pediatrics, 72*, 491. (28) Linna et al (1980) *Eur. J. Pediatr., 134*, 227. (29) Gurumurthy et al (1984) *Am. Rev. Resp. Dis., 129*, 58.

Morinamide

Causal relationship o

See 'Pyrazinamide'. Morinamide is said to be less hepatotoxic than pyrazinamide (1), but experience with the drug is limited. In a short review of this drug, jaundice was estimated to occur in 0.3–0.5% of patients. Serum aminotransferase levels were raised in approximately 2% (1).

(1) Dumon et al (1966) *Poumon Coeur, 22*, 671.

Protionamide

Causal relationship o/+

Elevated ALAT/ASAT levels are found varying from 3 to 13% (1–3). These studies mentioned jaundice in 2.5% (1) and 4% (3) of recipients, usually after more than 3 months of treatment. Dose–dependency was suggested by less frequently elevated liver enzyme levels at a dose of 500 mg/d (1).

(1) Several authors (1966) *Poumon Coeur, 22,* 665. (2) Rouques (1966) *Presse Méd., 74,* 2427. (3) Martin–Lalande et al (1966) *Rev. Tuberc. Pneum., 30,* 1233.

Pyrazinamide

—CO—NH₂

Causal relationship +

Pyrazinamide fell into disrepute as a first–choice agent despite its effectiveness, after early studies which showed a high incidence of abnormalities of bilirubin and BSP clearance (1–5) with overt hepatitis in up to 8%. Moreover, aminotransferase elevations were reported in up to 20% (6). Although most of these studies consisted of treatment with both pyrazinamide (usually over 50 mg/kg/d) and isoniazid, hepatic injury was largely ascribed to the former. An early study of several combination regimens demonstrated that combinations including a high–dose regimen of pyrazinamide (40 mg/kg/d) for prolonged periods (24 weeks) produced the highest incidence of liver dysfunction (11%) (4).

Several more recent studies suggest that pyrazinamide in lower doses, useful in combination regimens, does not appear to enhance the incidence of hepatic injury (7). On the other hand, the overall incidence of hepatic injury in several large studies seems slightly enhanced in the group treated with pyrazinamide–containing regimens (8, 10); daily regimens appear to have a higher incidence than thrice–weekly regimens (10). Moreover, the lower dose is probably not completely free from risk as illustrated by a case of fatal hepatic necrosis after 8 months of treatment with 25–30 mg/kg/d (9). According to Cohen et al (11), pyrazinamide is currently the major cause of hepatic injury associated with antituberculous therapy in South Africa despite use of a lower dose. Unfortunately, they do not provide data about the number of prescriptions.

Hepatic injury is hepatocellular; cholestasis is secondary to necrosis. Reproducibility in animals (5), dose dependence and absence of immunoallergic signs suggest an intrinsic toxic effect, although individual susceptibility seems to play a role. Structurally, the drug bears some resemblance to isoniazid and ethionamide, which suggests an analogous mechanism of injury.

(1) Campagna et al (1954) *Am. Rev. Tuberc., 69,* 334. (2) Düggeli (1956) *Schweiz. Z. Tuberk., 13,* 472. (3) McDermott et al (1954) *Am. Rev. Tuberc., 69,* 319. (4) US Public Health Service (1959) *Am. Rev. Resp. Dis., 80,* 627. (5) Yeager et al (1952) *Am. Rev. Tuberc., 65,* 523. (6) Hess et al (1970) *Prax. Pneumol., 24,* 486. (7) Hong Kong Tuberculosis Treatment Services/British Medical Research Council (1976) *Tubercle, 57,* 81. (8) Pretet et al (1980) *Rev. Fr. Mal. Resp., 8,* 307. (9) Danan et al (1981) *Lancet, 2,* 1057. (10) Hong Kong Chest Service/Medical Research Council (1981) *Lancet, 1,* 171. (11) Cohen et al (1983) *South Afr. Med. J., 63,* 960.

Thioacetazone

$CH_3-\overset{O}{\underset{\|}{C}}-NH-$⟨benzene ring⟩$-CH=N-NH-\overset{S}{\underset{\|}{C}}-NH_2$

Causal relationship o/+

Thioacetazone may cause hypersensitivity reactions such as fever, rash, Stevens–Johnson syndrome and blood disorders. Although largely abandoned in Western countries, it is still in use in Third World countries against tuberculosis and leprosy but almost invariably in combination with other antituberculous agents. Some cases of hepatocellular injury ascribed to thioacetazone alone were reported during its early years (1, 3, 4). Damage varied from foci of cell dropout (3) or steatosis (1) to extensive necrosis in combination with aplastic anemia (4).

Animal toxicity tests have been inconclusive, with both positive (8) and negative results (3) as regards hepatic injury. According to a small British study, the combination with isoniazid caused a higher incidence of hepatic injury than thioacetazone alone (5). Chronic malnutrition and anoxia were thought to predispose to hepatic injury (6). In 3 groups of comparable pediatric patients treated with isoniazid (10 mg/kg/d) and either streptomycin (I), thioacetazone (II) at 3–5 mg/kg/d, or p–aminosalicylic acid (III), significant ASAT/ALAT elevations, hepatomegaly in 18% and jaundice in 2.5% were noted in Group II. Milder or no signs of injury were present in Group III and I, respectively (2).

The currently used dose of 150 mg/d seems fairly safe. A large study comparing several dose regimens found an incidence of jaundice/hepatitis in approximately 0.7% on thioacetazone and isoniazid as well as on thioacetazone and streptomycin (7). However, no details were given about these cases.

(1) Böhm (1950) *Klin. Wochenschr., 28,* 548. (2) Gupta et al (1977) *Indian J. Med. Res., 65,* 327. (3) Klatskin (1975) In: Schiff (Ed), *Diseases of the Liver, 4th ed,* p 604. Lippincott, Philadelphia. (4) Csapó et al (1960) *Z. Klin. Med., 156,* 415. (5) Pines (1964) *Tubercle, 45,* 188. (6) Narang et al (1966) *Indian J. Tuberc., 31,* 77. (7) Miller et al (1970) *Bull. WHO, 43,* 107. (8) Savini (1950) *C.R. Soc. Biol., 144,* 1310.

Tiocarlide

$HN-$⟨benzene ring⟩$-O-CH_2-CH_2-\overset{CH_3}{\underset{CH_3}{CH}}$
$\underset{\|}{C}=S$
$HN-$⟨benzene ring⟩$-O-CH_2-CH_2-\overset{CH_3}{\underset{CH_3}{CH}}$

Causal relationship o

Elevated serum aminotransferase levels were found in 11 out of 246 patients, jaundice in 1 patient (1).

(1) Tobe et al (1966) *Poumon Coeur, 22,* 675.

I. URINARY TRACT CHEMOTHERAPEUTIC AGENTS

Sulfonamides are discussed in Section 14.G.

It is possible that these agents are occasionally administered in cases where the prodromal symptoms of acute hepatitis are wrongly ascribed to acute urinary tract infection. This fault may be made when symptoms are non–specific in patients with a well–known history of recurring urinary tract infections and in these cases subsequent jaundice may be falsely ascribed to the administered drug.

Urinary tract chemotherapeutic agents rarely cause liver injury. Dose–dependent toxic reactions are uncommon since these agents – unless renal impairment is present – are often rapidly excreted in the urine. Moreover, some of them are hardly metabolized by the liver (e.g. pipemidic acid). Nevertheless, pipemidic acid has also occasionally been associated with elevation of serum aminotransferase concentrations (1).

Most agents of this group have not been associated with clinically significant hepatic injury, with the exception of nitrofurantoin. Occasional elevations of liver enzyme concentrations have been reported with some of them, e.g. oxolinic acid (2), norfloxacin (4) and miloxacin (3).

(1) Several authors (1975) *Chemotherapy (Tokyo)*, *23*, 9. (2) Gleckman et al (1979) *Am. J. Hosp. Pharm.*, *36*, 1077. (3) *Chemotherapy (Tokyo)* (1978) *26*, *Suppl 4*. (4) Fujita et al (1983) *Chemotherapy (Tokyo)*, *31*, 278.

Cinoxacin

Causal relationship o

Elevated values for ALAT/ASAT and APh were found in approximately 1% of treated patients (1). Two cases of hepatitis were reported but no details were given (2).

(1) Scavone et al (1982) *Pharmacotherapy*, *2*, 286. (2) Sisca et al (1983) *Drugs*, *25*, 544.

Nalidixic acid

Causal relationship o

Cholestatic hepatitis (1) as well as a mainly hepatocellular pattern has been described, starting within 2 weeks after first intake (2); rash and eosinophilia were found (2). Lymphocyte stimulation tests were positive (2, 3).

(1) Rachel–Mohassel et al (1974) *Acta Med. Iran.*, *17*, 47. (2) Anonymous (1976) *Jpn. Med. Gaz., April 20*, 13. (3) Namihisa et al (1975) *Leber Magen Darm, 5*, 73.

Nitrofurantoin

Older literature (up till 1978) mentions approximately 20 cases of hepatic injury ascribed to the use of this urinary chemotherapeutic (1). The real figure can be expected to be higher because of underreporting and non–recognition. Moreover, only a minority of cases ever reaches publication. Acute cholestatic reactions have been reported more frequently than acute hepatocellular ones (1). However, it should be noted that ni-trofurantoin–induced cholestatic jaundice is not always due primarily to cholestatic hepatitis but may probably also result from obstruction of the common bile duct caused by edema of the pancreatic head, secondary to nitrofurantoin–induced pancreatitis (25). In cases reported, the onset ranged from 2 days to 5 months after starting therapy. In more than half of the patients fever accompanied hepatic injury; eosinophilia was even more frequent, while rash was present in one–third of the cases. Bio-chemically, patterns ranged from a cholestatic, via a mixed pattern, to predominantly hepatocellular injury (1). In a more recent case, signs of liver damage were accompanied by an acute lung reaction with severe dyspnea, chest pain, fever and chills starting 3 days after first intake (2). Other lesions which have been associated with the use of nitrofurantoin are granulomatous hepatitis (20) and focal nodular hyperplasia (21), the latter detected 7 months after initial intake.

In addition, several cases with a pattern of chronic active hepatitis have been reported (3–17, 24), especially from the U.S.A., Scandinavia and The Netherlands. Two other reports suggest chronic hepatitis; how-ever, no biopsy was performed in 2 cases (18, 19), while in 1 case a liver biopsy was normal (19). Most cases concern women, with only 1 excep-tion (7). The onset was insidious after 1 to several years of intermittent or continuous use but occasionally much faster (5, 16) in 1–2 months. Rash and fever were less frequently reported than with acute nitrofuran-toin–associated liver injury (10). Low–grade eosinophilia (3%) was pre-sent in most assessed cases (10). Pulmonary involvement was present in some patients (12–14, 16, 19). A rechallenge after normalization of liver enzyme levels was performed and found positive in some cases (3, 10, 13, 17, 24). In most patients in whom antinuclear factor and anti–smooth–muscle antibodies were assessed, these were positive; hypergammaglobu-linemia was frequent (10). HLA–B8 was positive in some patients (3, 15) but negative in another patient (9). Discontinuation led to improvement in most cases with clinical and biochemical normalization. Autoantibody levels declined but often remained positive. However, some patients showed beginning cirrhosis (4, 9, 10, 13, 15) and 3 died from hepatic fail-ure (4, 10).

Histology showed periportal 'piecemeal' necrosis, mononuclear infil-

191

tration, portal enlargement and fibrosis with, in some cases, cirrhotic changes and/or diffuse hepatocellular necrosis with bridging. A lymphocyte stimulation test, performed in 4 patients, was positive in 3 of them (11, 14, 19).

The mechanism of nitrofurantoin–induced hepatic injury is unknown, but immunoallergic signs in cases of acute liver injury and autoantibodies in the chronic form are consistent with a hypersensitivity reaction.

	Strong response (?)	Weak response (?)
Lung	Acute interstitial pneumonitis	Chronic interstitial pneumonitis
Lung+Liver		
Liver	Acute parenchymatous hepatitis	Chronic active hepatitis

FIG. 1 *Nitrofurantoin patterns. Lung and liver reactions may occur simultaneously. Note that there is a resemblance to viral hepatitis where strong responders develop acute hepatitis while weak responders develop chronic active hepatitis.*

It seems plausible that some hypersensitive patients react very strongly (acute form) to a complex of the drug/metabolite with lung and/or liver cells, while others show only a weak response (chronic form) (see Fig. 1). This may be superimposed on an intrinsic toxic effect of furan derivatives (23). An interesting structural resemblance exists between nitrofurantoin and dantrolene which may also cause both chronic active hepatitis and pleuropulmonary reactions (22).

(1) Zimmerman (1978) *Hepatotoxicity*, p 468. Appleton–Century–Crofts, New York. (2) McKelvie et al (1982) *Hosp. Pharm.*, *17*, 563. (3) Hatoff et al (1979) *Am. J. Med.*, *67*, 117. (4) Iwarsson et al (1979) *Scand. J. Gastroenterol.*, *14*, 497. (5) Strömberg et al (1976) *Br. Med. J.*, *2*, 174. (6) Fagrell et al (1976) *Acta Med. Scand.*, *199*, 237. (7) Miller et al (1982) *Ann. Intern. Med.*, *97*, 452. (8) Spoelstra et al (1981) *Ned. Tijdschr. Geneeskd.*, *125*, 61. (9) Vellenga et al (1981) *Ned. Tijdschr. Geneeskd.*, *125*, 63. (10) Sharp et al (1980) *Ann. Intern. Med.*, *92*, 14. (11) Black et al (1980) *Ann. Intern. Med.*, *92*, 62. (12) Selroos et al (1975) *Acta Med. Scand.*, *197*, 125. (13) Klemola et al (1975) *Scand. J. Gastroenterol.*, *10*, 501. (14) Bäck et al (1974) *Lancet*, *1*, 930. (15) Lindberg et al (1975) *Br. Med. J.*, *4*, 77. (16) Marsidi et al (1979) *Gastroenterology*, *76*, 1291. (17) Jokela et al (1967) *Gastroenterology*, *53*, 306. (18) Nolet (1981) *Ned. Tijdschr. Geneeskd.*, *125*, 59. (19) Lundgren et al (1975) *Scand. J. Gastroenterol.*, *56*, 208. (20) Strohscheer et al (1977) *Münch. Med. Wochenschr.*, *119*, 1535. (21) Anttinen et al (1982) *Acta Med. Scand.*, *211*, 227. (22) Faling et al (1980) *Ann. Intern. Med.*, *93*, 152. (23) Mitchell et al (1975) *Gastroenterology*, *68*, 392. (24) Hannon et al (1971) *Tijdschr. Geneeskd.*, *15*, 751. (25) Nelis (1983) *Gastroenterology*, *84*, 1032.

Phenazopyridine

H_2N —— NH_2 ... (structure) ... $N=N$

Causal relationship +

Approximately 20% of phenazopyridine is metabolized to paracetamol (7). Overdosage, however, is associated with hemolysis and renal failure rather than with liver damage.

Some cases of cholestatic jaundice and mildly elevated ASAT/ALAT levels were reported (1–3). Fever was prominent (1–3); rash (2) and eosinophilia were present in some cases (3). Onset was in the first week of use (1–3). Several challenges were immediately positive (1–3). Biopsy showed acute hepatitis with acidophilic bodies (2).

Clinical features favor an immunoallergic mechanism (1–3). The drug is however also hepatotoxic, according to cases of hepatic injury due to overdosage (4, 5) and according to animal toxicity tests (6).

(1) Hood et al (1966) *J. Am. Med. Assoc., 198,* 116. (2) Goldfinger et al (1972) *N. Engl. J. Med., 286,* 1090. (3) Badley (1976) *Br. Med. J., 2,* 850. (4) Cohen et al (1971) *Clin. Pediatr., 10,* 537. (5) Wander et al (1965) *Am. J. Dis. Child., 110,* 105. (6) Walton et al (1934) *J. Pharmacol. Exp. Ther., 51,* 200. (7) Johnson et al (1976) *Toxicol. Appl. Pharmacol., 37,* 371.

15. Contrast media

Introduction

With the exception of thorium–dioxide– and radium–224–induced (1) lesions, hepatic injury caused by radiological contrast media or radiopharmaceuticals usually concerns cholecystographic agents. Occasionally, elevations of liver enzyme concentrations are associated with other contrast media such as sodium diatrizoate (2), but it is not always clear whether the use of these agents is causative or coincidental.

Hepatic injury after cholangiography may be related to the contrast media employed or to the procedure itself, e.g. cholangitic sepsis after endoscopic retrograde cholangiopancreatography or bile leakage after percutaneous transhepatic cholangiography.

The occasional liver enzyme elevations which can be caused by all cholegraphic contrast media may be difficult to differentiate from underlying disease–related changes. However, a close temporal relationship will facilitate a correct diagnosis in most cases.

Bunamiodyl impairs excretion of BSP and indocyanine green and increases blood levels of unconjugated bilirubin. Older studies suggested inhibition of both the uptake of unconjugated (3) and the excretion of conjugated bilirubin (4, 5), probably via competition for the same pathway. Because of its toxicity to the kidneys, the use of this agent has been abandoned in most countries. Other orally administered agents such as iopanoic acid and the ipodate salts have largely the same effect on hepatic function.

The intravenous agents comprise salts of iodoxamic acid, iodipamide and ioglycamic acid. The latter was associated in 1 study with a high incidence of aminotransferase elevation (6). Although most patients had elevated values of aminotransferases and APh before administration, a sharp and marked elevation of aminotransferase levels after infusion strongly suggested a toxic effect of ioglycamic acid (6). Iodipamide is discussed below. The newer agents, iodoxamate and iotroxate, may also cause liver enzyme elevations, but this has been reported as more marked in the former, with signs of intrahepatic cholestasis, than in the latter (7).

(1) Mays (1980) *Monatschr. Kinderheilkd., 128,* 595. (2) Clark (1977) *Adv. Drug React. Bull.,* Oct., 232. (3) Berthelot et al (1966) *Am. J. Physiol., 211,* 395. (4) Billing et al (1963) *Ann. NY Acad. Sci., 111,* 319. (5) Dewey et al (1963) *Nature (Lon-*

don), *200*, 1176. (6) Winckler (1978) *Dtsch. Med. Wochenschr., 103*, 420. (7) Dohmen et al (1981) *Diagn. Imaging, 50*, 305.

Iodipamide

HN-CO-(CH₂)₄-CO-NH
I ⬡ I   I ⬡ I
  COOH HOOC
I   I

Causal relationship o/ +

Most cases of symptomatic hepatic injury due to cholecystographic media have been reported following intravenous injection of this agent. Nevertheless, it is rarely encountered. One patient developed periorbital edema and abdominal pain 1 day after infusion of 60 ml, followed within 3 days by very high ASAT and LDH elevation. There was mild eosinophilia. Subsequent improvement was rapid (1). In another case, rash and fever accompanied marked liver enzyme elevation after the fourth cholangiographic procedure (2). A third case presented with sneezing and chills, followed by fever, abdominal pain and marked elevation of aminotransferase levels in the serum. Peripheral eosinophilia was noted 9 days later and a macrophage migration inhibition test was positive (4). Others found no hypersensitivity phenomena, except for fever, and suggested a toxic effect (3). Readministration in 1 report was followed by a relapse (3).

Histology has shown centrilobular necrosis without portal inflammation (3), slight cellular pleomorphism and fatty infiltration (2).

According to 1 study, a dose–dependent effect may be demonstrated. A high–dose intravenous regimen produced abnormal ASAT values in 18.3% of 149 patients versus 8.7% of 126 patients on the lower dose (5). In a study of 25 patients, almost 50% reacted with a transient LDH$_5$ elevation within 24 hours after infusion of 40 ml methylglucamide iodipamide (6).

(1) Stillman (1974) *J. Am. Med. Assoc., 228*, 1420. (2) Imoto (1978) *Ann. Intern. Med., 88*, 129. (3) Sutherland et al (1977) *Ann. Intern. Med., 86*, 437. (4) Motoki et al (1979) *Am. J. Gastroenterol., 72*, 71. (5) Scholz et al (1974) *J. Am. Med. Assoc., 229*, 1724. (6) Hutton et al (1982) *Clin. Chim. Acta, 122*, 279.

Iopanoic acid

CH₃-CH₂-CH-COOH
         CH₂
I ⬡ I
  NH₂
I

Causal relationship o/ +

Iopanoic acid is an orally administered cholecystographic agent. In 1 case, chills and fever developed several hours after the intake of 3 g, followed by a morbilliform rash and eosinophilia on the 3rd day and jaundice on the 6th day. Complete recovery took 3 months. Histology demonstrated diffuse lobular mononuclear infiltration and extensive centrilobular and periportal necrosis (1).

(1) Klatskin (1975) In: Schiff (Ed), *Diseases of the Liver, 4th ed,* p 604. Lippincott, Philadelphia.

Thorium dioxide (Thorotrast)

ThO_2 (20–25%)   *Causal relationship* + +

Thorium dioxide was used very frequently as an X–ray contrast medium between 1928 and 1955 (11). It accumulates in the reticuloendothelial system, especially in liver ($\pm 70\%$) and spleen ($\pm 20\%$) where it remains demonstrable for the entire life of the individual. Its long physical and biological half–life has led to numerous cases of both hepatic and extrahepatic malignant diseases, usually appearing 20–30 years after administration. In Japan alone, 78 autopsy cases of thorium–dioxide–associated liver tumors had already been published between 1953 and 1980 (6). Liver disorders include fibrosis, cirrhosis, angiosarcoma, cholangiocarcinoma and hepatocellular carcinoma. Histology shows grey–brown particles, both free and in Kupffer cells surrounded by fibrosis. Cirrhosis is frequent (1). These particles, emitting 90% alpha–, 9% beta– and 1% gamma–rays, with a physical half–life of 1.41×10^{10} years, are held to be directly responsible for the abnormalities, although thorium dioxide, apart from its radioemission, has fibrinogenic properties (8). Da Silva Horta et al (2) demonstrated liver cirrhosis in 42 and angiosarcoma in 22 of 1107 thorium–dioxide–administered patients. Follow–up studies for more than 25 years in persons injected with this agent revealed incidences of primary liver tumors ranging from 15 to 16% of cases (3, 5), whereas 68% of autopsy cases had liver tumors (4). A 4– to 5–fold increased risk of death from liver cirrhosis or fibrosis appeared from these studies (3, 5). Most tumors are either cholangiocarcinoma or angiosarcoma. A Japanese study suggested a higher incidence of cholangiocarcinoma (6), but in a Portuguese study angiosarcoma was more frequent (7). Angiosarcoma developed later and in persons of higher age (6). According to Rubel et al (8) who studied 6 cases of cholangiocarcinoma, there was an increased incidence of benign and malignant thyroid disease in their cases. This has not been previously reported but needs confirmation since their group was too small. Although abandoned about 30 years ago, the issue of Thorotrast–induced lesions is still alive. Because of the long latent period, cases of liver tumors are still being reported (9, 10, 12–15). In 1 case veno–occlusive disease and peliosis hepatis without coexisting liver malignancy, 35 years after administration, were associated with thorium dioxide (16). The authors supposed that this might have been related to the protracted alpha–emitting effect of thorium dioxide deposits. Although the absence of malignancy may be difficult to prove, the presence of fibrosis with deposits suggested thorium dioxide as the cause.

196

The hepatic and extrahepatic malignancies, caused by thorium dioxide, comprise one of the most serious iatrogenic epidemics, especially since only one exposure is enough to cause the disease.

(1) Selinger et al (1975) *Gastroenterology, 68*, 799. (2) Da Silva Horta et al (1965) *Lancet, 2*, 201. (3) Mori et al (1983) *Health Phys., 44, Suppl 1*, 261. (4) Mori et al (1983) *Health Phys., 44, Suppl 1*, 281. (5) Van Kaick et al (1981) *Health Phys., 44, Suppl 1*, 299. (6) Yamada et al (1983) *J. Natl Cancer Inst., 70*, 31. (7) Saragoça et al (1982) In: *Abstracts, 17th Meeting, European Association for Study of the Liver, Gothenburg.* (8) Rubel et al (1982) *Cancer, 50*, 1408. (9) Zoppi et al (1982) *Schweiz. Med. Wochenschr., 112*, 1808. (10) Ghussen et al (1982) *Med. Welt, 50*, 1807. (11) Thomas et al (1984) *Med. Welt., 35*, 69. (12) Manning et al (1983) *Arch. Pathol. Lab. Med., 107*, 456. (13) Molla et al (1983) *Radiologia (Madrid), 25*, 41. (14) Mohr et al (1984) *Z. Gastroenterol., 22*, 153. (15) Irie et al (1984) *Acta Hepatol. Jpn., 34*, 221. (16) Dejgaard et al (1984) *Virchows Arch. Abt. A Pathol. Anat., 403*, 87.

16. Immunomodulators and immunosuppressants

Introduction

Immunomodulators are agents capable of enhancing or restoring immune competence. Although the Bacille Calmette Guérin (BCG) is usually included, it is not discussed here. Levamisole and interferon are discussed elsewhere.

Immunomodulators may aggravate underlying illness, at least in cases where an immunological component is responsible for injury. Treatment of HBsAg–positive carriers, for instance, may possibly cause elevation of aminotransferase levels through increased immunological destruction of virus–infected hepatocytes. Most immunomodulators may cause fever, sometimes up to 40°C, and mildly elevated serum aminotransferase levels which may be partly related to this – still unexplained – hyperpyrexia. Several of these agents have been associated occasionally with liver enzyme elevations, e.g. poly–I:C and lentinan (1). However, since these agents are often used as immunostimulants in cancer, the differential diagnosis may be difficult (see 'Antineoplastic Agents').

Immunosuppressants, which are also used as antineoplastic agents, are discussed in Chapter 17 (e.g. azathioprine, cyclophosphamide).

When liver enzyme elevations are noted during immunosuppressive therapy, one should also suspect the underlying disease. Several illnesses for which these agents are used have been suggested as a cause of liver injury, e.g. rheumatoid arthritis and systemic lupus erythematosus (2, 3), although they are usually mild and insignificant.

Corticosteroids – the most important immunosuppressants – may cause fatty change in hepatocytes. Only when high doses are employed can this lead to clinically significant steatosis, often combined with Cushing's syndrome (4–6). This effect is largely secondary to lipolysis, but enhanced lipogenesis possibly plays an additional role (7).

When administered in the early phase of acute viral hepatitis, the subsequent development of chronic active hepatitis is possibly more common (8). Whereas corticosteroids seem beneficial in the treatment of HBsAg–negative chronic active hepatitis (9), a controlled trial in HbsAg–positive cases suggested a detrimental effect (10). Clinical and biochemical remissions were less in the HBsAg–positive group, whereas treatment failures and deaths were higher than in the HBsAg–negative group treated with corticosteroids (11). Although aminotransferase levels may be lower, serum titers of DNA polymerase and serum HBsAg and the number of HBeAg–positive patients increase (12).

What treatment with corticosteroids may mean for the long–term survival of the HBsAg–negative group if treated for prolonged periods is uncertain, but concern has been expressed about the possible development of liver tumors in patients with long–standing autoimmune chronic liver disease (13). So far, there has been no convincing evidence for such an effect of immunosuppressants. However, malignancies arising in patients on long–term immunosuppressive therapy are a well–recognized event (7).

Bacterial and mycotic infections are possible during immunosuppressive therapy (7) and subsequent sepsis may cause liver injury.

Occasionally, corticosteroids have been suspected of causing peliosis hepatis when administered in high doses (14). Although these hormones resemble the sex hormones, such associations are still speculative.

(1) Descotes et al (1984) In: Dukes (Ed), *Side Effects of Drugs, Annual 8*, p 341. Excerpta Medica, Amsterdam. (2) Whaley et al (1977) *Clin. Rheum. Dis., 3*, 527. (3) Runyon et al (1980) *Am. J. Med., 69*, 187. (4) Alpers et al (1982) In: Schiff et al (Eds), *Diseases of the Liver, 5th ed*, p 813. Lippincott, Philadelphia. (5) Hill (1961) *N. Engl. J. Med., 265*, 318. (6) Jones et al (1965) *N. Engl. J. Med., 273*, 1453. (7) Von Eickstedt (1980) In: Dukes (Ed), *Meyler's Side Effects of Drugs, 9th ed*, p 643. Excerpta Medica, Amsterdam. (8) Singeisen et al (1977) *Schweiz. Med. Wochenschr., 107*, 1762. (9) Kirk et al (1980) *Gut, 21*, 78. (10) Lam et al (1981) *N. Engl. J. Med., 304*, 380. (11) Schalm et al (1976) *Gut, 17*, 781. (12) Scullard et al (1979) *Gastroenterology, 77*, 43A. (13) Burroughs et al (1981) *Br. Med. J., 282*, 273. (14) Asano et al (1982) *Acta Hepatol. Jpn., 32*, 860.

Cyclosporine A

One of the major representatives of a group of biologically active metabolites produced by *Tolypocladium inflatum Gams*   *Causal relationship* +

Hepatotoxicity seems less important than nephrotoxicity with this agent and the latter is often the dose–limiting factor (5). Hyperbilirubinemia occurred in 20% of cases (1, 2) as against 3% of cases on conventional therapy (1). Unfortunately, no details were given for the percentage of conjugated/unconjugated bilirubin or for liver enzymes. Hyperbilirubinemia occurred within 2 weeks of transplantation (2). Blood level dependence (> 400 ng/ml) is likely (2–4). On the other hand, in another study, in 209 recipients of renal transplants the incidence of liver injury was no higher in the group on cyclosporine and prednisone than in the control group on azathioprine and prednisone (3). Atkinson et al (6) held cyclosporine responsible for 34% of 28 hyperbilirubinemic episodes in 21 patients with allogenic marrow transplants. Hyperbilirubinemia was mainly conjugated and accompanied by moderate ALAT elevation. Some patients had an early increase accompanied by a rise in serum creatinine and cyclosporine concentrations whereas others showed a more gradual increase. The mechanism is still unknown, but direct toxicity is likely.

(1) European Multicentre Trial (1982) *Lancet, 1,* 57. (2) Laupacis et al (1981) *Lancet, 2,* 1426. (3) Canadian Multicentre Transplant Study Group (1984) *N. Engl. J. Med., 309,* 809. (4) Margreiter et al (1983) *Dialysis Transplant., 12,* 108. (5) Kennedy et al (1983) *Transplant. Proc., 15,* 471. (6) Atkinson et al (1983) *Transplant. Proc., 15,* 2761.

Frentizole

CH₃O ⬡ S NH-CO-NH ⬡
N

Causal relationship +

Several reports of hepatic injury (1–4) in a high percentage of patients suggest that this immunosuppressant has intrinsic toxic potential. Liver damage was reproducible in rats (3). ASAT/ALAT and APh elevations were reported in 30–70% of patients (1–4) treated for systemic lupus erythematosus (SLE) with 50–300 mg/d (3) or 4–6 mg/kg/d (2, 4). Jaundice (2) and ALAT elevations up to 2200 IU (4) often led to discontinuation of therapy. Onset was reported after 11–25 days of therapy, occasionally accompanied by fever (4). Biopsy in 2 patients showed chronic portal inflammation with fibrosis and focal necrosis (3). That untreated SLE may also show liver enzyme elevations is illustrated by a 29% incidence of aminotransferase elevation in the placebo–treated group (2).

(1) O'Duffy et al (1980) *Mayo Clin. Proc., 55,* 601. (2) Bang (1980) *Arthritis Rheum., 23,* 1388. (3) Sobharwal et al (1980) *Arthritis Rheum., 23,* 1376. (4) Kay et al (1980) *Arthritis Rheum., 23,* 1381.

17. Antineoplastic agents

A. Alkylating agents
  1. Nitrogen mustards
  2. Ethylenimine derivatives
  3. Alkylsulfonates
  4. Nitrosoureas
  5. Miscellaneous
B. Antimetabolites
  1. Folic acid antagonists
  2. Purine antagonists
  3. Pyrimidine antagonists
C. Antineoplastic antibiotics
D. Alkaloids
  1. Podophylline derivatives
  2. Vinca alkaloids
  3. Other alkaloids
E. Miscellaneous/Investigational

Introduction

It may be extremely difficult – or even impossible – to assess the causal relationship between signs of liver injury in cancer patients and a suspected antineoplastic agent (see Table 1). The underlying illness may be responsible, e.g. primary liver tumors, metastases or Hodgkin's disease, or therapy may be responsible, e.g. radiation, bone marrow transplanta-

TABLE 1 *Factors which may complicate the assessment of a causal relationship between hepatic injury and the use of a suspected drug*

Underlying illness (tumor, metastases)
Other antineoplastic agents
Other drugs (e.g. analgesics, antiemetics, antibiotics)
Radiation
Bone marrow transplantation
BCG vaccination (liver granulomas)
Total parenteral nutrition
Operative procedures (shock, anesthetics)
Viral/bacterial infections (transfusions, immunosuppression)
Aggravation of underlying non-malignant disease (e.g. cardiac failure)

tion ('graft versus host' reaction), total parenteral nutrition, other antineoplastic agents, antiemetics, analgesics and other concurrently used drugs. Immunosuppression may render the patient more susceptible to bacterial, mycotic and viral infections, the latter often secondary to multiple blood transfusions. In a study in 103 leukemic children in long–term remission, 70 developed chronic liver disease which proved to be related largely to viral hepatitis rather than to drug therapy (10). The cardiac function of the patient may be decompensated by anemia or fever with subsequent hepatic congestion. Moreover, cancer patients are operated upon relatively frequently, with the well–known risks of hepatic injury, especially in patients in poor general condition.

These factors may lead to both over– and underestimation of the hepatotoxic potential of antineoplastic agents. Only under optimal circumstances, i.e. a prospective and randomized double–blind trial, can data on hepatotoxicity be obtained. However, such studies cannot be performed with placebo as control and will miss the less frequent idiosyncratic form of liver injury.

As a rule, every antineoplastic agent is associated occasionally with liver enzyme or bilirubin elevations, but in relatively few agents has a hepatotoxic effect been proven. Well–known examples of the latter are methotrexate, mithramycin, mercaptopurine and colaspase (L–asparaginase).

The liver is relatively insensitive to antineoplastic agents, largely because these act preferentially on rapidly proliferating tissues such as bone marrow, hair roots and the gastrointestinal tract (2). Moreover, the liver may detoxify these agents, thereby preventing damage (1, 2). Naturally, the opposite can also occur.

Some regimens have been reported to potentiate the adverse effect of individual agents on the liver. Doxorubicin, for instance, seems to potentiate the hepatotoxic effect of mercaptopurine (3) and an analogous effect has been suggested for daunorubicin and tioguanine (4). A potentiating effect on radiation or vice versa has been suggested for vincristine (2, 5), actinomycin D (6, 7) and doxorubicin (8). Spiegel et al (9) also suggested a potentiating effect of cancer chemotherapy and haloalkane anesthesia.

Of great interest is the pattern of veno–occlusive disease which is ascribed with increasing frequency to antineoplastic drugs, e.g. dacarbazine, mitomycin, tioguanine, azathioprine, urethane and cytarabine (for references, see individual agents).

Although normal liver enzyme and function tests are not necessarily associated with a normal liver, regular evaluation is important. Liver enzyme assessment before starting therapy and subsequently every month is indicated. Serum protein assessment (e.g. asparaginase) or biopsy (e.g. methotrexate) may be important tools. Although nausea and abdominal pain are so common in cancer patients on chemotherapy that they can no longer serve as prodromal signs of hepatic injury, such complaints should be seriously investigated.

202

Finally, it should be remembered that antineoplastic agents may be dangerous to medical staff handling these agents daily in oncological wards, a matter which has been discussed previously (11). Sotaniemi et al (12) re–emphasized this issue by reporting liver injury with fibrotic changes in 3 head nurses who had handled large amounts of antineoplastic agents over several years.

(1) Ménard et al (1980) *Gastroenterology, 78,* 142. (2) Perry (1982) *Semin. Oncol., 9,* 65. (3) Minow et al (1976) *Cancer, 38,* 1524. (4) Penta et al (1977) *Ann. Intern. Med., 87,* 247. (5) Hansen et al (1982) *Acta Med. Scand., 212,* 171. (6) McVeagh et al (1975) *J. Pediatr., 87,* 627. (7) Jayabose et al (1976) *J. Pediatr., 88,* 898. (8) Kun et al (1978) *Cancer, 42,* 81. (9) Spiegel et al (1980) *Cancer Treat. Rep., 64,* 1023. (10) Locasciulli et al (1983) *Cancer, 52,* 1080. (11) Knowles et al (1980) *Br. Med. J., 2,* 589. (12) Sotaniemi et al (1983) *Acta Med. Scand., 214,* 181.

A. ALKYLATING AGENTS

These non–cell–cycle–specific agents act by alkylating and cross–linking guanine and possibly other bases in DNA, thereby inhibiting cell division.

The nitrosoureas and dacarbazine are the most frequently implicated alkylating agents in causing hepatic injury. The mechanism is unknown, but in cases of dacarbazine–associated injury there is evidence of an immunoallergic mechanism. Cases of veno–occlusive disease due to dacarbazine are convincing and worrying because of their unpredictability and rapidly fatal course. Despite the fact that some of these agents are activated in the liver by biotransformation to alkylating metabolites (e.g. cyclophosphamide) this does not seem to have much bearing on their liability to induce hepatic injury.

Besides the nitrosoureas mentioned below, semustine (7) and lomustine (CCNU) (1) have been associated with liver enzyme elevations, the latter also with an (unspecified) case of hepatic failure (6). A new agent, nimustine (ACNU), has also exhibited signs of hepatic injury (5). Amromin et al (2) attributed 2 cases of jaundice with focal necrosis, hydropic degeneration and fibrosis at autopsy to the use of uramustine. However, partial obstruction of the common bile duct was present in both cases (2). Triaziquone has occasionally been mentioned as a cause of cholestatic jaundice (3).

Several other alkylating agents have been associated occasionally with liver enzyme elevations, e.g. pentamethylmelamine (4), but, as far as we know, without clinically significant injury.

(1) Hansen et al (1971) *Cancer Res., 31,* 223. (2) Amromin et al (1962) *Gastroenterology, 42,* 401. (3) Klinge (1979) *Klinische Hepatologie,* p 6158. Thieme, Stuttgart. (4) Ihde et al (1981) *Cancer Treat. Rep., 65,* 755. (5) Kimura (1982) *Jpn. J. Pharmacol. Ther., 10,* 3787. (6) Hoogstraten et al (1975) *Med. Pediatr. Oncol., 1,* 95.

A.1. NITROGEN MUSTARDS

Chlorambucil

$$CH_2-CH_2-CH_2-COOH$$
$$CH_2-CH_2Cl$$
$$N$$
$$CH_2-CH_2Cl$$

Causal relationship o/ +

In a group of 181 patients with chronic lymphatic leukemia and Hodgkin's lymphoma, 22 cases of jaundice developed. Chlorambucil was held responsible in 6 patients who developed jaundice after treatment with 6–15 mg/d for $2^1/_2$–11 weeks. Histology showed hepatocellular necrosis, cholestasis, fibrosis and cirrhosis (1). In another case, rash and jaundice appeared after 15 days of treatment and disappeared 3 weeks after discontinuation; rechallenge induced a recurrence of rash and hepatomegaly (2). Hepatic injury is not a dominant side effect of this drug; the incidence is unclear. The Boston group found 1 'definite' (but unspecified) case in 144 chlorambucil–treated patients (3). Of interest is a recently reported HBsAg–negative case without cirrhosis who developed primary hepatocellular carcinoma after 10 years of treatment for Waldenström's macroglobulinemia (4). Although this may be a speculative report, it should be borne in mind that the carcinogenic potential of this drug appears to be considerable (5).

(1) Amromin et al (1962) *Gastroenterology, 42,* 401. (2) Koler et al (1958) *J. Am. Med. Assoc., 167,* 316. (3) Jick et al (1981) *J. Clin. Pharmacol., 21,* 359. (4) Renambot et al (1982) *Nouv. Presse Méd., 11,* 2418. (5) Amor et al (1980) *Clin. Rheum. Dis., 6,* 567.

Chlormethine

$$CH_2-CH_2Cl$$
$$CH_3-N$$
$$CH_2-CH_2Cl$$

Causal relationship o

Hepatic injury is trivial compared to the other side effects of this drug. An early report described extensive necrosis of the liver in 3 of 50 cases treated for Hodgkin's lymphoma. Aggravation of pre–existing jaundice occurred during treatment in 2 other cases (1). Other authors found no hepatic injury (2). Mild enzyme elevations, however, are common according to some authors (3).

(1) Dameshek et al (1949) *Blood, 4,* 338. (2) Zimmerman et al (1952) *J. Lab. Clin. Med., 40,* 387. (3) Hartmann et al (1981) *Cancer Treat. Rep., 65,* 327.

Cyclophosphamide

Causal relationship o/ +

Besides its use as an antineoplastic agent, cyclophosphamide is also employed as an immunosuppressant. Rare cases of hepatic injury have been ascribed to the use of this drug in the medical literature (1, 3–5). Pichlmayr (2) noted only occasional liver enzyme elevations or BSP retention in rats administered a lethal dose. No significant injury occurred in 30 patients (2). Besides liver enzyme elevations, which are sometimes marked (1), fatal, massive hepatic necrosis was reported in 1 patient, 2 months after operation for breast cancer (halothane narcosis) and in the subsequent 2 months of treatment with cyclophosphamide. No other causes were thought likely (4). In another report, a patient with systemic lupus erythematosus developed very high aminotransferase concentrations and jaundice 6 weeks after starting treatment with cyclophosphamide. This resolved after discontinuation. Two weeks after rechallenge, hepatic injury recurred (5).

(1) Walters et al (1972) *Med. J. Aust.*, *2*, 1070. (2) Pichlmayr (1965) *Klin. Wochenschr.*, *43*, 543. (3) Starzl et al (1971) *Surg. Gynecol. Obstet.*, *133*, 981. (4) Aubrey (1970) *Br. Med. J.*, *3*, 588. (5) Bacon et al (1982) *Ann. Intern. Med.*, *97*, 62.

Estramustine

Causal relationship o/ +

Estramustine is a combination of estradiol and normustine. It is concentrated in prostatic tissue where the carbamate linkage is split, liberating the estrogenic and alkylating moiety. In a study of 50 patients treated with 15 mg/kg/d for prostate carcinoma, 1 patient developed ASAT elevation and jaundice after 1 month of treatment. A rechallenge after normalization was followed by recurrence of abnormalities (1). In another study, jaundice and/or liver enzyme elevations developed in 2 patients with breast carcinoma, disappearing after discontinuation (2).

(1) Mittelman et al (1976) *J. Urol.*, *115*, 409. (2) Dawes (1982) *Cancer Treat. Rep.*, *66*, 581.

A.2. ETHYLENIMINE DERIVATIVES

Azetepa

Causal relationship o

Azetepa is a formerly used cytostatic related to thiotepa. One case of severe hepatocellular damage was ascribed to intravenous and intraperitoneal administration of this drug in a 76–year–old woman with ovarian carcinoma. Autopsy showed severe fatty metamorphosis of hepatocytes and necrosis of the peripheral zone, a pattern resembling acute phosphorus intoxication (1). The authors suggested a rapid breakdown of the molecule to inorganic phosphate with accumulation in the liver.

(1) Cochran et al (1969) *Med. Sci. Law, 9*, 202.

A.3. ALKYLSULFONATES

Busulfan

$$CH_3-O_2SO-(CH_2)_4-OSO_2-CH_3$$ *Causal relationship* o

Cholestatic jaundice in a patient with chronic granulocytic leukemia was ascribed to treatment with busulfan for 6 years. Histology showed marked centrilobular cholestasis, mild hepatocyte swelling and minimal leukemic infiltration (1). Another patient with a 'busulfan lung' caused by $4^1/_2$ years of treatment also showed hepatic injury with ascites and portal hypertension (2). Dimethylbusulfan was incriminated in a case of veno–occlusive disease (3).

(1) Underwood et al (1971) *Br. Med. J., 1*, 556. (2) Foadi et al (1977) *Postgrad. Med. J., 53*, 267. (3) Shulman et al (1980) *Gastroenterology, 79*, 1178.

A.4. NITROSOUREAS

Carmustine (BCNU)

Causal relationship o/ +

Liver enzyme elevations were noted in 26% of treated patients in 1 trial, appearing within 12–127 days after starting therapy (1). Other studies at comparable doses yielded much lower incidences (2, 3). Two cases of jaundice – one with concomitant pancytopenia – appeared 6 weeks after treatment with BCNU (40 mg/m²/d) and streptozocin (0.5 g/m²/d) for 5 days; there was pre–existing cirrhosis in 1 of these cases. Histology showed (sub)acute necrosis (4). More recently, veno–occlusive disease developed in 1 case 3 weeks after a 3–day course (500 mg/m²/d) and autologous bone marrow transplantation, with jaundice, hepatomegaly and ascites. Besides centri– and midzonal hemorrhagic necrosis, histology showed subintimal proliferation of loose fibrous tissue in the central veins; the larger sublobular veins were patent (5).

(1) De Vita et al (1965) *Cancer Res., 25,* 1876. (2) Walker et al (1970) *Cancer Chemother. Rep., 54,* 263. (3) Lessner et al (1974) *Cancer Chemother. Rep., 58, 407.* (4) Lokich et al (1974) *Clin. Pharmacol. Ther., 16,* 363. (5) McIntyre et al (1981) *Am. J. Clin. Pathol., 75,* 614.

Chlorozotocin

Causal relationship o/ +

Transient ALAT/ASAT elevations were observed in 25–33% of patients after intravenous doses over 120 mg/m² (1, 2). In 3 patients intrahepatic cholestasis developed after 1, 4 and 6 courses, respectively, with 225 mg/m² as a single dose at 6–weekly intervals (3). No immunoallergic symptoms were observed. Histology in 3 patients showed centrilobular cholestasis with minimal infiltration of leukocytes and mild hepatocellular degeneration.

(1) Taylor et al (1980) *Cancer, 46,* 2365. (2) Hoth et al (1979) *Cancer Treat. Rep., 63,* 17. (3) Belt et al (1980) *Cancer Treat. Rep., 64,* 1235.

Streptozocin

Causal relationship o/ +

Transaminase elevations have been variably reported (6–15%) (1, 2). In a study of patients with pancreatic islet–cell carcinoma, 67% had liver enzyme and/or bilirubin elevation, occurring 2–3 weeks after starting treatment. However, most patients had liver metastases (3).

(1) Stolinsky et al (1972) *Cancer, 30,* 61. (2) Schein et al (1974) *Cancer, 34,* 993. (3) Broder et al (1973) *Ann. Intern. Med., 79,* 108.

A.5. MISCELLANEOUS ALKYLATING AGENTS

Dacarbazine (DTIC)

$$CH_3 \backslash N-N=N$$

$$H_2N-C$$

Causal relationship o/ +

Besides transient and mild serum aminotransferase elevations during clinical trials in more than 50% of patients (1), several cases of severe hepatic injury have been reported (2–13). Most of these showed signs of a veno–occlusive syndrome (4–11, 13), characteristically starting during the second course of DTIC (200–250 mg/m²/d i.v. for 5 days) for malignant melanoma. In 2 of these cases, other antineoplastics were administered concurrently (6, 11). The clinical course with fever, hepatomegaly, ascites, shock and liver failure, high serum aminotransferases and coagulation disorders ended fatally in these cases. Peripheral eosinophilia was often present. Histology showed a varying degree of centrilobular, often hemorrhagic, necrosis, hepatic vein occlusion by thrombotic material and vascular infiltration with lymphocytes and many eosinophils. In none of the cases was tumor infiltration present. A recently described non–fatal case with a similar clinical picture but without vasculitis or thrombosis of the central veins (12) suggests the existence of more than 1 pattern. Electron microscopy in this case showed some resemblance to the early stages of phalloidin injury with microfilamentous changes, intracellular vacuoles, bleb formation and accumulation of electron–dense material in the pericanalicular ectoplasm (12).

(1) Johnson et al (1976) *Cancer Treat. Rep., 60,* 183. (2) Czarnetzki et al (1981) *Arch. Dermatol. Res., 270,* 375. (3) Sutherland et al (1981) *Cancer Treat. Rep., 65,* 321. (4) Greenstone et al (1981) *Br. Med. J., 282,* 1744. (5) Asbury et al (1980) *Cancer, 45,* 2670. (6) Lehrner et al (1978) *Ann. Intern. Med., 88,* 575. (7) Froschet et al (1979) *J. Cancer Res. Clin. Oncol., 95,* 281. (8) Balda et al (1980) *Münch. Med. Wochenschr., 21,* 122. (9) Voigt et al (1981) *Klin. Wochenschr., 59,* 229. (10) Runne et al (1980) *Dtsch. Med. Wochenschr., 105,* 230. (11) Hoghton et al (1979) *Cancer, 44,* 2324. (12) Dancygier et al (1983) *Hepato–Gastroenterology, 30,* 93. (13) Féaux de Lacroix et al (1983) *Cancer Treat. Rep., 67,* 779.

B. ANTIMETABOLITES

The antimetabolites are cell–cycle–specific agents. They act on the same enzymes as normal cellular metabolites, but arrest the metabolic process and inhibit the synthesis of nucleic acids. They antagonize folic acid, purine or pyrimidine.

The mechanism by which they cause hepatic injury is not well understood, but apparently their ability to interfere with DNA and RNA synthesis suffices to induce damage. In cases where steatosis is an important feature (e.g. methotrexate) it is assumed that inhibition of protein synthesis impairs lipid secretion by the hepatocytes. In fact, this has been demonstrated in azaserine–treated rats which had an increased total lipid content of liver cells, despite a decrease in lipogenesis (1).

Several antimetabolites have caused severe liver injury in a significant number of patients. In a group of 11 children on methotrexate and mercaptopurine an ultrastructural study showed disruption of rough and smooth endoplasmic reticulum, a variety of mitochondrial changes, steatosis, fibrosis and peroxisomal and lysosomal changes in all patients (12). Although one should be cautious in the interpretation of such uncontrolled studies, an intrinsic toxic effect is suggested by these data. Folic antagonists (e.g. methotrexate) and purine antagonists (e.g. mercaptopurine) have produced more conclusive evidence of a hepatotoxic effect, when employed in therapeutic doses, than pyrimidine antagonists (e.g. cytarabine).

Although aminopterin, now largely abandoned in favor of methotrexate, has not been associated with fibrosis and cirrhosis (as far as we know), its close structural resemblance to the latter suggests that it has the same potency.

Besides the purine antagonists mentioned below, related compounds have been incriminated, e.g. fluoroadenosine (2), buthiopurine (3) and chloropurine (4). The latter was associated in an older study with jaundice in over 40% of patients who had been treated with the drug for leukemia and lymphoma (4). Occasional reports of liver injury due to fluorouracil have been made, but these are inconclusive (5). Other pyrimidine antagonists have been occasionally associated with hepatic dysfunction, e.g. floxuridine (6, 11) and behenoyl–cytarabine (7). The latter – in combination with prednisone, mercaptopurine and daunorubicin – led to ASAT/ALAT elevations in 55%; 1 patient died due to hepatic injury (7). Some other agents (e.g. azaserine) have produced liver injury in dogs (8), mice and rats (1, 9). This effect was dose–dependent (8). Azauridine has caused fatty liver and necrosis in animals (10). Liver enzyme and/or bilirubin elevation has been reported after intra–arterial administration of fluorouracil and floxuridine combined with irradiation.

(1) Marchetti et al (1970) *Proc. Soc. Exp. Biol. Med., 133*, 30. (2) Stenfert Kroese (1968) In: Meyler et al (Eds), *Side Effects of Drugs, 6th ed,* p 444. Excerpta Medica, Amsterdam. (3) Stenfert Kroese (1972) In: Meyler et al (Eds), *Side Effects of Drugs, 7th ed,* p 598. Excerpta Medica, Amsterdam. (4) Ellison et al (1958) *Blood, 13,* 705. (5) Ménard et al (1980) *Gastroenterology, 78,* 142. (6) *The Extra Pharmacopoeia, 28th ed,* p 171. Pharmaceutical Press, London, 1982. (7) Yamada et al (1980) *Acta Haematol. Jpn., 43,* 1080. (8) Fleischman et al (1972) *Toxicol. Appl. Pharmacol., 22,* 595. (9) Sternberg et al (1957) *Cancer, 10,* 889. (10) Zimmerman (1978) In: *Hepatotoxicity,* p 523. Appleton–Century–Crofts, New York. (11) Barone et al (1982) *Cancer, 50,* 850. (12) Harb et al (1983) *Am. J. Pediatr. Hematol. Oncol., 5,* 323.

B.1. FOLIC ACID ANTAGONISTS

Dichloromethotrexate

Chlorinated derivative of methotrexate   *Causal relationship* o

Relatively little experience has been obtained with dichloromethotrex-
ate. In a recent study, 6 of 21 patients developed liver enzyme and/or bilirubin elevations, 1 of whom progressed to fatal hepatic failure. However, 3 of them had hepatocellular carcinoma (1).

(1) Tester et al (1980) *Cancer Chemother. Pharmacol., 8,* 305.

Methotrexate (MTX)

Causal relationship + +

Hepatic injury caused by MTX has been well–documented, especially
after treatment of leukemia, at autopsy (6), and during treatment of psoriasis (1–5, 8–18, 23). The causal relationship may be regarded as proven
despite the fact that there is usually some evidence of hepatic abnormalities in patients with psoriasis (2, 3, 5, 9, 12), probably due to alcohol use
and overweight rather than to the disease itself (8, 12). The pattern characteristically comprises macrovesicular steatosis and necrosis, followed
by periportal, portal–central and portal–portal bridging fibrosis and ultimately cirrhosis (13). Inflammatory cells are moderately present, mainly portal; liver cell carcinoma has been observed in fibrotic areas (20).
Frequencies of 25% for both fibrosis (14, 17) and cirrhosis (11) have been
reported. The onset is insidious. Symptoms are often absent even in advanced cases; immunoallergic signs are also absent. Although liver enzymes may show a mild elevation after the intake of a dose, they do not
reflect the severity of the damage (4, 8, 12, 15). Liver scanning (16) and
assessment of fasting bile acids (15) proved unreliable and inferior to
biopsy for the detection of injury. Low daily doses (2.5 mg) proved more
toxic than higher once–weekly doses (0.2–0.4 mg/kg) (3, 12, 17, 23). Duration of treatment (11, 17)/cumulative doses (> 2–4 g) (10) were related to
a higher incidence of fibrosis/cirrhosis. Zachariae et al (11) found a highly significant increase in the incidence of cirrhosis to over 25% of patients treated for more than 5 years. However, a large individual variation was demonstrated by the appearance of cirrhosis after cumulative
doses between 590 and 8105 mg (11). Risk factors mentioned in the literature are diabetes mellitus (4, 12) and obesity (4, 8–10, 12), alcoholism (8–
12, 18, 19), previous use of arsenicals (11, 19), decreased renal function
(11, 19), haloalkane anesthesia (21), abnormal pre–treatment histology

(9) and age (8, 9, 14). The A1 and B8 HLA–antigen combination seems to be more vulnerable (19). The mechanism is largely unknown; animal toxicity data have produced inconsistent results (7). An adverse effect on methionine biosynthesis and methylation processes has been suggested (24). Biopsies were recommended yearly (3, 14) or after every 1.5–2 g (11, 18). Recently, Roenigk et al (22) presented revised guidelines for MTX therapy in which they recommended repeat liver biopsies at intervals of 1.0–1.5 g cumulative doses.

(1) Muller et al (1969) *Arch. Dermatol., 100,* 523. (2) Berge et al (1970) *Br. J. Dermatol., 82,* 250. (3) Almeyda et al (1972) *Br. J. Dermatol., 87,* 623. (4) Roenigk et al (1971) *Arch. Dermatol., 103,* 250. (5) Shapiro et al (1970) *Gastroenterology, 58,* 1012. (6) Hutter (1960) *Cancer, 13,* 288. (7) Ménard et al (1980) *Gastroenterology, 78,* 142. (8) Nyfors et al (1976) *Acta Pathol. Microbiol. Scand., 84,* 253. (9) Nyfors et al (1976) *Acta Pathol. Microbiol. Scand., 84,* 262. (10) Nyfors (1977) *Acta Pathol. Microbiol. Scand., 85,* 511. (11) Zachariae et al (1980) *Br. J. Dermatol., 102,* 407. (12) Weinstein et al (1973) *Arch. Dermatol., 108,* 36. (13) Nyfors et al (1977) *Am. J. Surg. Pathol., 1,* 235. (14) Robinson et al (1980) *Arch. Dermatol., 116,* 413. (15) Lawrence et al (1983) *Clin. Chim. Acta, 129,* 341. (16) Geronemus et al (1982) *Arch. Dermatol., 118,* 649. (17) Dahl et al (1972) *Br. Med. J., 1,* 654. (18) Baker (1981) In: Davis et al (Eds), *Drug Reactions and the Liver,* p 257. Pitman Medical, London. (19) Zachariae et al (1980) *Ugeskr. Laeg., 142,* 2182. (20) Ruymann et al (1977) *J. Am. Med. Assoc., 238,* 2631. (21) Spiegel et al (1980) *Cancer Treat. Rep., 64,* 1023. (22) Roenigk et al (1982) *J. Am. Acad. Dermatol., 6,* 145. (23) Podurgiel et al (1973) *Mayo Clin. Proc., 48,* 787. (24) Barak et al (1984) *J. Am. Coll. Nutrit., 3,* 93.

B.2. PURINE ANTAGONISTS

Azathioprine

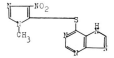

Causal relationship o/+

Azathioprine is used as an antineoplastic agent as well as an immunosuppressant. Cases of jaundice (1–7) with mild to moderate ASAT/ALAT elevations, suggesting a cholestatic to mixed pattern, have been ascribed to its use for renal transplantation (1), chronic active hepatitis (2), systemic lupus erythematosus (5, 20), scleroderma (6) and psoriasis (7). Some cases of hepatocellular injury after renal transplantation (8–13), where the drug was held responsible, were complicated by other possible causes associated with this condition, e.g. viral hepatitis, sepsis and exacerbation of underlying liver disease. An interesting recent observation is the association of hepatotoxicity with low pre–treatment values of IgA (18), but this needs confirmation.

Several cases of veno–occlusive disease were thought to be secondary to its use in renal transplant cases (14, 15) and chronic iridocyclitis (15). The first signs appeared after 8–23 months. The course was mostly fatal either due to hepatic failure or supervening pneumonia. Degott (16) observed 12 cases of peliosis hepatis, 3–17 months after renal transplantation, in a series of 500 patients (16). All had been treated with azathioprine and corticosteroids. Peliosis was present in 12 of 55 patients submitted to biopsy after transplantation against none of 138 during this procedure. The male/female ratio was 1:0.1 as against 1:0.5 in the whole group. Histology showed large and small blood cavities without endothelial lining and, in 4 patients, central vein walls thickened by subendothelial connective tissue. Unusually for veno–occlusive disease, the cavities were randomly distributed throughout the lobule. Another patient with peliosis hepatis, accompanied by jaundice appearing after 3 years on azathioprine and prednisone, was reported by Ross et al (21). Sinusoidal dilatation was demonstrated in dogs treated with azathioprine (17). Azathioprine is metabolized to mercaptopurine, a known hepatotoxin (see below) and it is possible that its hepatotoxic potential depends on the amount and speed of formation of mercaptopurine and subsequent breakdown products. Indeed, in 1 report of azathioprine cholestasis, a challenge with mercaptopurine was positive (2). Moreover, mercaptopurine and the related agent, tioguanine, have also been suspected of causing veno–occlusive disease and/or sinusoidal dilatation.

Immunosuppressants for severe viral hepatitis may be injurious. In 1 such case with severe bridging necrosis, azathioprine improved symptoms but probably promoted viral replication, with subsequent chronic active hepatitis and cirrhosis after 10 months (19). Lee et al (22) suggested that prolonged immunosuppression may have led to primary hepatocellular carcinoma in 1 of their patients with Crohn's disease treated with prednisolone and azathioprine; no underlying liver disease was detected histologically, clinically or serologically. Although it is obviously impossible to extrapolate from individual cases, such a suggestion has also been made with regard to other immunosuppressants and merits serious consideration.

(1) Sparberg et al (1969) *Gastroenterology, 57,* 439. (2) Davis et al (1980) *Postgrad. Med. J., 56,* 274. (3) Freise et al (1976) *Dtsch. Med. Wochenschr., 101,* 1223. (4) Corley et al (1966) *Am. J. Med., 41,* 404. (5) Drinkard et al (1970) *Medicine, 49,* 411. (6) Rosenthal et al (1971) *J. Am. Med. Assoc., 216,* 2011. (7) Greaves et al (1970) *Br. Med. J., 2,* 237. (8) Malekzadeh et al (1972) *J. Pediatr., 81,* 279. (9) Briggs et al (1973) *Arch. Intern. Med., 132,* 21. (10) Millard et al (1973) *Transplantation, 16,* 527. (11) Rashid et al (1973) *Arch. Intern. Med., 132,* 29. (12) Berne et al (1975) *Surg. Gynecol. Obstet., 141,* 171. (13) Zardey et al (1972) *J. Am. Med. Assoc., 222,* 690. (14) Marubbio et al (1975) *Gastroenterology, 69,* 739. (15) Weitz et al (1982) *Virchows Archiv Abt. A Cell Pathol., 395,* 245. (16) Degott et al (1978) *Gut, 19,* 748. (17) Stuart et al (1967) *Ann. Surg., 165,* 325. (18) Harvey et al (1983) *Br. Med. J., 287,* 534. (19) Sagnelli et al (1983) *Infection, 11,* 31. (20) De Pinho et al (1984) *Gastroenterology, 86,* 162. (21) Ross et al (1972) *Pathol. Eur., 7,* 273. (22) Lee et al (1983) *Hepato–Gastroenterology, 30,* 188.

Mercaptopurine

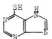
Causal relationship +

Jaundice was reported to occur in 16 of 38 patients treated with this agent, as against 1 of 11 not receiving the drug; all had leukemia (1). Other studies confirmed a high incidence of hepatic injury, varying from 7 to 53% (2, 5–7, 13). Cholestasis (1, 3) and hepatocellular injury (1, 3, 4, 10) were reported, the latter often fatal. In some cases a causal relationship was confirmed by a positive rechallenge (1). Besides cholestasis and focal or extensive necrosis on biopsy one report suggests sinusoidal dilatation (4). The onset of injury varied from 2 weeks to 2 years after starting therapy (1). Einhorn et al (1) claimed that doses in excess of 2.5 mg/kg/d are more likely to produce hepatic injury. Jaundice was often accompanied by leukopenia and oral ulceration. An important individual variation in susceptibility appears from their data. The high incidence, absence of immunoallergic signs and reproducibility in animals (8, 9) favor a direct toxic effect of mercaptopurine. Adults seem more vulnerable to this effect (12). On the other hand, acute overdosage does not seem to have much effect on the liver (17). In treatment of chronic active hepatitis up to 50% of patients developed jaundice in 1 series (14). It should be realized, however, that at the time of this report it was difficult to distinguish between viral and non–viral forms and that immunosuppressants such as mercaptopurine may possibly have facilitated viral replication. Indeed, there are several reports in the literature of aggravation of hepatic injury in cases of chronic active hepatitis (11, 14–16).

(1) Einhorn et al (1964) *J. Am. Med. Assoc., 188*, 802. (2) Ellison et al (1959) *Ann. Intern. Med., 51*, 322. (3) McIlvanie et al (1959) *Blood, 14*, 80. (4) Clark et al (1960) *Br. Med. J., 1*, 393. (5) Farber (1954) *Ann. NY Acad. Sci., 60*, 412. (6) Frei et al (1958) *Blood, 13*, 1126. (7) Gaffney et al (1954) *Ann. NY Acad. Sci., 60*, 478. (8) Philips et al (1953) *Proc. Am. Assoc. Cancer Res., 1*, 42. (9) Clarke et al (1953) *Cancer Res., 13*, 593. (10) Klatskin (1975) In: Schiff (Ed), *Diseases of the Liver, 4th ed*, p 604. Lippincott, Philadelphia. (11) Krawitt et al (1967) *Arch. Intern. Med., 120*, 729. (12) Acute Leukemia Group B (1961) *Blood, 18*, 431. (13) Coffey et al (1972) *Cancer Res., 32*, 1283. (14) Mackay et al (1964) *Lancet, 1*, 899. (15) Arter et al (1966) *Aust. Ann. Med., 15*, 222. (16) Mackay et al (1967) *Postgrad. Med., 41*, 72. (17) Hendrick et al (1984) *Lancet, 1*, 277.

Tioguanine

Causal relationship o/ +

Liver enzyme elevations and cholestatic jaundice have been reported (1, 6). Several cases of veno–occlusive disease have been reported during combined use of tioguanine with cytarabine in 3 patients (2, 5) and methotrexate in 2 others (3, 4). Discontinuation of both drugs led to clinical and histological recovery or improvement (3, 4). A fatal course was observed in other patients (2, 5). In 1 of these reports, histological abnormalities were restricted to centrilobular congestion while the presence of subintimal fibrous tissue and vein narrowing were not mentioned, although the acute onset of ascites, abdominal pain and fever 3 months after starting treatment with 120 mg/kg/d were compatible with veno–

occlusive disease (4). D'Cruz et al (7) noted a pattern resembling veno–occlusive disease in 3 children on daunorubicin, cytarabine and tioguanine. They were maintained on tioguanine alone without aggravation. Renewed intake of the original regimen was followed by a relapse and the authors suggested an interaction between tioguanine and cytarabine and/or daunorubicin. It should be noted that there is an interesting structural resemblance to azathioprine which has also been incriminated of causing veno–occlusive disease.

(1) Council on Drugs (1967) *J. Am. Med. Assoc., 200*, 619. (2) Griner et al (1976) *Ann. Intern. Med., 85,* 573. (3) Gill et al (1982) *Ann. Intern. Med., 96,* 58. (4) Krivoy et al (1982) *Ann. Intern. Med., 96,* 788. (5) Satti et al (1982) *J. Clin. Pathol., 35,* 1086. (6) Milligan et al (1982) *Cancer, 50,* 836. (7) D'Cruz et al (1983) *Cancer, 52,* 1803.

B.3. PYRIMIDINE ANTAGONISTS

Azacitidine

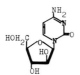

Causal relationship o

Non–dose–related elevation of serum aminotransferase and bilirubin levels was observed in 5 of 22 patients treated for metastatic tumors with $275–850$ mg/m^2 s.c. for 10 days (1). Three died in hepatic coma but showed hepatic metastases. In a study of 24 leukemic adults treated with azacitidine and zorubicin 15 developed ASAT and APh elevations. Five patients became jaundiced. However, before treatment 8 patients already had elevated aminotransferase levels (2). Liver enzyme elevations in other studies varied from 1 to 30% (3, 4), which illustrates the complexity of assessing the causal relationship in patients with malignancy. Administration to dogs in high doses produced necrosis and steatosis (5).

(1) Bellet et al (1974) *Cancer Chemother. Rep., 58,* 217. (2) Peterson et al (1982) *Cancer Treat. Rep., 66,* 563. (3) Valez–Garcia et al (1977) *Cancer Treat. Rep., 61,* 1675. (4) Armitage et al (1977) *Cancer Treat. Rep., 61,* 1721. (5) Cihak et al (1966) *Coll. Czech. Chem. Commun., 31,* 3015.

Cytarabine

Causal relationship o/ +

Clinical trials in patients with leukemia revealed an incidence of 5–7%

in hepatic function test abnormalities (1). Some studies mentioned a higher percentage of 46% (4) or more (5). In the former study, treatment was discontinued in 12 patients with subsequent normalization whereas in 10 patients abnormalities disappeared despite continuation. A rechallenge, performed in 1 case, was positive (4). Another study noted mild and transient aminotransferase elevation in 4 of 7 patients (5). According to Herzig et al (6), 43 of their 57 patients treated with high doses had mildly/moderately abnormal liver chemistry. Severe hepatotoxicity was encountered only with the highest dose. Pizzuto et al (7) described 2 cases with aminotransferase and bilirubin elevation starting after the first cycle of cytarabine, vincristine and prednisone. The second cycle, given after near–normalization, caused a serious relapse. Vincristine alone produced no adverse effect.

Combined use of cytarabine and tioguanine (2, 3) and multiple chemotherapy and irradiation (6) have been associated with the development of veno–occlusive disease. An important role in the causation of this condition for all antimetabolites was suggested by Woods et al (6). Nevertheless, it is clear that other antineoplastic agents (e.g. dacarbazine) may also cause veno–occlusive disease.

(1) Official Literature on New Drugs (1970) *Clin. Pharmacol. Ther.*, *11*, 155. (2) Griner et al (1976) *Ann. Intern. Med.*, *85*, 573. (3) Satti et al (1982) *J. Clin. Pathol.*, *35*, 1086. (4) Goodell et al (1971) *Clin. Pharmacol. Ther.*, *12*, 599. (5) Hryniuk et al (1972) *J. Am. Med. Assoc.*, *219*, 715. (6) Herzig et al (1983) *Blood*, *62*, 361. (7) Pizzuto et al (1983) *Med. Pediatr. Oncol.*, *11*, 287.

Pseudoisocytidine

Causal relationship o

Dose–related hepatic injury was observed in 1 study (30–180 mg/kg, 5–day course). Prolongation of the prothrombin time was noted in most patients, whereas ASAT elevations occurred in 12 of 21 patients. One patient showed severe periportal necrosis at autopsy while another had cirrhosis. Patients with metastases of the liver, however, were not excluded from this study. According to the authors, high doses caused the same pattern of injury in monkeys (1).

(1) Woodcock et al (1980) *Cancer Res.*, *40*, 4243.

C. ANTINEOPLASTIC ANTIBIOTICS

Most antibiotics are assumed to interfere with nucleic acids by inhibit-

215

ing transcription and/or translation. A subsequent decrease in protein synthesis may cause steatosis and/or necrosis of liver cells. Others act as antimetabolites (e.g. azaserine) or as alkylating agents (e.g. streptozocin). Several have a very complicated structure.

These agents show a wide variety in ability to cause hepatic injury. On the one hand, there is mithramycin which may cause aminotransferase elevations in up to 100% of recipients, while, on the other hand, the anthracycline derivatives daunorubicin and doxorubicin seem to be without any significant hepatotoxic effect.

Some other agents, not discussed below, have been associated with liver enzyme elevations, usually mild (e.g. azotomycin) (1). Calvacin and puromycin have caused necrosis and steatosis, respectively, in animals but are used in man rarely or not at all (2).

(1) Carter (1968) *Cancer Chemother. Abstr., 1,* 207. (2) Zimmerman (1978) *Hepatotoxicity,* p 523. Appleton–Century–Crofts, New York.

Aclacinomycin A (ACM–A)

Causal relationship o/ +

Aclacinomycin A is an anthracycline derivative related to doxorubicin/ daunorubicin. ALAT/ASAT and/or APh elevations developed in 4 of 15 patients, only when high doses (3.5–4 mg/kg) were employed (1). Elevation of aminotransferase levels recurred after readministration (2) in 1 study.

(1) Ogawa et al (1979) *Cancer Treat. Rep., 63,* 931. (2) Van Echo et al (1982) *Cancer Treat. Rep., 66,* 1127.

ANTHRACYCLINE DERIVATIVES (except aclacinomycin A)

Doxorubicin

216

Daunorubicin

Causal relationship o

Doxorubicin (adriamycin) and daunorubicin form stable complexes with DNA and interfere with the synthesis of nucleic acids. The main concern with these agents is their adverse effect on heart and bone marrow. In animals, only mild liver cell changes have been demonstrated (1). No unequivocal cases of hepatic injury have been ascribed to these drugs, although hepatic venous congestion secondary to their cardiotoxicity seems a possible cause of occasional liver enzyme elevations. Penta et al (2) mentioned daunorubicin as the common denominator in 13 cases of suspected drug–induced hepatic injury. All patients had leukemia and used several other cytostatics. The total dose of daunorubicin varied from 180 to 450 mg/m^2. Minow et al (3) suggested an enhanced hepatotoxic effect of 6–mercaptopurine by interaction with doxorubicin. In fact, in rabbits blood levels of the former were higher when they were pretreated with doxorubicin (4). In some cases of veno–occlusive disease (5) and acute hepatic vein thrombosis (6, 7) daunorubicin and doxorubicin, respectively, were possibly co–responsible. One report suggested that doxorubicin may enhance radiation–induced liver injury or vice versa (8).

(1) Bertazolli (1972) *Toxicol. Appl. Pharmacol., 21,* 287. (2) Penta et al (1977) *Ann. Intern. Med., 87,* 247. (3) Minow et al (1976) *Cancer, 38,* 1524. (4) Pannuti et al (1974) *Riv. Patol. Clin., 29,* 169. (5) Griner et al (1976) *Ann. Intern. Med., 85,* 578. (6) Houghton et al (1979) *Cancer, 44,* 2324. (7) Lehrner et al (1978) *Ann. Intern. Med., 88,* 575. (8) Kun et al (1978) *Cancer, 42,* 81.

Bleomycin

Glycopeptide antibiotic isolated from
Streptomyces verticillus   *Causal relationship* o

Like many other antineoplastic antibiotics, bleomycin inhibits RNA formation and subsequently protein synthesis. Hepatic injury has been demonstrated in animals treated with a high dose (1, 2); hepatic injury, however, does not seem very significant in man, in contrast to the drug's potential to cause lung reactions. One report of hyperbilirubinemia of a transient nature occurring in 30% of patients after administration of bleomycin in combination with vinblastine (3) has not yet been confirmed. In a study of almost 1200 patients, no hepatic injury could be attributed to bleomycin (4).

(1) Umezawa et al (1967) *Cancer, 20,* 891. (2) Tamura et al (1967) *Fol. Pharmacol. Jpn., 63,* 346. (3) Samuels et al (1975) *Cancer Chemother. Rep., 59,* 563. (4) Blum et al (1973) *Cancer, 31,* 903.

Chromomycin A3

Main part of an antibiotic complex
produced by *Streptomyces griseus*   *Causal relationship* o/ +

Chromomycin derivatives produce steatosis and cellular degeneration in animal toxicity tests (1); chromomycin A3 induces also hepatic injury in man. Indeed, mild ASAT and/or APh elevations were reported in 6 of 43 patients with metastatic cancer treated with 1–1.6 mg/m²/d i.v. on 5 alternate days. Recovery occurred in the drug–free period (2). Kovach et al (4) noted abnormal ASAT and/or APh values in 7 of 38 cases, especially in patients on the highest dose (1.1 mg/m²/d x 5) (4). However, in another study (0.25–1.5 mg/m²/d, 5 alternate days) no liver enzyme elevations were reported (2).

(1) Zimmerman (1978) *Hepatotoxicity,* p 523. Appleton–Century–Crofts, New York. (2) Reynolds et al (1976) *Cancer Treat. Rep., 60,* 125. (3) Samal et al (1978) *Cancer Treat. Rep., 62,* 19. (4) Kovach et al (1973) *Cancer Treat. Rep., 57,* 341.

Dactinomycin

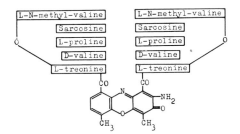

Causal relationship o

In therapeutic doses this drug is toxic mainly to the bone marrow and gastrointestinal tract; initially, only a slight increase in hepatic lipids was reported (1). Especially the combination with irradiation was held responsible for enhanced toxicity and more recently some cases of hepatic injury have been ascribed to this combination in children with Wilms' tumor (2, 3). Sudden hepatomegaly, abnormal liver function and filling defects on the liver scan suggested metastases, but spontaneous normalization took place after discontinuation. Biopsy showed non–specific changes (3) or mild necrosis and periportal fibrosis (2). The authors suggested a potentiation of dactinomycin and radiation on liver tissue. However, vincristine, administered concurrently, may also have been responsible. Another case with filling defects showed signs of veno–occlusive disease, with occlusion of central veins by connective tissue and centrilobular sinusoidal congestion. Although other cytostatics were used concomitantly, discontinuation of dactinomycin alone resulted in improvement while other drugs were continued (4). According to Abramson et al (5), the filling defects reflect response to therapy and should not be automatically interpreted as metastatic disease.

218

(1) Zimmerman (1978) *Hepatotoxicity*, p 523. Appleton–Century–Crofts, New York. (2) Jayabose et al (1976) *J. Pediatr., 88*, 898. (3) McVeagh et al (1975) *J. Pediatr., 87*, 627. (4) Callihan et al (1983) *ASCO Abstr., 76*. (5) Abramson et al (1984) *Radiology, 150*, 701.

2′–Deoxycoformycin

A nucleoside analog produced by
Streptomyces antibioticus   *Causal relationship* o

Severe hepatic injury and fever developed in 2 out of 26 pediatric patients with acute lymphoblastic anemia. Onset was 1 to several days after starting the antineoplastic course (0.75 mg/kg/d). One patient developed ascites and died. Histology showed centrilobular fatty changes (1).

(1) Poplack et al (1981) *Cancer Res., 41*, 3343.

Mithramycin

Causal relationship + +

Moderate to marked liver enzyme elevations do occur with a very high incidence of up to 50–100% (1–3, 5, 7) during treatment of both Paget's disease and neoplasms. In a study of 58 patients treated with 10–50 μg/kg/d for a variety of advanced neoplasms, up to 100% of assessments of liver enzymes and/or function tests were abnormal! (7). Histology showed centrilobular vacuolization, resembling fatty change, and necrosis. Of this group 27% died, due either to hepatic or renal toxicity or to bleeding disorders (7). Also, other studies showed liver enzyme elevations in 100% of patients treated with 25–50 μg/kg/d (3) and with 15–37.5 μg/kg/d (1). In another study (5) of 14 patients, all showing bilirubin and liver enzyme elevations, 6 had centrilobular hemorrhagic necrosis. One case of acute hepatic necrosis, accompanied by a bleeding syndrome after a 4–day course (25 μg/kg/d), ended fatally (4). Hepatic injury proved reproducible in dogs and monkeys at a dose of 100 μg/kg/d. Mice and rats were insensitive (6).

(1) Ream et al (1968) *J. Am. Med. Assoc., 204*, 96. (2) Ansfield et al (1969) *Oncology, 23*, 283. (3) Foley et al (1972) *J. Urol., 108*, 439. (4) Fraisse et al (1980) *Ann. Méd. Interne, 131*, 281. (5) Koons et al (1966) *Bull. Johns Hopk. Hosp., 118*, 462. (6) Morrison et al (1967) *Toxicol. Appl. Pharmacol., 11*, 468. (7) Kennedy (1970) *Am. J. Med., 49*, 494.

Mitomycin

H₃C... (chemical structure)

Causal relationship o/ +

Liver function abnormalities/liver enzyme changes have been observed in up to 23% of patients (1), mostly mild and not always clearly attributable to the drug. In some patients, more serious hepatocellular damage has been reported (2, 3). In dogs, large doses (110 mg/m^2 over 2 weeks) induced focal necrosis, cholestasis and fatty change (4). Studies in mice suggested that concurrent administration of fumaric acid reduced the incidence of renal and hepatic histological abnormalities (7).

Recently, several cases of veno–occlusive disease were reported after use of high doses of mitomycin followed by autologous bone marrow transplantation (5). Dose–dependency was suggested by an increasing incidence (60 mg/m^2, 3 of 14 patients, 75 mg/m^2, 2 of 9 patients; 90 mg/m^2, 2 of 3 patients; all on 3–day courses). This increase, however, was not significant. Onset varied between 15 and 70 days after mitomycin treatment. Three patterns were observed: asymptomatic, symptomatic but stable, and progressive liver failure (in 3 of 7 cases). Although other cytostatics had been used previously, liver disturbances were related in time to mitomycin use (5). Autopsy findings in 3 of these patients showed central and sublobular vein narrowing, due to edema, and a loose subintimal network of reticulum fibers (6). Sixteen comparable cases, treated with other cytostatics (16 patients) and autologous bone marrow transplantation (10 patients), showed none of these changes (6). One case of veno–occlusive disease was noted in a 39–year–old female, 2 months after starting mitomycin (cumulative dose: 72 g). No radiation, transplantation or other causative factors were present (8).

(1) Ménard et al (1980) *Gastroenterology, 78*, 142. (2) Moertel et al (1968) *J. Am. Med. Assoc., 204*, 1045. (3) Kenis et al (1964) *Chemotherapia, 8*, 114. (4) Philips et al (1960) *Cancer Res., 20*, 1354. (5) Lazarus et al (1982) *Cancer, 49*, 1789. (6) Gottfried et al (1982) *Hum. Pathol., 13*, 646. (7) Kuroda et al (1982) *Gann, 73*, 656. (8) Sakaguchi et al (1983) *Acta Hepatol. Jpn, 24*, 1036.

Rufocromomycin

(chemical structure)

Causal relationship o

Three cases of centrilobular necrosis were noted in a study of 57 patients treated for leukemia, Hodgkin's disease or sarcomas. These were attributed by the authors to too high a dose and a decrease was followed by improvement (1). Chauvergne et al (2) observed 2 cases of hepatic injury (unspecified) in a study of 166 patients.

(1) Jacquillat et al (1965) *Presse Méd., 73*, 2003. (2) Chauvergne et al (1966) *Bull. Cancer (Paris), 53*, 229.

D. ALKALOIDS

With the probable exception of indicine N–oxide and related pyrrolizidine derivatives currently being investigated for their antineoplastic properties, the alkaloids seem relatively non–toxic to the liver.

Although not yet documented, as far as we know, indicine N–oxide may be expected to cause veno–occlusive disease.

D.1. PODOPHYLLINE DERIVATIVES

Etoposide

Teniposide

Causal relationship o

These drugs (etoposide and teniposide) are related to podophyllotoxin and are used in the treatment of hematological malignancy and several solid tumors. As a spindle poison, they block cell division in the meta-

221

phase. One study showed incidental ASAT elevation in 4 of 24 patients treated with teniposide (1), whereas another study showed transient bilirubin and ASAT/APh elevations in 2 of 12 patients (1–1.5 g/m^2) (2). Two cases of a mixed to hepatocellular type of injury were noted in patients receiving high doses of etoposide for refractory germinal neoplasms. Each patient received a cumulative dose of 6800 mg/m^2; jaundice and liver enzyme elevations occurred 3 weeks after the last dose, followed by spontaneous resolution. Histology in 1 case showed diffuse necrosis with periportal and centrilobular infiltration with many eosinophils (3).

(1) Muggia et al (1971) *Cancer Chemother. Rep.*, *55*, 575. (2) Van Echo et al (1980) *Cancer Clin. Tr.*, *3*, 325. (3) Johnson et al (1983) *Cancer Treat. Rep.*, *67*, 1023.

D.2. VINCA ALKALOIDS

Vinblastine   **Vincristine**

R = CH$_3$ R = CHO

Vindesine

Causal relationship o

The vinca alkaloids (vinblastine, vincristine and vindesine) bind to tubulin of cellular microtubules and arrest cellular mitosis in the metaphase. Their main adverse effects are on the central nervous system. In high doses they induce ultrastructural changes in the hepatocytes of rats (1, 2), mainly microtubular. With exception of an initial report of patchy liver necrosis at autopsy in 5 patients (3) and an unspecified remark about destructive changes in bile ducts (4) no hepatotoxicity has been reported in man, when employed in therapeutic doses. Overdose in 1 case (25 mg)

222

with vincristine caused severe neurotoxic damage. Hepatic injury appeared 3 days after intake (5). In another case, vincristine was suspected of having a potentiating effect on radiation–induced lesions. Fatal liver injury developed 1 week after termination of radiation and vincristine (6). One study noted severe toxicity in 10 of 35 patients on this combination (7), being fatal in 1 case. It was suggested that radiation delayed the transit of vincristine through the liver and its excretion into bile. Because it is often given in combination regimens and in complicated clinical cases, it is difficult to prove or disprove its innocence. Of course, this holds true for most cytostatics.

(1) Kovacs et al (1977) *Arzneim.–Forsch., 27,* 825. (2) Rollason et al (1983) *J. Pathol., 140, 91. (3) Costa et al (1962) Cancer Chemother. Rep., 24,* 39. (4) Zimmerman (1978) *Hepatotoxicity,* p 523. Appleton–Century–Crofts, New York. (5) Thomas et al (1982) *Cancer Treat. Rep., 66,* 1967. (6) Hansen et al (1982) *Acta Med. Scand., 212,* 171. (7) Perry (1982) *Semin. Oncol., 9,* 65.

D.3. OTHER ALKALOIDS

Indicine N–oxide

A pyrrolizidine alkaloid N–oxide
isolated from *Heliotropum indicum*   *Causal relationship* o/ +

As may be expected, indicine N-oxide proved hepatotoxic in animals (1). Metabolic conversion to indicine aggravates its hepatotoxic effect. A clinical trial in 37 patients (1–9 g/m^2 every 4 weeks) with various malignant disorders demonstrated elevation of ASAT, ALAT and/or bilirubin concentrations in 7 patients, 3 of whom had abnormal pre–treatment values (1). Letendre et al (2) treating 10 patients with acute lymphocytic and non–lymphocytic leukemia (3 g/m^2/d x 5) noted jaundice and fatal hepatic failure in 2 patients while 3 others showed reversible aminotransferase elevation. An earlier study by these authors revealed mild ASAT elevation in 3 of 44 courses (2).

   Massive hepatic necrosis in a 5–year–old boy with acute myelocytic leukemia appeared 2 days after intravenous administration of a single dose of 5.6 g. No thrombosis was seen, either in the portal venous radicles or in the central veins, but sinusoids were dilated and engorged with erythrocytes (3).

(1) Ohnuma et al (1982) *Cancer Treat. Rep., 66,* 1509. (2) Letendre et al (1981) *Cancer, 47,* 437. (3) Cook et al (1983) *Cancer, 52,* 61.

E. MISCELLANEOUS/INVESTIGATIONAL

The miscellaneous group of antineoplastic agents comprises a wide variety of compounds as regards their structure and mechanism of action.

The most unequivocal hepatotoxin of this group is colaspase, which has caused liver dysfunction in 50% or more of recipients.

Many investigational agents do not pass preclinical toxicity testing. Toxicity to bone marrow, kidneys or heart often precludes clinical use. Some drugs have been abandoned because of a high incidence of jaundice in early clinical trials, e.g. 4,4'-diaminodiphenylamine (1). Several drugs currently under investigation have been associated with signs of hepatic injury, e.g. acronine (2), ACNU (3), 1-octadecyl-2-methylglycero-3-phosphocholine (4), mitoxantrone (7), mitoguazone (8), tricyclic nucleoside phosphate (9) and IMPY (10). These associations have still to be determined.

Quelamycin, triferric doxorubicin, seems to cause iron toxicity either due to excessive unbound iron in the drug preparation or to iron-chelated doxorubicin (5). Hepatocellular damage and fatty change were observed in 4 of 6 patients (40 mg/m² x 2–3 i.v.), while all patients had mild to moderate hemosiderosis after 2–8 courses (5). Liver fibrosis was present in 1 patient.

(1) Denman et al (1960) *Br. Med. J., 1,* 482. (2) Scarffe et al (1983) *Cancer Treat. Rep., 67,* 3. (3) Kimura (1982) *Jpn. Pharmacol. Ther., 10,* 3787. (4) Berdel et al (1982) *Cancer, 50,* 2011. (5) Brugarolas et al (1979) *Cancer Treat. Rep., 63,* 909. (6) Imoto et al (1979) *Ann. Intern. Med., 91,* 129. (7) Paciucci et al (1983) *Cancer Res., 43,* 3919. (8) Perry et al (1983) *Cancer Treat. Rep., 67,* 91. (9) Mittelman et al (1983) *Cancer Treat. Rep., 67,* 159. (10) Neidhart et al (1980) *Cancer Treat. Rep., 64,* 251.

Aminoglutethimide

Causal relationship +

Aminoglutethimide is an analog of the hypnotic, glutethimide. It is used mainly in the treatment of metastatic breast cancer for its blocking effect on the production of adrenal steroids. γ–GTP elevations have been reported in more than 50% of recipients (1), while transient elevations of aminotransferases were seen in up to 8% of patients (2). Cases of cholestatic jaundice (3, 4) have been observed. Fever (4), rash (3, 4), eosinophilia (3) and a prompt reaction to rechallenge (4) suggested immunoallergy.

(1) Nagel et al (1982) *Cancer Res., 42, Suppl,* 3442s. (2) Savaraj et al (1980) *Med. Pediatr. Oncol., 8,* 251. (3) Gerber et al (1982) *Ann. Intern. Med., 97,* 138. (4) Perrault et al (1984) *Ann. Intern. Med., 100,* 160.

Amsacrine (m–AMSA)

H₃CO / NHSO₂CH₃ structure...

H_3CO — — $NHSO_2CH_3$

Causal relationship o/ +

Transient ASAT and APh elevations were reported in patients treated with 50–150 mg/m²/d i.v. for 5 days (1). Hyperbilirubinemia, predominantly conjugated, seems to occur fairly frequently (1–3) and was reported in up to 25% of patients (2). In 1 study (100–200 mg/m²/d x 5–7, i.v.), 16 of 45 patients with several forms of leukemia developed APh elevation (3). Hyperbilirubinemia was frequent; 1 patient died due to hepatic failure. Histology showed severe centrilobular necrosis and fatty degeneration (3). Other cases of hepatic failure have been reported, developing within 1 month after starting therapy (5, 6). Preclinical studies in dogs demonstrated significant hepatotoxicity (4).

(1) Slevin et al (1981) *Cancer Chemother. Pharmacol., 6,* 137. (2) Arlin et al (1981) *Cancer Clin. Trials, 4,* 317. (3) Lawrence et al (1982) *Cancer Treat. Rep., 66,* 1475. (4) Henry et al (1980) *Cancer Treat. Rep., 64,* 855. (5) Appelbaum et al (1982) *Cancer Treat. Rep., 66,* 1863. (6) Panasci et al (1982) *Cancer Treat. Rep., 66,* 1596.

L–Asparaginase (colaspase)

An enzyme produced by several bacteria and fungi

Causal relationship + +

Hepatic dysfunction is one of the most significant side effects of L–asparaginase. In a study of almost 300 adults and children on this drug, several liver function tests and liver enzymes in serum became abnormal (see Table 2) (5). These figures were largely confirmed by another study (6). Plasma levels of albumin, ceruloplasmin, haptoglobin, transferrin, cholesterol and other serum proteins are depressed (1, 5). Interference with coagulation homeostasis with hemorrhage and/or thrombosis may occur

TABLE 2 *Liver function abnormalities and enzyme changes in patients treated with L-asparaginase (5)*

	Children (%)	Adults (%)
BSP retention	57	84
Albumin decrease	71	82
ASAT elevation	46	63
APh elevation	31	47
5-NT elevation	15	26
Bilirubin elevation (total)	29	51
PTT prolongation	18	
Fibrinogen decrease	97	

in 1–6% of patients, usually during the first weeks of therapy (1, 5). Histology showed fatty change (3, 4). In a study of 31 postmortem cases, who
had received L–asparaginase for various hematological malignancies, 27
(87%) had steatosis of varying degree of severity up to 261 days following
the last dose (4). The severe form was mostly present in patients treated
with the high–dose regimen (4000 IU/m^2/d or 20,000 IU/m^2/wk). Fatty
change was most prominent in the peripheral zone (4). Other studies
noted lower but still significant degrees of steatosis in almost 50% or
more of recipients (5, 6).

The mechanism of hepatic injury is unclear but must be sought in association with the drug's capacity to influence protein synthesis. Hence,
the frequently encountered hypersensitivity reactions are probably not
related to the hepatotoxic effects of the drug. Most likely steatosis results from decreased lipoprotein synthesis with subsequent decreased fat
egress, but the exact mechanism remains enigmatic. A recently tested (in
mice) glutaminase–free asparaginase from *Vibrio succinogenes* was suggested to be less hepatotoxic than the usual *E. coli* type; according to the
authors, hepatic injury in man secondary to asparagine and glutamine
depletion may be prevented by these agents (2).

(1) Cairo (1982) *Am. J. Pediatr. Hematol. Oncol., 4*, 335. (2) Durden et al (1983)
Cancer Res., 43, 1602. (3) Haskell (1981) *Cancer Treat. Rep., 65, Suppl 4*, 57. (4)
Pratt et al (1971) *Cancer, 28*, 361. (5) Oettgen et al (1970) *Cancer, 25*, 253. (6) White-
car et al (1970) *N. Engl. J. Med., 282*, 732.

Cisplatin

Cl\   /NH₃
    >Pt<
Cl/   \NH₃
                                                    Causal relationship +

Most studies noted mild and transient ALAT/ASAT elevations in a relatively low number of cases (1–4) despite an often high concentration of
cisplatin in the liver (4). One study reported an overall incidence of 34%
(5). The incidence seems to be dose–related and varies from 29% after administration of 40–50 mg/m^2 to 92% at 100 mg/m^2, both in a 2–24–hourly
infusion (5). ALAT/ASAT elevations reached their maximum during the
first 5 days and returned to normal within 9 days (5). A symptomatic case
of hepatic injury was seen by Cavelli et al (6). Two weeks after every
course, the patient had liver enzyme and bilirubin elevation with mild
jaundice. Both cholestasis, fatty change and minimal necrosis were seen
on biopsy.

(1) Jacobs et al (1978) *Cancer, 42*, 2135. (2) Hayes et al (1977) *Cancer, 39*, 1372. (3)
Lippman et al (1973) *Cancer Chemother. Rep., 57*, 191. (4) Hill et al (1975) *Cancer
Chemother. Rep., 59*, 647. (5) Vermorken et al (1982) *Neth. J. Med., 25*, 270. (6) Ca-
valli et al (1978) *Cancer Treat. Rep., 62*, 2125.

Hydroxycarbamide (hydroxyurea)

H$_2$N–CO–NHOH   *Causal relationship +*

Hydroxycarbamide, an inhibitor of DNA synthesis, has been used as both antineoplastic and antipsoriatic agent. Rare cases of mildly elevated liver enzymes have been reported (1). In 1 convincing case of considerable ASAT elevation (up to x18 normal), accompanied by fever, discontinuation resulted in complete recovery within 1 week. Rechallenge was followed almost immediately by high fever and re–elevation of hepatic enzymes, thereby strongly suggesting an immunoallergic mechanism (2).

(1) Thurman et al (1963) *Cancer Chemother. Rep., 29*, 103. (2) Heddle et al (1980) *Med. J. Aust., 1*, 121.

ICRF–187   *Causal relationship* o/+

Mild, transient ASAT elevations were observed during a 3–day course (500–1800 mg/m^2/d) (1, 2), peaking on the 8th day (2), in 3 of 23 patients (2). ALAT/ASAT elevations have been seen in dogs (3).

(1) Natale et al (1983) *Cancer Treat. Rep., 67*, 311. (2) Von Hoff et al (1981) *Cancer Treat. Rep., 65*, 249. (3) Koeller et al (1981) *Cancer Treat. Rep., 65*, 459.

Procarbazine

Causal relationship o

The frequency and importance of extrahepatic side effects outweigh the relatively mild problem of drug–induced hepatic injury. Jaundice was observed in 1 of 94 patients, with various malignancies, treated with procarbazine alone (1). Jaundice was also observed in another study, in 1 case after 10 days of treatment. The injury was hepatocellular (2). Procarbazine is a hydrazine derivative and may therefore be suspected of hepatotoxicity. A role in the development of hepatic angiosarcoma has been suggested (3), but this is still speculative.

(1) Kenis et al (1966) *Eur. J. Cancer, 2*, 51. (2) Zarrilli et al (1966) *Clin. Ter., 39*, 123. (3) Daneshmend et al (1979) *Lancet, 2*, 1249.

Spirogermanium

Causal relationship o

Hepatitis was observed in a patient with pre–existing liver disease (no further details given). Normalization of ALAT/ASAT levels occurred after discontinuation (1). Other studies have not shown hepatic toxicity (2, 3).

227

(1) Budman et al (1982) *Cancer Treat. Rep.,66,* 173. (2) Schein et al (1980) *Cancer Treat. Rep., 64,* 1051. (3) Weiselberg et al (1982) *Cancer Treat. Rep., 66,* 1675.

Urethane

$$C \underset{\displaystyle OC_2H_5}{\overset{\displaystyle NH_2}{=}} O$$

Causal relationship o/ +

Urethane is no longer used as an antineoplastic agent. Several cases of fatal hepatic damage have been ascribed to use of the drug (1–4). Usually injury was discovered 10–20 months after starting therapy (1, 3, 4). A pattern resembling veno–occlusive disease (3, 4, 6) was observed, with jaundice, hepatomegaly and ascites as clinical signs. Histology showed perisinusoidal fibrosis and fibrosis with thrombosis of the central veins (6). In another case, cirrhosis appeared after 6 years of therapy (7). Animal toxicity testing suggested damage to the central vein with secondary centrilobular edema, sinusoidal wall disruption and sinusoidal extravasation of blood cells. The authors concluded that vascular changes in urethane poisoning were much more important than direct parenchymal damage (5).

Methyl carbamate, an agent structurally related to urethane, has been reported as a cause of 4 cases of severe bridging necrosis (6). A rechallenge was positive in at least 3 of these patients.

(1) Flanagan (1955) *Arch. Intern. Med., 96,* 277. (2) Hazlett et al (1955) *Blood, 10,* 76. (3) Meacham et al (1952) *Am. J. Clin. Pathol., 22,* 22. (4) Ohler et al (1950) *N. Engl. J. Med., 243,* 984. (5) Doljanski et al (1944) *Am. J. Pathol., 20,* 945. (6) Brodsky et al (1961) *Am. J. Med., 30,* 976. (7) Jonstam (1961) *Acta Med. Scand., 170,* 701.

18. Diuretics

A. Thiazides
B. Carbonic anhydrase inhibitors
C. Aldosterone inhibitors
D. Miscellaneous

Introduction

Diuretics are often used in combination with other drugs in elderly patients and this clinical setting may complicate the assessment of a causal relationship with hepatic injury.

Hepatic complications from diuretics are 3–fold. Firstly, these agents, especially the highly potent ones (e.g. furosemide), may precipitate hepatic encephalopathy. Secondly, there is some epidemiological evidence that they are associated with an enhanced incidence of gallbladder disease. The significance of this association, however, has not yet been elucidated. Thirdly, diuretics, with the exception of tienilic acid, are a very rare cause of hepatic injury. Although some of them are toxic in animal tests when given in high doses (e.g. furosemide), in therapeutic doses in man most diuretics appear to cause a mainly cholestatic to mixed pattern of injury as an idiosyncratic effect of unknown mechanism. Rarely, liver enzyme elevations or symptomatic hepatic injury have been ascribed to less commonly used diuretics such as amiloride (1), methylclothiazide (2), indapamide (3) and bumetanide (4).

(1) Heffernan (1968) *Lancet, 1*, 361. (2) Anonymous (1979) *Jpn. Med. Gaz., 16*, 12. (3) Butaeye et al (1979) *Nouv. Presse Méd., 8*, 1516. (4) Murchison et al (1975) *Br. J. Clin. Pharmacol., 2*, 87.

A. THIAZIDES

Chlorothiazide

Causal relationship o

Cholestatic hepatitis was reported in 1 case after 2 weeks of treatment, with recovery in 2 months. Jaundice was the only sign observed (1). One case was reported of a primary biliary cirrhosis–like pattern with peri-portal necrosis and fibrosis, expanded portal tracts with granulomata and bile duct proliferation. There was extensive bile stasis. This hepatic injury was discovered after more than 2 years of treatment with chloro-thiazide (2).

The epidemiological association observed between acute cholecystitis and the use of thiazide–containing drugs (3) has been challenged (4) and needs confirmation.

(1) Drerup et al (1958) *N. Engl. J. Med., 259,* 534. (2) Huseby (1964) *Am. J. Dig. Dis., 9,* 439. (3) Rosenberg et al (1980) *N. Engl. J. Med., 303,* 546. (4) Porter et al (1981) *N. Engl. J. Med., 304,* 954.

Chlortalidone

Causal relationship o

Cholestatic hepatitis, starting after several weeks of treatment, was re-ported in a pregnant (!) woman (3rd trimester); she recovered fully after discontinuation of treatment. Biopsy showed central bile accumulation and scattered areas of cell drop–out with a mild portal and lobular lym-phocytic infiltrate; there was bile duct proliferation (1).

(1) Klatskin (1975) In: Schiff (Ed), *Diseases of the Liver, 4th ed,* p 604. Lippincott, Philadelphia.

Metolazone

Causal relationship o

An occasional case is reported in the medical literature (1). Hepatomega-ly was discovered 12 weeks after starting treatment. Rash and peripheral eosinophilia were absent. Biopsy showed portal granulomas with small epithelioid cells. Focal collections of eosinophils and plasma cells were present. No other causes (e.g. sarcoidosis, tuberculosis, fungi etc.) were found.

(1) McMaster et al (1981) *Lab. Invest., 44,* 61.

Polythiazide

Causal relationship o

Four patients developed 'non–specific drug–induced hepatitis with cho-

230

lestasis' (1) defined as (peri)portal inflammation with mainly lympho-cytes and histiocytes, a frequent admixture of neutrophils and eosino-phils, piecemeal necrosis, mild intralobular necrosis and prominent cho-lestasis (no further details were given) (1).

(1) Popper et al (1965) *Arch. Intern. Med., 115,* 128.

Quinethazone

Causal relationship o/+

Cholestatic jaundice appeared after 7 weeks of treatment (1). Biopsy showed centrilobular bile staining of hepatocytes, cellular unrest and a mild portal infiltrate of mononuclear cells; scattered eosinophils were observed in the sinusoids. Rechallenge was positive within 1 week (1).

(1) Hutchison et al (1946) *Curr. Ther. Res., 6,* 199.

Trichlormethiazide

Causal relationship o

An occasional case of hepatic injury is reported in the literature (1). A pattern of hepatosplenomegaly, lymphadenopathy and peripheral eosino-philia appeared 1 week after starting treatment. Bone marrow biopsy re-vealed granulomas. Liver biopsy showed non–caseating epithelioid cell granulomas with central nuclear fragmentation. No other causes (sarcoi-dosis, tuberculosis, fungi etc.) were found.

(1) McMaster et al (1981) *Lab. Invest., 44,* 61.

B. CARBONIC ANHYDRASE INHIBITORS

Acetazolamide

Causal relationship o

An occasional case of hepatic injury has been reported in a patient who developed jaundice and rash 1 month after starting therapy for glauco-ma. The combination of hepatic injury, dehydration, circulatory failure and renal failure was fatal. Histology showed intracellular and canalicu-lar cholestasis and widespread patchy steatosis. A mediastinal Hodgkin's lymphoma was found but not held responsible for the fatal reaction (1). See also 'Sulfonamides'.

(1) Kristinsson (1967) *Br. J. Ophthalmol., 51,* 348.

Methazolamide

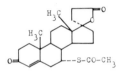

Causal relationship o

One case of cholestatic hepatitis was observed with jaundice, rash and subsequent pure red cell aplasia (1). Onset occurred within $2^1/_2$ weeks after initial intake, with normalization in 1 year. Biopsy showed marked cholestasis and bile thrombi in dilated canaliculi; there was mononuclear portal infiltration. Injury occurred despite concurrent use of prednisone. See also 'Sulfonamides'.

(1) Krivoy et al (1981) *Arch. Intern. Med., 141,* 1229.

C. ALDOSTERONE INHIBITORS

Spironolactone

Causal relationship o/ +

Asymptomatic and moderate elevation of ALAT/ASAT and APh was observed in a patient with secondary hyperaldosteronism after 2 months of treatment (300 mg/d); normalization occurred within 8 weeks after discontinuation. Biopsy showed hepatocellular unrest, rare foci of cellular infiltration and mild portal fibrosis (1). Retreatment, $1^1/_2$ years later, with 200 mg/d resulted in elevated liver enzymes after 1 month. Recovery occurred in 6 weeks after discontinuation.

(1) Shuck et al (1981) *Ann. Intern. Med., 95,* 708.

D. MISCELLANEOUS DIURETICS

Etacrynic acid

Causal relationship o/ +

Hepatocellular injury with mild jaundice starting after 2 weeks therapy

232

was reported in an emaciated patient with congestive heart failure; normalization occurred 3 weeks after discontinuation. Biopsy showed chronic venous congestion with dilated veins and congested sinusoids with minimal necrosis. In addition, a pattern of diffuse focal necrosis was observed (1). Rechallenge was positive twice (7 and 1 week latency time) with coma after the second challenge; the patient died 1 week later. Although there was a clear temporal relationship underlining a causal role for etacrynic acid, the underlying cardiac failure was probably partly responsible for the injury.

(1) Datey et al (1967) *Br. Med. J., 2,* 152.

Furosemide

Causal relationship o/ +

High doses (approximate threshold > 100 mg/kg) induced centrilobular necrosis in mice; pretreatment with phenobarbital changed necrosis from centrilobular to midzonal. Toxicity was related to the free fraction of furosemide, which expanded after saturation of plasma proteins (1). However, the incidence of furosemide–induced hepatic injury is low when it is given in a therapeutic dose. Several cases of jaundice have been reported, either unspecified (2) or secondary to a high dose and accompanied by severe dehydration (3, 7); more recently, liver enzyme elevations and jaundice were reported in 2 patients treated with therapeutic doses (3). In 1 of these patients reinstitution on methylclothiazide was again followed by mild liver enzyme elevation.

The increased risk of side effects in patients with liver cirrhosis (4), e.g. electrolyte disturbances, volume depletion and hepatic coma, is of course well–known.

Some reports of cholelithiasis in premature infants treated for respiratory distress syndrome with total parenteral nutrition and furosemide are interesting (5, 6). The mechanism is unknown and the association with furosemide may be coincidental. Nevertheless, furosemide appears to have some effect on biliary secretion, as demonstrated in dogs where it stimulated biliary secretion and its components by 75–150% (8).

(1) Mitchell et al (1975) *Gastroenterology, 68,* 392. (2) Dargie et al (1975) In: Dukes (Ed), *Meyler's Side Effects of Drugs, 8th ed,* p 483. Excerpta Medica, Amsterdam. (3) Anonymous (1979) *Jpn. Med. Gaz., 16,* 12. (4) Naranjo et al (1979) *Clin. Pharmacol. Ther., 25,* 154. (5) Whitington et al (1980) *J. Pediatr., 97,* 647. (6) Callahan et al (1982) *Radiology, 143,* 437. (7) Burmeister et al (1972) *Med. Klin., 67,* 1401. (8) Wallach et al (1983) *J. Clin. Pharmacol., 23,* 401.

Tienilic acid (ticrynafen)

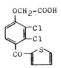

Causal relationship + +

Many cases have been reported (1–12), mainly of hepatocellular injury, acute as well as chronic. Lafey et al (12) described 37 French cases. The average duration of therapy till the onset of overt disease was 106 days (range 9 days–$3\frac{1}{2}$ years) in the French cases but 4 weeks (range 2–8 weeks) in a series of possible cases reported to the FDA (3). Digestive complaints, pruritus and fever were prodromal in 60–70% (3, 12); 75% were women in the French study (12) but 44% in the FDA cases. Rash/eosinophilia was not encountered except in 1 case (4). A lymphocyte stimulation test was negative (1), but leukocyte migration inhibition (8) and basophil degranulation testing (9) were positive. Rechallenge was positive (1–5, 9–12), in some cases in 24 hours. The reaction was fatal in 14% (12); other fatal cases have also been described (2). The incidence of hepatitis due to this agent was estimated at 0.002–0.02% (7, 13). Biopsy showed, besides mostly diffuse necrosis, a pattern of chronic active hepatitis (2, 4, 5, 12); cirrhosis (2, 5, 12) may be present. Cholestasis (6–9) seems secondary to necrosis. A peculiar feature is the presence of a serum liver/kidney Type 2 microsomal antibody, differing from the more usual type (2, 4, 5, 12), which was considered as specific for tienilic acid (12, 15). In a large analysis of 340 probable and possible cases reported to the FDA and the manufacturer, Zimmerman et al (16) largely confirmed the picture described above (see Table 1). Comparison of the demographic characteristics of the population exposed to tienilic acid with the group developing hepatic injury suggested a higher risk for females over 60 years (16). Unfortunately, they did not analyse the 'possible' and 'likely' cases separately.

The mechanism is unknown. Fever, accelerated reaction to rechallenge, the liver/kidney Type 2 antibody and the apparent dose–independence seem compatible with an immunoallergic reaction. The often–long latent period favors metabolic idiosyncrasy, especially in view of the absence of rash and eosinophilia in most cases. In fact, evidence for a reactive metabolite was obtained from experiments in perfused rat liver (14).

This drug was withdrawn by the manufacturers in some countries because of several reports of fatalities.

(1) Groussin et al (1979) *Méd. Chir. Dig., 8,* 463. (2) Poupon et al (1980) *Nouv. Presse Méd., 9,* 1881. (3) *ADR Highlights, 17 Jan.,* 1980. (4) Eugène et al (1980) *Nouv. Presse Méd., 9,* 1885. (5) Pariente et al (1981) *Gastroénterol. Clin. Biol., 5,* 567. (6) Schumacher et al (1981) *Med. Welt, 32,* 402. (7) Manier et al (1982) *Am. J. Gastroenterol., 77,* 401. (8) Simon et al (1981) *Ouest Méd., 34,* 721. (9) Mechali et al (1980) *Thérapie, 35,* 197. (10) Bousquet et al (1980) *Thérapie, 35,* 205. (11) Manigand et al (1980) *Gaz. Méd. Fr., 87,* 395. (12) Lafay et al (1983) *Gastroenterol. Clin.*

TABLE 1 *Clinical, biochemical and histological data from a study of 340 tienilic-acid-associated cases of hepatic injury*

Dosage	250 mg/d	80%	
	500 mg/d	20%	
Onset	<30 days therapy	ca. 10%	⎫
	30-150 days	ca. 80%	⎬ (192 cases)
	>150 days	ca. 10%	⎭
Symptoms, signs	Jaundice	48%	⎫
	Rash	3.4%	⎪
	Fever	15%	⎬ (87 likely cases)
	Nausea/vomiting	38%	⎪
	Viral-like illness	8%	⎭
	Eosinophilia	1.5% (340)	
Fatality	All cases	7.3% (340)	
	Jaundiced cases	10.2% (246)	
ALAT ≥ ASAT		75% (150)	
ASAT > 300 IU		80%	⎫ (322)
ASAT > 1000 IU		38%	⎭
Positive rechallenge		94% (16)	
Histology: Acute pattern		74%	⎫
	Spotty panlobular necrosis/degeneration	18.5%	⎪
	Submassive (zone 2+3)	51.9%	⎪
	Massive (zone 1+2+3)	3.7%	⎬ (27)
	Chronic pattern	26%	⎪
	Chronic active hepatitis	7.4%	⎪
	Cirrhosis	14.8%	⎪
	Undetermined	3.7%	⎭

( ) number of cases on which the percentage is based. Adapted from Zimmerman et al (16) (91/249 possibly/likely related to intake).

Biol., 7, 523. (13) McMahon (1983) *J. Am. Med. Assoc., 249*, 481. (14) Zimmerman et al (1982) *Hepatology, 2*, 255. (15) Homberg et al (1984) *Clin. Exp. Immunol., 55*, 561. (16) Zimmerman et al (1984) *Hepatology, 4*, 215.

Trometamol

$H_2N-C\begin{smallmatrix} CH_2OH \\ -CH_2OH \\ CH_2OH \end{smallmatrix}$

Causal relationship +

Trometamol in concentrated solution is highly alkaline and may cause phlebitis and vasospasm when injected into small veins. In 22 of 67 new-

born infants with respiratory distress syndrome, administration of trometamol (1.2 M, pH 10.2) and bicarbonate into the umbilical vein against
acidosis caused severe hepatic damage. Histology at autopsy showed extensive periportal hemorrhagic liver necrosis. Those receiving the solution via the umbilical artery or bicarbonate alone via the umbilical vein
were not affected (1). However, in some other cases injection into the umbilical artery caused severe hemorrhagic multisystem necrosis, being fatal in 1 of them (2). These problems are to be expected when the solution
is too alkaline and/or too rapidly injected.

(1) Goldenberg et al (1968) *J. Am. Med. Assoc., 205,* 81. (2) Rehder et al (1974)
Arch. Dis. Child., 49, 76.

19. Sex hormones

A. Sex hormones
B. Sex hormone antagonists

A. SEX HORMONES

The 3 groups of sex hormones are estrogens, androgens and progestogens of which estradiol, testosterone and progesterone are the main natural representatives. Several synthetic analogs have been produced to facilitate oral treatment, to enhance the effect, to dissociate various physiological effects or to associate these effects. In most cases this has been done by removal or substitution of alkyl and other groups at the C–17 and/or C–19 position.

Both natural and synthetic sex hormones are metabolized by the mixed–function oxidase system; by competition and induction they may interact with the metabolism and thus with the effect of several endogenous and exogenous substances. This subject is not discussed here, with the exception of precipitation of porphyria.

Natural androgens and progestagens do not have a cholestatic effect, at least not in physiological conditions and amounts. However, markedly increased levels of natural estrogens in the last trimester of pregnancy, in combination with individual susceptibility, are held responsible for cholestasis of pregnancy (1).

Most experience regarding liver dysfunction has been obtained from the use of orally administered synthetic estrogens and androgens as contraceptive and anabolic agents, respectively. Both groups have been demonstrated as a cause of dose–dependent cholestasis, whereas progestagens are usually devoid of such effects (5).

Sex steroids inhibit BSP excretion both in animals (2, 4) and in man (1, 3). Uptake or conjugation is not affected (1, 2). This is secondary to the chemical configuration of the molecule rather than to the androgenic, estrogenic or progestational potency of the compounds (3). For enhanced BSP retention, C–3 oxylation (C–3 ketone group > C–3 hydroxyl group) (3) and C–17 alkylation (methyl group > longer side–chain) (4) are important. Saturation of the A–ring (see Fig. 1 and Table 1) reduces BSP retention (4). Hydroxylation or methoxylation at C–1 or C–2 decreases BSP retention (2). Glucuronidation of C–16 and/or C–17 of estrogens and testosterone produces compounds which markedly inhibit bile flow in rats (6).

In high therapeutic doses, androgens may lead to a high incidence of jaundice. During treatment of 254 cases of aplastic anemia, treated with a high dose (1–2.5 mg/kg/d oxymetholone, metenolone, metandienone or norethandrolone) for 10–20 months, overt jaundice was noted in 17.3%, while in 18.2% liver function tests or liver enzymes were abnormal. Fifty percent of abnormalities occurred within the first 4 months and 80% before the 10th month (7). On the other hand, Westaby et al (8) found no cases of jaundice in 60 patients on long–term therapy with methyltestosterone (150 mg/d), although 1 patient had biochemical evidence of cholestasis; 19 patients incidentally had elevated ASAT levels which were unrelated to duration of therapy. In a study of 13 patients treated with 100–400 mg/d of danazol or 1–5 mg/d of stanozolol, a moderate elevation of aminotransferase levels occurred in 3. Histology was not considered significant except for giant mitochondria and intracanalicular bile pigment without marked cholestasis (96). According to an older study, 24 of 31 patients with methyltestosterone–associated jaundice developed this sign between 1 and 6 months after starting therapy. It was also evident from these data that impairment of BSP excretion starts immediately after first intake (9).

High doses of estradiol, a natural estrogen, causes BSP retention in animals (2) and man (1). Especially the 17–ethinyl substituted derivatives have a cholestatic effect (5).

Removal of the C–19 methyl group and addition of a C–17 ethinyl group to progesterone has produced progestagens which may cause cholestatic jaundice, e.g. norethynodrel and norethisterone. This may be partly explained by transformation in vivo to estrogens (5). One report even mentioned jaundice in up to 6% of recipients (35) and estimated the incidence from several studies at 2–3%. These synthetic progestagens also reduced BSP excretion and bile flow in animals (5).

Cholestatic jaundice in users of oral contraceptives is of course much rarer than in users of androgens for aplastic anemia or other conditions. The dose of estrogen in oral contraceptives is much lower and the incidence of this effect has been estimated at 1:4000 in Sweden and other high–incidence areas (e.g. Chile) versus 1:10,000 cases elsewhere (5). Patients with recurrent intrahepatic cholestasis (10), cholestasis of pregnancy (11), Dubin–Johnson syndrome (12) or underlying liver diseases such as primary biliary cirrhosis (13) are more likely to react with cholestatic jaundice to oral contraceptives.

Clinically (5, 13) the syndrome may start with malaise, anorexia and nausea, usually during the first or second cycle. Pruritus is frequent and may be the only sign. Conjugated bilirubin in the serum may be very high but usually remains below 170 μmol/l. The APh level is usually markedly elevated. Mild to moderate ASAT/ALAT elevations are frequent but may be normal in the characteristic pattern of pure cholestasis. Occasionally very high aminotransferase levels suggest serious hepatic necrosis (15).

Histology shows bile plugging and intracellular bile pigment, mainly centrilobular. Hepatocytes are otherwise normal or show mild degenera-

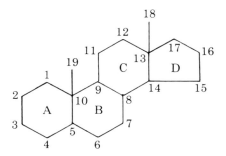

FIG. 1 *Structural formula of the sex hormones.*

TABLE 1 *Structural differences of some important sex hormones*

	A-ring (double bonds)	C-3	C-17	C-19 (present,+; absent,−)
Androgens				
Testosterone	C_4-C_5	=O	-OH	+
Methyltestosterone	C_4-C_5	=O	-OH	+
			...CH_3	
Norethandrolone	C_4-C_5	=O	-OH	−
			...C_2H_5	
Estrogens				
Estradiol	C_1-C_2,C_3-C_4, C_5-C_{10}	-OH	-OH	−
Ethinylestradiol	C_1-C_2,C_3-C_4, C_5-C_{10}	-OH	-OH	−
			...$C{\equiv}CH$	
Progestins				
Progesterone	C_4-C_5	=O	-CO-CH_3	+
Norethisterone	C_4-C_5	=O	-H	−
			...$C{\equiv}CH$	
Ethinylestrenol	C_4-C_5		-OH	−
			...$C{\equiv}CH$	

tion; sometimes necrosis of single cells is present. Inflammatory cells are absent or scarce. Although usually rapidly reversible, prolonged choles-tasis may occur despite discontinuation of the drug (13). Although cho-lestasis is considered to be characteristic for oral contraceptives, occa-sional studies suggest that a hepatitic component may be frequent (16).

Noteworthy is a recent report on non–alcoholic steatohepatitis induc-ed by high doses of synthetic estrogens for several months to years for the treatment of prostate carcinoma. None of the patients used excessive amounts of alcohol. Histology showed steatonecrosis, intralobular neu-trophils and prominent centrilobular fibrosis (36).

The *mechanism* is probably analogous for all sex steroids. Most data suggest that compositional changes in membrane lipids may be responsi-ble for estrogen–induced cholestasis. A change in the membrane choles-terol/phospholipid molar ratio, phospholipid polar head group composi-tion and/or in the degree of saturation and branching of fatty acids may affect membrane fluidity (37), with a secondary decrease in biliary excre-tory function. Inhibition of $(Na^+ + K^+)$–ATPase is probably not the pri-mary cause, as was previously thought, but secondary to this change in membrane fluidity (38). In an in–vitro perfused rat liver system, infusion of sodium taurocholate prevented estrogen–induced cholestasis, proba-bly by increased micellar solubilization, and facilitated biliary excretion of the estrogen (14). Elias et al (105) suggested that increased tight–junc-tion permeability could facilitate reflux of biliary constituents from bile to plasma via the paracellular pathway; however, according to Jaeschke et al (104) altered permeability of this pathway may be the cause of *a*–naphthylisothiocyanate–induced cholestasis but is not the primary event in ethinylestradiol cholestasis.

Several vascular complications have been associated with the use of sex steroids. Sinusoidal dilatation has been noted both in patients on high–dose androgens for several years (17) and in oral contraceptive us-ers (16, 18–20). The localization was mainly periportal to midzonal (18–20). A study in rats on ethinylestradiol suggested that constriction in Zone III of Rappaport and subsequent increased pressure in Zone I ac-counted for the predominance of dilatation in the latter zone (21). Paradi-nas et al (17), also found centrilobular sinusoidal dilatation and did not note a particularly zonal preponderance; their study was in androgen–treated patients however, which may possibly produce a different pat-tern. These authors found subendothelial accumulation of hepatocytes in the central veins up to the point of complete obliteration and suggest-ed this as a causative factor (17).

Besides mild to moderate hepatomegaly, sinusoidal dilatation hardly produces any symptoms and little is known about its prevalence. In a study of biopsies of 155 oral contraceptive users, sinusoidal dilatation was noted in 73 (40.7%) (16), which at least suggests that sinusoidal dila-tation may be more common than was previously thought.

Peliotic changes are often seen in areas of sinusoidal dilatation (16–18). Usually, however, blood–filled cavities are randomly distributed throughout the liver (22). Peliosis hepatis has been associated most fre-quently with androgens (8, 17, 23–30). In some of these cases non–C–17–alkylated compounds had been used (23, 26, 30). Peliosis hepatis has been associated occasionally with progestagens (30) and estrogens alone (25, 33). Frank *peliosis hepatis* has rarely been associated with oral contra-ceptives alone (79), but peliotic changes are common in patients with oral–contraceptive–associated liver tumors.

Hemangiomas have occasionally been associated with use of oral con-

240

traceptives (34), but a causal relationship remains speculative.

The *Budd–Chiari syndrome* has been associated with oral contraceptive use in a number of cases. It manifests as abdominal pain, ascites and hepatomegaly which may present acutely or insidiously, depending on the number of obliterated veins and rapidity of onset. Tsung et al (39) reported a case and reviewed the literature. Of the 18 cases reported only 6 recovered. The remaining 12 died 3 weeks to $1\frac{1}{2}$ years after the first symptoms. The latent period between first intake of oral contraceptives and first symptoms varied from 2 weeks to 8 years. In 9 patients, not only the large hepatic veins were affected; histology showed a veno–occlusive disease–like pattern with intimal proliferation and fibrosis with necrosis, sinusoidal dilatation and erythrocyte extravasation in the centrilobular area (39, 40). Additional cases have been reported since, mainly with analogous features (41, 42) including one associated with a progestagen (51). In one of these cases a hepatic adenoma was present (41), as was noted previously (40). One study demonstrated antibodies against ethinylestradiol in 7 patients with oral–contraceptive–associated Budd–Chiari syndrome and suggested a role in the formation of immune–complexes with subsequent thrombosis (42).

Jacobs (103) associated hepatic artery thrombosis, and subsequent infarction, with the intake of oral contraceptives. According to the author, concurrent use of propranolol could have contributed to infarction by a decrease in blood flow. Another case with infarction and bile lake formation was reported by Peterson et al (111).

Although not proven, there can be little doubt that use of oral contraceptives may increase the incidence of *hepatocellular adenomas*. Previously a rare tumor, more than 100 cases were reported within 5 years (19, 43) after the first report of this association (44). Two studies (45, 46) demonstrated that the duration of use was related to an increased relative risk. However, their estimation was different, varying from a relative risk of 16.3 (45) to 503 (46), both after 85 months or more. Vana et al (47) demonstrated that the age distribution of women with benign liver tumors in oral contraceptive users showed a clear peak in the 26–30 year group, whereas in non–users the tumors occurred largely in older women.

In a compilation of the literature Klatskin (19) compared 79 cases of oral–contraceptive–associated adenomas with 138 liver adenomas not related to these agents. Besides a preponderance in the middle–aged group, oral contraceptive users had larger and more frequently ruptured or hemorrhagic tumors.

Regression after discontinuation has been reported on several occasions (19, 43, 49, 50), although progressive growth may nevertheless take place (48). Androgens have also been associated with adenomas (8), even after use of non–C–17–alkylated derivatives (100).

Unlike adenomas which consist of (sometimes encapsulated) areas of more or less normal liver cells without bile ducts or septa and with thin–walled vessels, focal nodular hyperplasia is a lobular tumor with a large central scar with fibrous septa radiating to the periphery. The fibrous areas contain bile ductules and thick–walled blood vessels and sometimes mononuclear infiltration. Liver cells look normal (13, 32). Focal nodular hyperplasia has never been a very rare lesion and is often found in men, sometimes ascribed to the use of androgens (110). It is not so closely related to hormone use as the adenoma (13). Series published before and after the introduction of oral contraceptives showed mainly analogous epidemiological features (32). It is not impossible, however, that oral contraceptives have some effect on pre–existing focal nodular hyperplasia, since these were larger in users who presented more frequently with bleeding (19). Sometimes discontinuation of oral contraceptives leads to apparent regression of focal nodular hyperplasia (98, 99). A potentially confounding factor, however, is the fact that they may show overlapping features with the adenomas (32). A small sample from a large nodule may mimic adenoma.

The association between sex hormones and hepatocellular carcinoma is still in doubt. Gala et al (53) reviewed 25 reported oral–contraceptive–associated cases. The average age of the patients was 31 years, which may be expected of oral contraceptive users but is uncommon for this type of cancer. The average duration of oral contraceptive use was 5.34 years (range 0.5–12 years). The clinical presentation was the usual for this type of cancer, but serum a–fetoprotein was elevated in only 1 of 13 patients. In some patients metastases were demonstrated (53, 97). Focal nodular hyperplasia was present in 4 patients. The prognosis seems better than for non–oral–contraceptive–associated hepatocellular carcinoma (53). There are several reasons for suspecting a relationship between these tumors and oral contraceptive use, e.g. the uncommon presentation of the tumor in young female patients without cirrhosis, the less frequently elevated a–fetoprotein level, long survival, less metastatic disease, localization amid adenomas (19, 54–56) or focal nodular hyperplastic areas (57) and reproducibility in animals (52). On the other hand, there is some doubt about whether 'steroid hepatocellular carcinoma' is a real carcinoma since a histological distinction between adenoma and carcinoma may be very difficult in these cases (32). Moreover, the epidemiological evidence for an association is still not conclusive (58). According to a recent study an etiological association is lacking since the apparent increase in hepatocellular carcinomas in young women could be explained by the presence of cases of fibrolamellar ('scirrhous') carcinoma in this age group (59). The incidence of this tumor is high in young adults of both sexes and this could coincide with oral contraceptive use (59). On the other hand, Henderson et al (101) demonstrated a highly significant difference in the incidence and duration of oral contraceptive use in a group of women with hepatocellular carcinoma when compared with age–matched neighborhood controls; however, their study was small. In an analysis of mortality rates over the last 24 years, there was a small but consistent increase in the number of women with primary liver cancer in the 20–39 year age–group. This increase, however, was not

242

seen in other countries (102). It is clear that, despite the continuing reporting of cases in oral contraceptive users (61, 62, 97) and in men treated with estrogens for prostate carcinoma (63, 64), an association may be suspected but is far from clear. Other malignant tumors occasionally associated with oral contraceptives are angiosarcoma (65, 66), cholangiocarcinoma (60, 64, 67–70) and hepatoblastoma (71). A relationship has still to be proven.

Cases of hepatocellular carcinoma or tumors resembling hepatocellular carcinoma have also been associated with androgens, several of recent date (72–78, 109). Cap et al (76) described a case of a 10–year–old boy who died after rupture and shock due to a hepatocellular carcinoma ascribed to 5 years of intermittent therapy (76). Also, in androgen–associated cases, a–fetoprotein is often negative (80). Although the malignant potential has been doubted (52), some reports mentioned metastases (81, 82). Besides carcinomas reports concerning angiocarcinoma (83) and cholangiocarcinoma (32, 78) have appeared. One of these mentioned both cholangiocarcinoma and hepatocellular carcinoma in 1 patient (78), which is not surprising since mixed forms exist and differentiation may sometimes be difficult.

The mechanism of a carcinogenic effect of sex steroids is largely unknown. Several studies favor a tumor–promoting effect rather than initiation (84, 85), possibly due to failure to establish normal intercell contact and loss of normal contact inhibition (86) and/or by an increase in mitotic activity (85). One should however realize that these effects occur at 200–fold the usual contraceptive dose. In a study in rats all sex steroids had a tumor–promoting effect (84). In some studies the development of preneoplasms, hyperplastic nodules and hepatocellular carcinomas in rats fed with oral contraceptives for 1–2 years suggests a possible initiating effect (52, 106).

Women on long–term oral contraceptive use showed a 2–fold higher incidence of surgically confirmed gallbladder disease than non–users (87). An analogous increase was observed in postmenopausal women taking estrogens (88). A comparison between 2 groups of 50 women (similar age and parity; one group with, the other without gallstones) demonstrated a significantly higher incidence of oral contraceptive use (89). Bennion et al (90) demonstrated increased cholesterol saturation and a change in bile acid composition. In the bile there is an increase in cholesterol concentration and a decrease in the concentration, pool size (especially chenodeoxycholate) and synthesis rate of bile acids during oral contraceptive use (91). From a study in which individual bile acids were assessed, it appeared that the newer 'low–estrogen' pills are also able to change the bile composition by a marked increase in cholic acid pool size and synthesis, whereas other bile acids showed a minor decrease (108). A large case–control study of long–term oral contraceptive use suggested no overall incidence of gallbladder disease (cholelithiasis and cholecystitis); however, the development and presentation of the disease in susceptible women may be accelerated (92).

243

Progestagens and their metabolites induce aminolevulinic acid synthetase in animal hepatocyte cultures (93, 94), apparently more strongly than androgens and estrogens (94). Nevertheless, all sex steroids including estrogens may probably precipitate porphyria in man (95). Most hepatic porphyrias may probably be precipitated, e.g. acute intermittent porphyria and porphyria cutanea tarda. In the latter group, inhibition by estrogens/oral contraceptives of a hereditarily decreased activity of uroporphyrinogen–decarboxylase was suggested (107).

(1) Kappas (1968) N. Engl. J. Med., 278, 378. (2) Gallagher et al (1966) Medicine, 45, 471. (3) DeLorimer et al (1965) Arch. Intern. Med., 116, 289. (4) Lennon (1966) Steroids, 7, 157. (5) Metreau et al (1972) Digestion, 7, 318. (6) Meyers et al (1981) J. Pharmacol. Exp. Ther., 218, 63. (7) Pecking et al (1980) Nouv. Rev. Fr. Hématol., 22, 257. (8) Westaby et al (1977) Lancet, 2, 261. (9) Zimmerman (1963) Ann. NY Acad. Sci., 104, 954. (10) De Pagter et al (1976) Gastroenterology, 71, 202. (11) Orellana–Alcalde et al (1966) Lancet, 2, 1278. (12) Cohen et al (1972) Gastroenterology, 62, 1182. (13) Sherlock (1980) In: Farber et al (Eds), Toxic Injury of the Liver, Part B, p 597. Marcel Dekker, New York. (14) Adinolfi et al (1984) Hepatology, 4, 30. (15) Ockner et al (1968) N. Engl. J. Med., 276, 331. (16) Mölleken (1979) Zbl. Allg. Pathol. Pathol. Anat., 123, 195. (17) Paradinas et al (1977) Histopathology, 1, 225. (18) Winkler et al (1975) Scand. J. Gastroenterol., 10, 699. (19) Klatskin (1977) Gastroenterology, 73, 386. (20) Camilleri et al (1981) Gastroenterology, 80, 810. (21) Raufman et al (1980) Gastroenterology, 79, 1174. (22) Zafrani et al (1983) Arch. Intern. Med., 143, 495. (23) Burger et al (1952) Am. J. Clin. Pathol., 22, 569. (24) Bernstein et al (1971) N. Engl. J. Med., 284, 1135. (25) Naeim et al (1973) Arch. Pathol. Lab. Med., 95, 284. (26) Bagheri et al (1974) Ann. Intern. Med., 81, 610. (27) Groos et al (1974) Lancet, 1, 874. (28) Nadell et al (1977) Arch. Pathol. Lab. Med., 101, 405. (29) Taxy (1978) Hum. Pathol., 9, 331. (30) Karasawa et al (1979) Acta Pathol. Jpn., 29, 457. (31) Contostavlos (1973) Lancet, 1, 1200. (32) Portmann et al (1981) In: Davis et al (Eds), Drug Reactions and the Liver, p 290. Pitman Medical, London. (33) Puppala et al (1979) Postgrad. Med. J., 65, 277. (34) Kositchek et al (1970) Calif. Med., 113, 70. (35) Langlands et al (1975) Lancet, 1, 584. (36) Seki et al (1983) Gastroenterol Jpn., 18, 197. (37) Schreiber et al (1983) Hepatology, 3, 607. (38) Simon et al (1980) J. Clin. Invest., 65, 851. (39) Tsung et al (1980) J. Clin. Lab. Sci., 10, 518. (40) Alpert (1976) Hum. Pathol., 7, 709. (41) Pees et al (1983) Med. Welt, 34, 722. (42) Beaumont et al (1982) J. Med., 13, 339. (43) Warren et al (1979) Drug Intell. Clin. Pharm., 13, 680 (Part I), 741 (Part II). (44) Baum et al (1973) Lancet, 2, 926. (45) Edmondson (1976) N. Engl. J. Med., 294, 470. (46) Rooks et al (1979) J. Am. Med. Assoc., 242, 644. (47) Vana et al (1977) J. Am. Med. Assoc., 238, 2154. (48) Mariconi (1979) Gastroenterology, 77, 1319. (49) Steinbrecher et al (1981) Dig. Dis. Sci., 26, 1045. (50) Bühler et al (1982) Gastroenterology, 82, 775. (51) Girardin et al (1983) Gastroenterology, 84, 630. (52) Imai (1983) Acta Hepatol. Jpn., 24, 182. (53) Gala et al (1983) J. Surg. Oncol., 22, 11. (54) Neuberger et al (1980) Lancet, 1, 273. (55) Tesluk et al (1981) Arch. Pathol. Lab. Med., 105, 296. (56) Kerlin et al (1983) Gastroenterology, 84, 994. (57) Davis et al (1975) Br. Med. J., 4, 496. (58) Vana et al (1979) NY State J. Med., 49, 321. (59) Goodman et al (1983) Hepatology, 2, 440. (60) Porter et al (1981) Pharmacotherapy, 1, 160. (61) Shar et al (1982) Cancer, 49, 407. (62) Gatewood Dudley et al (1982) Diagn. Gynecol. Obstet., 4, 301. (63) Rosinus et al (1981) Schweiz. Med. Wochenschr., 111, 1139. (64) De Pagter et al (1979) Ned. Tijdschr. Geneeskd., 123, 881. (65) Shi et al (1981) Med. J. Aust., 1, 473. (66) Monroe et al (1981) J. Am. Med. Assoc., 246, 64. (67) Slaoui et al (1980) Nouv. Presse Méd., 9, 456. (68) Ellis et al (1978) Lancet, 1, 207. (69) Littlewood et al (1980) Lancet, 1, 310. (70) Caggiano et al (1980) Lancet, 2, 365. (71) Meyer et al (1974) Lancet, 2, 1387. (72) Treuner et al (1980) Med. Welt, 31, 952. (73) Cocks (1981) Med. J. Aust., 2, 617. (74) Zevin et al (1981) Nephron, 29, 274. (75) Messner et al (1981)

Nouv. Presse Méd., 10, 2904. (76) Cap et al (1983) *Bratisl. Lek. Listy, 79*, 1. (77) Malt et al (1983) *World J. Surg., 7*, 247. (78) Turani et al (1983) *Isr. J. Med. Sci., 19*, 332. (79) Schönberg (1982) *J. Reprod. Med., 27*, 753. (80) Sugiyama et al (1982) *Acta Hepatol. Jpn., 23*, 927. (81) Farrell et al (1975) *Lancet, 1*, 430. (82) Mokrihisky et al (1977) *N. Engl. J. Med., 296*, 1411. (83) Falk et al (1979) *Lancet, 2*, 1120. (84) Desser–Wiest (1981) *Onkologie (Basel), 3*, 120. (85) Wanless et al (1982) *Lab. Invest., 46*, 313. (86) Sweeney et al (1981) In: Davis et al (Eds), *Drug Reactions and the Liver*, p 304. Pitman Medical, London. (87) Boston Collaborative Drug Surveillance Program (1973) *Lancet, 1*, 1399. (88) Boston Collaborative Drug Surveillance Program (1974) *N. Engl. J. Med., 290*, 15. (89) Howat et al (1975) *J. Intern. Med. Res., 3*, 59. (90) Bennion et al (1976) *N. Engl. J. Med., 294*, 189. (91) Pertsemlidis et al (1971) *Gastroenterology, 66*, 565. (92) Royal College of General Practitioners (1982) *Lancet, 2*, 957. (93) Kappas et al (1968) *Ann. NY Acad. Sci., 151*, 842. (94) Edwards et al (1975) *J. Biol. Chem., 250*, 2750. (95) Zimmerman et al (1966) *Arch. Intern. Med., 118*, 229. (96) Cicardi et al (1983) *J. Allergy Clin. Immunol., 72*, 294. (97) Horii et al (1982) *Hepato–Gastroenterology, 29*, 187. (98) Ross et al (1976) *Ann. Intern. Med., 85*, 203. (99) Scott et al (1984) *J. Am. Med. Assoc., 251*, 1461. (100) Carrasco et al (1984) *Ann. Intern. Med., 100*, 316. (101) Henderson et al (1983) *Br. J. Cancer, 48*, 437. (102) Forman et al (1983) *Br. J. Cancer, 48*, 349. (103) Jacobs (1984) *Arch. Intern. Med., 144*, 642. (104) Jaeschke et al (1983) *Gastroenterology, 85*, 808. (105) Elias et al (1983) *Eur. J. Clin. Invest., 13*, 383. (106) Machnik et al (1983) *Exp. Pathol., 24*, 183. (107) Doss et al (1983) *Dtsch. Med. Wochenschr., 108*, 1857. (108) Van der Werf et al (1984) *Gastroenterology, 86*, 1286. (109) Chandra et al (1984) *Arch. Pathol. Lab. Med., 108*, 168. (110) Alberti–Flor et al (1984) *Am. J. Gastroenterol., 79*, 150. (111) Peterson et al (1984) *Am. J. Roentgenol., 142*, 1155.

B. SEX HORMONE ANTAGONISTS

Sex hormone antagonists, mainly antiestrogens, have only occasionally been associated with hepatic injury, with the exception of cyclofenil which appears to give rise to a higher incidence of liver injury than the other members of the group. These agents are derivatives of chlorotrianisene and exert their effect by interacting with estrogen receptor sites. They have a very weak estrogenic effect and lack the hepatotoxic potential of the sex hormones. However, there is some evidence that they may cause hepatic injury as an idiosyncratic effect (1).

(1) Olsson et al (1983) *Gut, 24*, 260.

Clomiphene

Causal relationship o

Liver function abnormalities may occur during treatment with this ovulation–inducing agent (1).

Melamed et al (2) described hepatoblastoma of the mixed type in a 15–month–old girl, born to a mother who had been treated for sterility with clomiphene, FSH and LH. *a*–Fetoprotein, extremely elevated before operation, decreased after operation and was still undetectable 1 year after operation. The association with clomiphene is of course still speculative since these tumors may occur spontaneously in this age group (3). The same considerations apply to a 25–year–old woman in whom a liver cell adenoma was detected after 24 months of treatment. She had never been on oral contraceptives and no other causes were found (4).

(1) *The Extra Pharmacopoeia, 28th ed,* p 1401. Pharmaceutical Press, London, 1982. (2) Melamed et al (1982) *N. Engl. J. Med., 307,* 820. (3) Balistreri et al (1982) In: Schiff et al (Eds), *Diseases of the Liver, 5th ed,* p 1265. Lippincott, Philadelphia. (4) Carrasco et al (1984) *N. Engl. J. Med., 310,* 1120.

Cyclofenil

H$_3$C–CO–O–⟨⟩–C–⟨⟩–O–OC–CH$_3$

Causal relationship +

In a double–blind crossover study in 11 scleroderma patients 4 had to be withdrawn because of liver dysfunction during treatment with cyclofenil (1). Høgh et al (2) reported on a 9–year–old child with scleroderma, treated with 600 mg/d, in whom symptomless ASAT/ALAT elevation was detected after 4 months of treatment. Rechallenges were positive on several occasions despite dose reduction to 200 mg/d. In a review of 30 cases (3) from Sweden, a mostly mild hepatocellular pattern of injury emerged. The reaction started in 80% in 1–4 months after starting treatment. Low–grade fever (13%), gastrointestinal symptoms (66%) and pruritus (33%) were the main symptoms. In some cases there was arthropathy (7%) and/or slight eosinophilia (10%). Histology showed viral hepatitis–like injury with scattered foci of necrosis with mononuclear infiltration, occasional centrilobular cholestasis and granulomas in 1 case. The authors suggested an incidence of 1.3% and indicated the analogy to the high incidence of steroid–induced liver damage in Sweden (3).

(1) Gibson et al (1983) *Br. J. Rheum., 22,* 218. (2) Høgh et al (1983) *Acta Derm.– Venereol., 63,* 445. (3) Olsson et al (1983) *Gut, 24,* 260.

Tamoxifen

H$_3$C\
 \ N–H$_2$C–H$_2$C–O–⟨⟩–C≡C–⟨⟩\
H$_3$C/\
                                C$_2$H$_5$

Causal relationship o/ +

Hepatotoxicity is not a common feature of the adverse reaction pattern of this antiestrogen, although some cases of a cholestatic or a mixed pattern of injury have been reported (2, 3). In one of these cases a rechallenge was positive (3). Biopsy showed swollen hepatocytes and cholestasis (3).

246

An interesting but tentative case–report about tamoxifen–induced peliosis hepatis was recently published (1). The patient had been treated for breast carcinoma for 2 years. Shortly after admission with pain radiating to the abdomen the right liver lobe ruptured and she died in shock despite operation. At autopsy 2 liters of unclotted blood were found in the abdomen. Many areas of blue hemorrhage and hemorrhagic cysts were found. Histology showed peliosis hepatis with cysts; these were not lined with endothelium but with connective tissue and they communicated with sinusoids.

(1) Loomus et al (1983) *Am. J. Clin. Pathol., 80,* 881. (2) Agrawal et al (1981) *Ann. Intern. Med., 141,* 1240. (3) Blackburn et al (1984) *Br. Med. J., 289,* 288.

20. Dermatological agents

A. Antipsoriatic agents
B. Miscellaneous

Introduction

Although liver injury such as fatty change and/or non–specific reactive changes have been associated with psoriasis *per se* (1), some authors have suggested that factors such as age, overweight and alcohol intake are responsible to a far greater extent than psoriasis (2).

Several orally administered antipsoriatic agents, including methotrexate which is discussed elsewhere, may cause liver injury. Whereas methoxsalen appears to induce occasionally an immunoallergic type of reaction, the vitamin–A derivatives, isotretinoin and etrenitate, probably exert their injurious effect through intrinsic toxicity, analogous to their parent compound. Although these agents seem to be safer because of their therapeutic efficacy at relatively low doses (3), the same pattern of injury may be expected as for vitamin A, especially when high doses are employed. Unfortunately, little is known about the long–term effects on the liver of these agents.

The use of topically administered agents rarely leads to liver injury. Even when hepatotoxic agents (e.g. selenium sulfide) are used, absorption is usually not sufficient to produce hepatic injury. Of course, this will depend on the concentration, the extent of application, and the potency of the drug to penetrate the skin. Apparently, some drugs are able to do so and occasionally cause liver enzyme elevations, e.g. podophyllin resin (4). Boric acid has caused liver damage when used on inflamed or otherwise damaged skin areas and has been largely abandoned as an antiseptic for human use. Chlorhexidine (5) and benzylalcohol (6) may cause liver dysfunction or necrosis after ingestion but probably not after topical use.

(1) Almeyda et al (1972) *Br. J. Dermatol., 87,* 623. (2) Nyfors et al (1976) *Acta Pathol. Microbiol. Scand., 84,* 253. (3) Orfanos (1979) *Schweiz. Med. Wochenschr., 109,* 1909. (4) Nater et al (1984) In: Dukes (Ed), *Meyler's Side Effects of Drugs, 10th ed,* p 254. Elsevier, Amsterdam. (5) Gershanik et al (1982) *N. Engl. J. Med., 307,* 1384. (6) Massano et al (1982) *Lancet, 1,* 289.

A. ANTIPSORIATIC AGENTS

Etretinate

Causal relationship +

Liver enzyme elevations have been reported in several studies (1–4), varying from 10% (1, 2) to 25% (3) while one study showed no significant alterations in ASAT/ALAT levels (4). However, in the latter study the total serum bilirubin level was significantly elevated. Cases of liver injury have been described (3, 5–7, 10, 11), mostly with biochemical and/or histological evidence of mild to moderate hepatocellular necrosis. A positive rechallenge was performed in some of them (7, 10). One of the latter patients was treated with isotretinoin without reactivation (7). In 1 of the cases the localization was centrilobular with parenchymal degeneration (5). In 2 other cases, chronic active hepatitis was possibly related to the intake of etretinate (8). The onset of hepatic injury, or rather its detection, occurs mostly after several months of therapy but can be after 1 month (10). Immunoallergic signs are absent, with the exception of eosinophilia in 1 patient which did not recur after rechallenge (10). In a study by Glazer et al (9) liver biopsies were evaluated prior to starting therapy and after a 6–months course on 0.75 mg/kg/d. Five of 20 patients showed morphological changes. Three showed progressive steatosis, 2 liver cell necrosis and progressive fibrosis. However, most of these 20 patients had an abnormal pre–treatment histology. Perisinusoidal lipid deposition in Ito cells or fibrosis as seen with vitamin A intoxication was not observed. It would seem advisable to check liver enzyme and serum triglyceride levels 2–3 weeks after starting therapy, after 6 weeks and then monthly if prolonged treatment is thought necessary.

(1) Kaplan et al (1983) *J. Am. Acad. Dermatol., 8*, 95. (2) Fontan et al (1983) *Arch. Dermatol., 119*, 187. (3) Foged et al (1982) *Dermatologica, 164*, 395. (4) Orfanos et al (1979) *Dermatologica, 159, 62*. (5) Thune et al (1980) *Dermatologica, 160*, 405. (6) Schmidt et al (1981) In: *Retinoids*, p 359. Springer Verlag, Berlin. (7) Van Voorst Vader et al (1984) *Dermatologica, 168*, 41. (8) Frederiksson (1978) *Dermatologica, 157, Suppl 1*, 13. (9) Glazer et al (1982) *J. Am. Acad. Dermatol., 6*, 683. (10) Weiss et al (1984) *Arch. Dermatol., 120*, 104. (11) Paskaleva et al (1983) *Dermatol. Venerol. (Sofia), 12*, 40.

Isotretinoin

Causal relationship o/ +

Isotretinoin is said to be less toxic than tretinoin (1), of which it is the stereoisomer. Serum aminotransferase levels were found to be transiently elevated in 2 of 14 patients treated for acne with 1–3.3 mg/kg/d for 4 months (2). In another study 76 patients with acne, divided into 3 groups, were treated with 0.1, 0.5 and 1 mg/kg/d, respectively, for 16 weeks (3). Mean ASAT levels rose in the 0.5 and 1 mg/kg/d groups but only with the highest dose to an abnormal value. In a study of 523 patients (mean: 109 mg/d; for 150 days) liver function abnormalities were noted in 10% (7). One author found significant γ–GT elevations with 0.8 mg/kg/d for 3 months (4). Ott et al (5) found liver enzyme elevations in 7–13% of patients during 12 months of treatment with 40 mg/d. In a study of 17 patients with myelodysplastic syndromes, treated with a single daily dose (up to 125 mg/m^2), the 2 patients on the highest dose showed reversible hepatic injury with bilirubin and aminotransferase elevation (6).

(1) *The Extra Pharmacopoeia, 28th ed,* p 490. Pharmaceutical Press, London, 1982. (2) Peck et al (1979) *N. Engl. J. Med., 300,* 329. (3) Jones et al (1983) *Br. J. Dermatol., 108,* 333. (4) Lyons et al (1982) *Br. J. Dermatol., 107,* 591. (5) Ott et al (1982) *Ann. Dermatol. Venereol., 109,* 849. (6) Gold et al (1983) *Cancer Treat. Rep., 67,* 981. (7) Windhorst et al (1982) *J. Am. Acad. Dermatol., 6,* 675.

Methoxsalen

Causal relationship +

Methoxsalen is used for the treatment of psoriasis in combination with ultraviolet A (PUVA). Some older studies failed to show liver function abnormalities (1, 2). More recently, a case was reported in which serum aminotransferase elevations and fever accompanied methoxsalen administration (3). Readministration was again followed by ASAT elevation; a challenge with methoxsalen without ultraviolet A was also positive, with re–elevation of ASAT/ALAT. Fever followed immediately on every challenge (3). In another case, fever and hepatic enzyme elevation occurred after the 15th PUVA treatment. Normalization occurred within 5 days after stopping PUVA. Subsequent rechallenge with PUVA was positive. Topical treatment with methoxsalen remained uneventful (4).

(1) Fitzpatrick et al (1958) *J. Am. Med. Assoc., 167,* 1586. (2) Tucker (1959) *J. Invest. Dermatol., 32,* 277. (3) Bjellerup et al (1979) *Acta Derm.–Venereol., 59,* 371. (4) Pariser et al (1980) *J. Am. Acad. Dermatol., 3,* 248.

B. MISCELLANEOUS DERMATOLOGICAL AGENTS

Povidone–iodine

Complex of polyvinylpyrrolidone and iodine   *Causal relationship o*

Liver damage may occur in patients with extensive burns treated with topical administration of this agent (1). High serum levels of iodide were present at the same time (1), suggesting a causal effect. Povidone itself is probably not absorbed and, if these cases of injury were drug–induced, it should have been caused by the iodide. In fact, iodide has caused centrizonal necrosis in animal toxicity tests (2, 3), but data on the human liver are lacking. Severe burning may be a cause of liver enzyme elevations, but these are mainly mild or moderate.

(1) Lavelle et al (1974) *Pharmacologist, 16,* 208. (2) Webster et al (1957) *J. Pharmacol. Exp. Ther., 120,* 171. (3) Lavelle et al (1975) *Toxicol. Appl. Pharmacol., 33,* 52.

Tannic acid

Consists of derivatives of flavanols
(condensed tannins) and of
hydrolyzable tannins   *Causal relationship* o/ +

Tannic acid has been used both in the treatment of burns and as an additive to barium enemas to inhibit mucin secretion, to stimulate contraction and to promote adhesion of barium to the mucosal surface. Its use in burns was abandoned after the occurrence of severe centrizonal necrosis in treated patients (1–5). Although severely burned patients may show signs of mild or moderate liver damage, tannic acid was probably the causative agent since a hepatotoxic effect could be reproduced in animals (2–5). The effect probably depends on the extent of the areas involved and on individual susceptibility. When added to barium enemas at a concentration of 2%, it caused hepatic necrosis in children (6–9).

(1) Wells et al (1942) *N. Engl. J. Med., 226,* 629. (2) Forbes et al (1943) *Surg. Gynecol. Obstet., 76,* 612. (3) Barnes et al (1943) *Lancet, 2,* 218. (4) Hartman et al (1943) *Ann. Surg., 118,* 402. (5) Baker et al (1943) *Ann. Surg., 118,* 417. (6) Editorial (1964) *Br. Med. J., 1,* 997. (7) McAllister et al (1963) *Radiology, 80,* 765. (8) Refshauge (1964) *Med. J. Aust., 1,* 739. (9) Lucke et al (1963) *Can. Med. Assoc. J., 89,* 1111.

21. Gastrointestinal agents

A. Laxatives
B. Other gastrointestinal agents

Introduction

Contrary to what is widely believed, several laxatives may be absorbed in amounts sufficient to cause systemic effects. Oxyphenisatine is the well–known example of a laxative that may cause hepatic injury. With this agent it was recognized for the first time that a drug could cause chronic active hepatitis. This was followed by its withdrawal from the market in several countries. Similar phenisatins may cause the same reaction. For instance, triacetyldiphenolisatin caused chronic active hepatitis and cirrhosis in several patients. A rechallenge in 14 patients was positive (2). Another laxative which has been suspected of causing hepatic injury is quinoloyl–methylen–diphenol (1); even liquid paraffin has been suspected (3).

The problem with laxatives is their almost compulsive and often unadmitted use, which can make it difficult to make a diagnosis. When asking the patient for his or her drug intake, it is important to enquire specifically about the use of these agents since most patients do not consider them as drugs.

The rare association of hepatic injury with the use of anti–ulcer drugs mostly concerns the H_2–antihistamines, which are discussed in Chapter 5. Besides the anti–ulcer drugs discussed below, pirenzepine, a new selective antimuscarinic drug, has occasionally been associated with mild ASAT/ALAT elevation (4).

(1) Wiegelmann et al (1975) *Arzneim.–Forsch.*, *25*, 949. (2) Lindner et al (1975) *Dtsch. Med. Wochenschr.*, *100*, 2530. (3) Blewitt et al (1977) *Gut*, *18*, 476. (4) Giorgi–Conciato et al (1982) *Scand. J. Gastroenterol., Suppl 81*, *17*, 1.

A. LAXATIVES

Dantron

Causal relationship o/ +

Chronic active hepatitis was discovered in a patient after the use of Doxi-

dan (dantron 50 mg + dioctyl calcium sulfosuccinate 60 mg) for 1 year
(1 caps./d). Symptoms started after the dose had been increased (4 caps./
d). There was concurrent leukopenia and eosinophilia. Recovery occurred within 1 month after discontinuing treatment (1). Besides the histology of chronic active hepatitis, a biopsy using a special technique showed
IgE deposits, especially in Kupffer cells. Rechallenge with each compound separately was negative, but was positive with the combination.

(1) Tolman et al (1976) *Ann. Intern. Med.*, *84*, 290.

Dioctyl sulfosuccinate

Causal relationship o

This anionic surfactant with wetting, dispersing, detergent and emulsify-
ing properties may break the gastric mucosal barrier and facilitate gastrointestinal absorption or hepatocyte uptake of drugs, thereby enhancing their activity and possibly toxicity (1).
   In 1 patient with chronic active hepatitis (see 'Dantron'), signs of liver
injury recurred only after readministration of both dantron and dioctyl
sulfosuccinate but not with each agent separately (2). In–vitro testing
suggested an analogous effect for the combination with oxyphenisatine
(3).

(1) *The Extra Pharmacopoeia, 28th ed,* p 1439. Pharmaceutical Press, London,
1982. (2) Tolman et al (1976) *Ann. Intern. Med.*, *84*, 290. (3) Dujovne et al (1972)
Clin. Pharmacol. Ther., *13*, 602.

Oxyphenisatine

Causal relationship + +

After about 40 years of seemingly innocuous use of oxyphenisatine–containing laxatives, Reynolds et al (1) published the first cases of liver injury, soon followed by numerous reports summing up over 100 cases in 1978
(2). Besides acute liver disease (16), mainly chronic injury was reported.
In fact, for the first time it was recognized that a drug could cause chronic active hepatitis and several cases were reported (3–12, 15, 20). The onset of these cases was often insidious and in several of these beginning
or advanced cirrhosis was present (3, 4, 9, 11, 15, 17, 20). Discontinuation
was mostly favorable unless irreversible damage was already present.
Sometimes the reaction took a fatal course (5, 8, 20). Fever (16) and eosi-

nophilia (1) are uncommon. The appearance of hepatic injury was mostly after 6–12 months and sometimes after several years of use. A causal relationship with the drug was proven by a positive reaction to rechallenge (1, 3, 4, 6, 10–14, 20) within days to weeks. A lymphocyte stimulation test was negative (16), but Morizane (18) saw leukocyte migration inhibition in the presence of oxyphenisatine. An interesting finding is the high prevalence of antibodies against double–stranded DNA in cases of suspected drug–induced chronic active hepatitis (19); some of these were possibly caused by oxyphenisatine. This report, however, needs further confirmation.

Since most preparations also contained dioctyl sodium sulfosuccinate, the latter has been suggested to play a contributory role. Dujovne et al (21) noted in Chang cell cultures that sodium dioctyl sulfosuccinate was cytotoxic, both alone as well as in combination with oxyphenisatine. Nevertheless, oxyphenisatine alone has also caused liver injury (4, 6) and a challenge with oxyphenisatine alone was positive in 1 case (6). The drug has been abandoned in most countries, but not in all as demonstrated by more recent reports of hepatic injury (15, 17).

(1) Reynolds et al (1970) *J. Am. Med. Assoc., 211,* 86. (2) Zimmerman (1978) In: *Hepatotoxicity,* p 544. Appleton–Century–Crofts, New York. (3) Gjone et al (1972) *Scand. J. Gastroenterol., 7,* 395. (4) Gjone et al (1973) *Lancet, 1,* 421. (5) Goldstein et al (1972) *Aust. NZ J. Med., 2,* 320. (6) Mallory et al (1971) *N. Engl. J. Med., 285,* 1266. (7) Reynolds et al (1972) *Am. J. Gastroenterol., 57,* 566. (8) Saltos et al (1972) *Aust. NZ J. Med., 4,* 386. (9) Willing (1971) *Med. J. Aust., 1,* 1179. (10) Reynolds et al (1971) *N. Engl. J. Med., 285,* 813. (11) Cooksley et al (1973) *Aust. NZ J. Med., 3,* 124. (12) Dietrichson (1975) *Scand. J. Gastroenterol., 10,* 617. (13) Fischer et al (1972) *Am. J. Gastroenterol., 58,* 58. (14) McHardy et al (1970) *J. Am. Med. Assoc., 211,* 83. (15) Delchier et al (1979) *Nouv. Presse Méd., 8,* 2955. (16) Pearson et al (1971) *Lancet, 1,* 994. (17) Schmitz et al (1983) *J. Méd. Strasbourg, 14,* 155. (18) Morizane (1978) *Gastroenterol. Jpn., 13,* 281. (19) Caruana et al (1983) *Lancet, 1,* 776. (20) Goldstein et al (1973) *Dig. Dis., 18,* 177. (21) Dujovne et al (1972) *Clin. Pharmacol. Ther., 13,* 602.

B. OTHER GASTROINTESTINAL AGENTS

Povidone

Causal relationship o/+

This mixture of synthetic polymers of 1–vinyl–2–pyrrolidone is used as a vehicle to retard the absorption of active ingredient. It is not itself absorbed from the gastrointestinal tract. When injected intravenously or intramuscularly for prolonged periods, it is stored in the reticuloendothelial system where it may cause hepatosplenomegaly as one of its signs (1, 2). Kupffer cells are swollen and vacuolar, containing an amorphous substance (2). This substance has a granular pattern when seen under the electron microscope (1). In 1 case, liver cirrhosis was present; Kupffer cells and histiocytes stained purple with alcoholic congo–red in this case (3).

(1) Bert et al (1972) *Sem. Hôp. Paris, 48*, 1809. (2) Fossati et al (1972) *Rev. Fr. Endocrinol. Clin., 13*, 57. (3) Kanetaka et al (1973) *Acta Pathol. Jpn., 23*, 617.

Omeprazole

Causal relationship o

Omeprazole is a substituted benzimidazole with a potent inhibitory effect on gastric acid secretion. This drug does not act on cholinergic or histamine H_2–receptors but probably on the proton pump in the secretory membrane of the parietal cell (1). Mostly mild and transient aminotransferase elevations were noted in 10 of 32 patients (20–60 mg/d) in 1 study (1). However, this was challenged by others (2) and a subsequent study by the first group in 60 volunteers failed to confirm their earlier results (3).

(1) Gustavsson et al (1983) *Lancet, 2*, 124. (2) Sharma et al (1983) *Lancet, 2*, 346. (3) Lööf et al (1984) *Lancet, 1*, 1347.

Tritiozine

Causal relationship o/ +

Tritiozine is an anti–ulcer drug with antisecretory properties. It is not an anticholinergic. In 1 study of 271 patients (1200 mg/d), 8 showed significant serum aminotransferase elevations (1). Cases of acute parenchymatous hepatitis have been ascribed to this drug (2, 3). A rechallenge after normalization was positive (2).

(1) Pellegrini (1979) *J. Int. Med. Res., 7*, 452. (2) Cruz et al (1983) *Rev. Esp. Enferm. Apar. Dig., 63*, 188. (3) Martin et al (1984) *Gastroenterol. Hepatol., 7*, 141.

22. Psychopharmacological agents

A. Neuroleptics
  1. Phenothiazines
  2. Thioxanthenes
  3. Butyrophenones
  4. Miscellaneous
B. Hypnotics/Sedatives/Anxiolytics
  1. Benzodiazepines
  2. Barbiturates
  3. Alcohols/Aldehydes
  4. Carbamates/Miscellaneous
C. Antidepressants
  1. Monoamine oxidase (MAO) inhibitors
  2. Tricyclics
  3. Tetracyclics/Miscellaneous
D. Psychostimulants

Introduction

There is no known relationship between psychiatric disease *per se* and hepatic injury, although one may speculate that in isolated cases psychiatric disease is secondary to hepatic illness. Psychostimulants, however, are abused by a group with a high incidence of needle–transmitted hepatic disease, which should be realized when evaluating case–histories of suspected drug–induced hepatic injury in this group.

Neuroleptics Although chlorpromazine was very often reported as a cause of hepatic injury during its early years of use, data on the incidence were unreliable and probably exaggerated. Especially in these early years viral causes of hepatic injury were impossible to disprove in the reports.

Most data were derived from spontaneous reports in the literature or from reports to monitoring centers and it is well known that this is influenced by many factors. Reporting increases markedly if attention is drawn to a previously unknown adverse reaction, while well–known reactions are less often reported.

The previously accepted assumption that phenothiazines with an aliphatic side–chain (e.g. chlorpromazine) are a more frequent cause of hepatic injury than those with a piperazine (e.g. prochlorperazine, fluphenazine) and piperidine (e.g. thioridazine, mepazine) side–chain was recently challenged by Jones et al (1). Although more frequently reported to the FDA (proportion of reports of hepatic injury versus reports of other side effects: aliphatics 6.8%, piperidines 4.9%, piperazines 1.5%) (2), statistical analysis of the Medicaid data in 2 states demonstrated no difference in relative risk for the different derivatives (1). Although there was a large difference in prevalence of hepatic disease, the data from both states were consistent.

All phenothiazines and related compounds have been associated occasionally with signs of hepatic injury, either mild or severe, including less frequently used agents, e.g. levomepromazine (7), triflupromazine (7) and clomacran (16).

Thioxanthenes and butyrophenones have rarely been associated with symptomatic hepatic injury. Mild liver enzyme elevations are probably as frequent with these agents as with phenothiazines. In a study comparing clozapine, perazine and haloperidol there was no significant difference between these drugs as regards hepatic enzyme elevations (3). In another study comparing fluphenazine decanoate, flupentixol decanoate and fluspirilene, mild hepatic function abnormalities were frequent in all groups (4). Mildly abnormal liver function tests seem to be frequent during neuroleptic treatment (3, 5, 6, 12). For ethical reasons, however, a placebo group is never included in such studies and long–term studies often lack a control group treated with other neuroleptics. This makes some results difficult to interpret, especially if other drugs have been used concurrently.

Also, most non–phenothiazine neuroleptics have been associated occasionally with mild liver enzyme elevations, as have less frequently used drugs, e.g. lenperone (8), melperone (13) and molindone (14).

Hypnotics/Sedatives/Anxiolytics Benzodiazepines have been rarely incriminated as a cause of hepatic injury. There is an incidental report of peliosis hepatis and adenomas in mice exposed to oxazepam (9), but as far as we know this has not been confirmed. Barbiturates are well–known enzyme–inducing agents. There has been some concern about a possible association with liver tumors in man, especially during long–term use as an anticonvulsant (10), but this has not yet been substantiated. Nevertheless, it should be borne in mind that barbiturates have marked tumor–promoting capacity when given in high doses in animal toxicity tests (15).

Hepatic injury due to alcohol/aldehydes and carbamates is rare if therapeutic doses are employed.

Antidepressants Of the antidepressants, MAO inhibitors are a significant cause of hepatic injury. Their use has markedly declined, but there seems to be some renewed interest in them. In some countries (e.g. France) they are still in use on a relatively large scale. There is no convincing evidence for a marked difference in hepatotoxicity of the individual agents, with the possible exception of tranylcypromine which has a different structure. With the exception of the latter, these agents share the hydrazine moiety (HN–NH) which may be converted to alkylating metabolites.

Tricyclics are a rare cause of symptomatic hepatic injury, which is mostly of a mixed to cholestatic pattern. A possible exception is amineptine which has been associated relatively frequently with hepatic injury. Most tricyclics and related compounds have been associated occasionally with mild liver enzyme elevations, e.g. clomipramine (17), doxepin (18), trimipramine (17), nortriptyline (17) and maprotiline (19). Mild liver enzyme elevations have also been noted occasionally during treatment with citalopram (20) and amoxapine (21), with the latter also as part of a malignant neuroleptic syndrome (22).

Of the tetracyclics and other antidepressants, nomifensine and zimelidine are of interest. Nomifensine is a frequent cause of fever which is often associated with liver enzyme elevations. Although the incidence is unknown, it seems to be higher than that of the tricyclics. Zimelidine caused fever, headache, muscle/joint pain and liver enzyme elevations in several patients. In some cases this was followed by a Guillain–Barré syndrome with sensory and/or motor loss. For this reason the manufacturer withdrew the drug worldwide from the market.

Psychostimulants The psychostimulants occasionally cause liver enzyme elevations, but these are mostly mild. Since many of these agents are very often employed by drug abusers, it is difficult to prove or disprove an eventual adverse effect on the liver because of frequent hepatic disease from other causes in this group.

Although no longer used as a medicinal agent, it is worth noting that cocaine in high doses causes hepatic injury in animals (23), possibly by enhanced production of norcocaine nitroxide, a potentially hepatotoxic metabolite (25). In man, this psychostimulant has been associated occasionally with hepatic injury (24).

Cinanserin, a serotonin antagonist used in the treatment of mania and schizophrenia, has been associated with liver tumors in animals (11).

(1) Jones et al (1983) *Psychopharmacol. Bull., 19,* 24. (2) Jones et al (1982) *Clin. Pharmacol. Ther., 31,* 237. (3) Bauer et al (1983) *Pharmacopsychiatrie, 16,* 23. (4) Nolen et al (1978) *Bull. Coord. Commun. Biochem. Onderz. NZR, 11,* 69. (5) Pietzcker et al (1981) *Arch. Psychiatr. Nervenkr., 229,* 315. (6) Degkwitz et al (1976) *Nervenarzt, 47,* 81. (7) Rees (1966) *Abst. World Med., 39,* 129. (8) Digiacomo et al (1977) *Curr. Ther. Res., 22,* 605. (9) Fox et al (1974) *Res. Commun. Chem. Pathol. Pharmacol., 8,* 841. (10) Schneiderman (1974) *Lancet, 2,* 1085. (11) *The Extra Pharmacopoeia, 28th ed,* p 1695. Pharmaceutical Press, London, 1982. (12) Goncalves et al (1977) *Pharmacopsychiatria, 10,* 36. (13) Kirkegaard et al (1981) *Arzneim.–Forsch., 31,* 737. (14) Forsell et al (1977) *Hosp. Pharm., 12,* 419. (15) Schwarz et al (1983) *Cancer Lett., 21,* 17. (16) Ruiz et al (1979) *Neurol. Neurocir. Psiquiatr., 20,* 13. (17) Anonymous (1981) *Jpn. Med. Gaz., 18(8),* 9. (18) Pinder et al (1977) *Drugs, 13,* 161. (19) Moldawsky (1984) *J. Clin. Psychiatry, 45,* 178. (20) Lindegaard Pedersen (1982) *Psychopharmacology, 77,* 199. (21) Ine et al (1982) *Drugs, 24,* 1. (22) Steele (1982) *Am. J. Psychiatry, 139,* 1500. (23) Kloss et al (1982) *Toxicol. Appl.*

Pharmacol., *64*, 88. (24) Acker et al (1983) *Am. J. Obstet. Gynecol.*, *146*, 220. (25) Rauckman et al (1982) *Mol. Pharmacol.*, *21*, 458.

A. NEUROLEPTICS

A.1. PHENOTHIAZINES

Chlorpromazine

Causal relationship + +

Chlorpromazine was the first phenothiazine neuroleptic to be used extensively. Its ability to cause cholestatic hepatitis is one of the most often cited examples of drug–induced hepatic injury.

Mild liver enzyme elevations have been reported to occur varying from 10% (1) to 42% (2). Dickes et al (2) performed serial studies of liver function in 50 patients on chlorpromazine and found mild BSP excretion and APh abnormalities in 42% which were transient in 26% despite continuation of therapy (2). Some older studies estimated the incidence of jaundice between 0.6% and 2% (12–14), some even up to 5% (3). More recent studies suggest a lower incidence of approximately 0.1% (15). It is not clear whether older reports were biased or whether the incidence is declining, as previously suggested (27).

The occurrence of cholestatic hepatitis is well known although cases where necrosis predominated have been reported on several occasions (1, 9–11). More than 90% of cases developed within the first 5 weeks of therapy (3) with a mean of 15 days in one study (4). Prodromal signs occurred in 70–80% and were either influenza–like or gastrointestinal (3, 4). Peripheral eosinophilia occurred in 60% (3) to 73% (4). Rash was infrequent and estimated at 3–5% (3, 4), although one study mentioned rash in 5 of 11 cases (5). Concurrent agranulocytosis has been reported in some cases (6–8). Besides mostly moderate ASAT/ALAT and APh elevations a considerable rise in serum bilirubin and cholesterol levels occurred. In one study normalization took longer than 12 weeks in approximately 20% (4). Rechallenge performed in some cases yielded a prompt reaction (2, 14). In one study 80% responded to a rechallenge (14).

Cross–sensitivity with other phenothiazines is rare (4) but has been reported (21). Patch tests and intracutaneous tests were inconsistent or negative (14). A lymphocyte stimulation test has been both positive (25) and negative (26).

The symptomatic cases showed no sex preponderance; the female/male ratio showed a wide variation but did not demonstrate unequivocal figures (4). There appeared to be no dose–dependence (4).

In a number of the prolonged cases (≥ 6 months) a pattern resembling primary biliary cirrhosis (PBC) emerged with continuous/intermittent jaundice, xanthomata, bone thinning, steatorrhea, very high levels of cholesterol and APh, and less marked hyperbilirubinemia/aminotransferasemia (4, 16–20). Although the prognosis is better than in cases of PBC, some of them ended in biliary cirrhosis (19, 20). In one report of cholestatic hepatitis, chronic active hepatitis developed after a year (22).

In a study of 36 patients with phenothiazine–associated hepatic injury Ishak et al (4) quantified the histological features as follows: hepatocellular and canalicular cholestasis, centrilobular and/or midzonal (80–100%), cellular unrest (100%), Kupffer cell hypertrophy (97%), focal necrosis (70%), acidophilic bodies (58%), eosinophils in sinusoids (64%), and a spotty portal infiltrate in 56% of the cases. Lymphocytes were present in the portal area in 89% of the cases, while neutrophils and eosinophils were seen in this area in 64% and 61% of cases respectively. In the 16 cases where peripheral eosinophils were found to be increased (73%), 6 had a predominantly portal eosinophilic infiltrate. All 16 cases had sinusoidal eosinophils. In the chronic cases, piecemeal necrosis, pseudoxanthomatous change, moderate portal inflammation and destruction of interlobular ducts were present. According to these authors, inflammation was less marked than in cases of PBC, and lymphoid follicles and active segmental or concentric destruction of bile ducts, often surrounded by granulomas, were absent. Copper pigmentation seemed to be less marked in these cases. Most reported chronic cases were described at a time when antimitochondrial antibodies were not yet assessed and data on this test in chlorpromazine–associated cases of PBC–like damage are lacking as far as we know.

The mechanism of injury is presumed to be a combination of mild toxicity and immunoallergy, as is the case with many other drugs. Mild liver function abnormalities in a large percentage of patients (see above) and a dose–related effect of chlorpromazine on hepatic enzyme release in in–vitro studies, impairment of bile secretion in isolated perfused rat liver systems, and inhibition of enzymes in isolated liver plasma membranes favor an intrinsic toxic effect (23).

Chlorpromazine inhibits $(Na^+ + K^+)$–ATPase and Mg^{2+}–ATPase in isolated rat liver plasma membranes (24). Glutathione and other sulfhydryls may block this inhibition (24). The 7,8–dihydroxy metabolite produces much stronger inhibition (23) whereas sulfoxide metabolites cause less inhibition than the parent compound (24). In a perfused rat liver system the 7,8–dihydroxy metabolite had a much stronger cholestatic effect than chlorpromazine (23).

Since an accelerated reaction to rechallenge, eosinophilia, dose–independence and a usual latent period of 1–6 weeks after starting treatment are prominent features in a number of cases, an additional immunoallergic component is likely.

Although such reactions cannot usually be reproduced in animals, a recent study has shown both humoral and secretory antibodies to chlorpromazine in rats. Preimmunization with a chlorpromazine–protein con-

260

jugate aggravated periportal glycogen loss and centrilobular fatty change (27). It should be noted, however, that the dose was high and that the pattern in man is different.

(1) Bloom et al (1975) *Am. J. Psychiatry, 121,* 788. (2) Dickes et al (1957) *N. Engl. J. Med., 256,* 1. (3) Zimmerman (1963) *Ann. NY Acad. Sci., 104,* 904. (4) Ishak et al (1972) *Arch. Pathol., 93,* 283. (5) Cohen (1956) *Am. J. Psychiatry, 113,* 115. (6) Hodges et al (1955) *J. Am. Med. Assoc., 158,* 114. (7) Jeub et al (1956) *Minn. Med., 39,* 740. (8) Cheongvee et al (1967) *Br. J. Clin. Pract., 21,* 95. (9) Lomas et al (1955) *Lancet, 1,* 1144. (10) Elliot et al (1956) *Am. J. Psychiatry, 112,* 940. (11) Romeo et al (1981) *Rass. Med. Int., 2,* 105. (12) Cares et al (1957) *Am. J. Psychiatry, 114,* 318. (13) Lamas et al (1955) *Lancet, 1,* 1144. (14) Hollister (1957) *Am. J. Med., 23,* 870. (15) Jick et al (1981) *J. Clin. Pharmacol., 21,* 359. (16) Levine et al (1966) *Gastroenterology, 50,* 665. (17) Read et al (1961) *Am. J. Med., 31,* 249. (18) Bolton (1967) *Am. J. Gastroenterol., 48,* 497. (19) Walker et al (1966) *Gastroenterology, 51,* 631. (20) Meyers et al (1957) *Trans. Assoc. Am. Physicians, 70,* 243. (21) Herron et al (1960) *Gastroenterology, 38,* 87. (22) Russell et al (1973) *Br. Med. J., 1,* 655. (23) Boyer (1981) In: Davis et al (Eds), *Drug Reactions and the Liver,* p 64. Pitman Medical, London. (24) Samuels et al (1978) *Gastroenterology, 74,* 1183. (25) Namihisa et al (1975) *Leber Magen Darm, 5,* 73. (26) Sarkany (1967) *Lancet, 1,* 743. (27) Mullock et al (1983) *Biochem. Pharmacol., 32,* 2733.

Cyamemazine

Causal relationship o

Cholestatic jaundice appeared 2 days after starting treatment with cyamemazine, trihexyphenidyl and barbiturates. There were no other symptoms. Recovery occurred in 3 weeks after discontinuation of all drugs (1). Hepatic failure was reported in a heroin addict with a malignant neuroleptic syndrome (2).

(1) Rager et al (1983) *Presse Méd., 12,* 1941. (2) Bleichner et al (1981) *Lancet, 1,* 386.

Fluphenazine

Causal relationship o/ +

Liver function abnormalities have been variously reported; especially the enanthate form has been associated with a higher incidence (1). Only occasional cases of cholestatic (2) and hepatocellular (1) jaundice have been reported. In the latter case the patient was a drug–abuser in whom withdrawal and reinstitution of fluphenazine coincided (?) with a fluctuation in liver enzyme levels. Another report mentioned jaundice in 1 patient in a study of approximately 90 cases (3). Kennedy (4) pointed out the danger of depot preparations. His patient developed jaundice 17 days after the first dose and remained very ill for 4 months. Treatment with haloperidol was followed by a sharp rise in serum ALAT concentration (4). Before starting treatment with a depot preparation he recommends testing the drug by oral administration.

(1) Snyder (1980) *Am. J. Gastroenterol., 73,* 336. (2) Walters et al (1963) *Am. J. Psychiatry, 120,* 81. (3) NIMH Psychopharmacology Service Center Collaborative Study Group (1964) *Arch. Gen. Psychiatry, 10,* 246. (4) Kennedy (1983) *Br. J. Psychiatry, 143,* 312.

Metopimazine

Causal relationship o

This phenothiazine with a piperidine side–chain was held responsible for 1 case of centrilobular necrosis accompanied by intracellular cholestasis, bile plugging and marked eosinophilic infiltration. The onset was 4 weeks after starting treatment with symptoms of abdominal pain, fever and jaundice. Complete recovery occurred within 4 weeks after discontinuation. No other causes were found (1).

(1) Arnau et al (1983) *Gastroenterol. Hepatol., 6,* 93.

Pecazine (mepazine)

Causal relationship o

Two unspecified cases of jaundice were reported in a group of 37 patients (5.4%) appearing after 16 and 32 days, respectively (1).

(1) Mitchell et al (1957) *Br. Med. J., 1,* 204.

Perazine

Causal relationship o

In an open study of 33 schizophrenic patients who had been treated continuously for more than 10 years (mean 18 ± 2.1), an assessment of liver enzymes demonstrated mild ALAT/ASAT elevations in 30% of cases. In the patients with high plasma levels (70–280 ng/ml) there was a higher incidence of liver enzyme elevations than in patients with low levels (10–70 ng/ml). This difference was statistically significant (1). In a comparative study (mean 41–48 days) of clozapine (mean 200.5 mg/d), perazine (mean 289 mg/d) and haloperidol (mean 18.4 mg/d) incidental elevation of one liver enzyme (ASAT, ALAT, or γ–GT) occurred in 29.2%, 25.4% and 28.5% respectively (2).

(1) Pietzcker et al (1981) *Arch. Psychiatr. Nervenkr., 229*, 315. (2) Bauer et al (1983) *Pharmacopsychiatria, 16*, 23.

Perphenazine

CH$_2$–CH$_2$–CH$_2$–N⟨ ⟩N–CH$_2$–CH$_2$OH

Causal relationship o

Cook et al (1) briefly mentioned 1 case of intrahepatic cholestasis with jaundice appearing 56 days after starting treatment with 24 mg/d. The patient recovered in 3 weeks after discontinuation. Berkowitz et al (2) described a patient with cholestatic jaundice starting 2 months after stay in a mental institution where he was treated with 24 mg/d. Biopsy showed cholestasis with only minimal periportal infiltration and cellular change. According to Ayd (3) jaundice has been reported rarely and less frequently than with chlorpromazine (3).

(1) Cook et al (1965) *Lancet, 1*, 175. (2) Berkowitz et al (1961) *Am. J. Dig. Dis., 6*, 160. (3) Ayd (1964) *Dis. Nerv. Syst., 25*, 311.

Prochlorperazine

CH$_2$–CH$_2$–CH$_2$–N⟨ ⟩N–CH$_3$

Causal relationship o/ +

Several cases of cholestatic jaundice (1–5) have been described, appearing 5 days (3) to 4 months (4) after starting treatment. Recovery was reported to vary between 3 weeks (4) and 3 months (3). Peripheral eosinophilia was noted in some cases (4, 5). Histology showed cholestasis with a mild mononuclear infiltrate (3, 5). One case of prolonged cholestasis showed features resembling those of primary biliary cirrhosis (1). In 2 other cases, severe hepatocellular necrosis had a fatal course (6, 7). In one of these cases this severe reaction was attributed to an interactive effect with iproniazid (6).

(1) Ishak et al (1972) *Arch. Pathol., 93*, 283. (2) Weinstein et al (1959) *J. Am. Med. Assoc., 170*, 1663. (3) Solomon et al (1959) *Am. J. Med., 27*, 840. (4) Deller et al (1959) *Br. Med. J., 2*, 93. (5) Mechanic et al (1957) *N. Engl. J. Med., 259*, 778. (6) Capron et al (1980) *Gastroentérol. Clin. Biol., 4*, 123. (7) McFarland (1963) *Am. J. Clin. Pathol., 40*, 284.

Promazine

CH₂-CH₂-CH₂-N(CH₃)₂ structure (phenothiazine)

Causal relationship o/ +

Cholestatic jaundice (1–3) has been reported, appearing within 2 days (1) to 2 weeks (3) after starting treatment. Resolution took place within 1–2 months after discontinuation. Concurrent fever (2, 3), eosinophilia (3) and urticaria (3) were compatible with an immunoallergic mechanism. Cross–sensitivity with chlorpromazine was noted in some studies (2, 3) but was reported to be absent by others (4, 5). Histology showed bile staining and canalicular stasis in the centrilobular area and periportal mononuclear and eosinophilic infiltration (2).

(1) Kemp (1957) *Gastroenterology, 32,* 937. (2) Herron et al (1960) *Gastroenterology, 38,* 87. (3) Waitzkin (1957) *N. Engl. J. Med., 257,* 276. (4) Ishak et al (1972) *Arch. Pathol., 93,* 283. (5) Hollister (1957) *Am. J. Med., 23,* 870.

Thioridazine

CH₂-CH₂- piperidine structure (phenothiazine with S-CH₃)

Causal relationship o/ +

Some cases of a cholestatic or mixed (1–4) pattern of hepatic injury have been noted, either mild (1, 2) or with jaundice (2–4). Abnormalities appeared within 4 days (2), but in other cases in 5 months or more (1, 3, 4) after starting treatment. In 2 cases the same but milder reaction appeared after the use of chlorpromazine (2). In 1 patient with jaundice appearing after 15 months of treatment, the same reaction had occurred 17 years previously during use of chlorpromazine (3). Histology, reported in 1 (alcoholic) patient, showed cholestasis and mild portal fibrosis (4).

(1) Block (1962) *Am. J. Psychiatry, 119,* 77. (2) Reinhart et al (1966) *J. Am. Med. Assoc., 197,* 767. (3) Kristensen (1975) *Tidsskr. Nor. Laegeforen, 95,* 1910. (4) Barancik et al (1967) *J. Am. Med. Assoc., 200,* 175.

Trifluoperazine

CH₂-CH₂-CH₂-N piperazine N-CH₃ structure (phenothiazine with CF₃)

Causal relationship o/ +

Cases of cholestatic hepatitis have been reported, appearing after approximately 2 weeks of use. There was jaundice with mild ASAT/ALAT elevations (1, 2). Concurrent rash (2) and eosinophilia (1, 2) were noted.

264

Recovery occurred within 1 month after discontinuation. Histology showed moderate hepatocellular bile accumulation, occasional bile plugging, focal degeneration, and a moderate portal mononuclear infiltrate (1). Klatskin (3) mentioned 1 case of biliary cirrhosis, possibly related to trifluoperazine but without giving further details.

(1) Kohn et al (1961) *N. Engl. J. Med.*, *264*, 549. (2) Margulis et al (1968) *Can. Med. Assoc. J.*, *98*, 1063. (3) Klatskin (1975) In: Schiff (Ed), *Diseases of the Liver*, *4th ed*, p 604. Lippincott, Philadelphia.

Thioproperazine

Causal relationship o

Rarely cases of hepatic injury have been reported, starting after one (1) to several months (2) of treatment. There were no immunoallergic symptoms. Centrilobular necrosis and cholestasis were seen with dense mononuclear infiltration of the portal area (2). A lymphocyte stimulation test was positive (2).

(1) Denber et al (1960) *Dis. Nerv. Syst.*, *1*, 39. (2) Opolon et al (1969) *Presse Méd.*, *20*, 2041.

A.2. THIOXANTHENES

Chlorprothixene

Causal relationship o

Cholestatic jaundice was observed after 8 days of treatment. However, concurrent pneumococcal septicemia and bronchopneumonia as well as the use of other drugs complicated this case (1).

(1) Ruddock et al (1973) *Br. Med. J.*, *1*, 231.

Clopenthixol

Causal relationship o

In an open study in 58 patients on a maximum dose of 300 mg/d, 11 patients showed an increase in serum ALAT concentrations and 6 in total bilirubin but no details were given of time, duration or height of the values (1).

(1) Yaryura–Tobias et al (1970) *Curr. Ther. Res., 12,* 271.

Tiothixene

Causal relationship o

Mildly elevated aminotransferase levels (mostly transient) were observed in 9.5% of 136 patients. The relationship to dosage was not mentioned (1).

(1) Overall et al (1969) *Clin. Pharmacol. Ther., 10,* 36.

A.3. BUTYROPHENONES

Halopemide

Causal relationship o

Halopemide resembles haloperidol but is claimed to have a different pharmacological and clinical profile. An open study in 11 schizophrenic patients showed ESR elevation in 10 patients after 1 week of treatment and mild serum aminotransferase elevation in 3 patients (1), but both were transient.

(1) Nolen et al (1981) *Pharmakopsychiatr. Psychopharmakol., 14,* 21.

Haloperidol

Causal relationship +

Haloperidol–induced hepatic injury is probably very rare (1), although high doses (100 mg/d) administered to 10 patients for 3 months caused elevation of alkaline phosphatase levels in 7 of these (2). In another study doses of up to 32 mg/d were associated with ASAT elevation in 4 of 20 men (no further details) (6). Normal doses are not associated with significant changes in liver enzymes but minor elevations may be frequent (7). Occasional cases of cholestatic jaundice have been described (3, 4) in which fever and jaundice appeared within 5 weeks after starting treatment. Rash (3) and eosinophilia (4) may point to an immunoallergic reaction in these cases. In 1 patient the course was chronic; marked portal and bridging fibrosis and hepatocellular unrest were still present 2 years after discontinuation of the drug (4). The other patients showed cholestasis with or without mild necrosis and marked eosinophilic portal inflammation (3).

One recent case showed predominantly hepatocellular injury (5). Histology revealed chronic active hepatitis with portal–portal and portal–central bridging. An accidental rechallenge was positive. LE cells were present in this patient. Several autoantibodies were present and a lymphocyte stimulation test was positive in the presence of haloperidol (5). In a case of fluphenazine–associated jaundice, treatment with haloperidol was followed by marked ASAT elevation, which suggests possible cross–sensitivity (8).

(1) Ayd (1972) *Dis. Nerv. Syst., 3,* 459. (2) McCreadie et al (1977) *Br. J. Psychiatry, 131,* 310. (3) Fuller et al (1977) *West. J. Med., 127,* 515. (4) Dincsoy et al (1982) *Gastroenterology, 83,* 694. (5) Nagasaka et al (1981) *Acta Hepatol. Jpn., 22,* 1176. (6) Gerlach et al (1974) *Acta Psychiatr. Scand., 50,* 410. (7) Bauer et al (1983) *Pharmacopsychiatria, 16,* 23. (8) Kennedy (1983) *Br. J. Psychiatry, 143,* 312.

Pimozide

Causal relationship o

Pimozide is a diphenylbutylpiperidine, structurally similar to the butyrophenones. Liver function abnormalities have been reported with its use (1). Ansseau et al (2) reported a malignant neuroleptic syndrome and mild liver enzyme elevations, 3 days after starting treatment with pimozide (4 mg/d) and nomifensine (75 mg/d). A 4–fold elevation of conjugated bilirubin suggested cholestatic hepatitis, but a biopsy was not performed and jaundice was not mentioned. The authors suggested an interactive effect of nomifensine with pimozide as the cause of the malignant neuroleptic syndrome (2).

(1) *The Extra Pharmacopoeia, 28th ed,* p 1552. Pharmaceutical Press, London, 1982. (2) Ansseau et al (1980) *Acta Psychiatr. Belg., 80,* 600.

A.4. MISCELLANEOUS NEUROLEPTICS

Clozapine

Causal relationship o

Elevated ASAT concentrations were found in 7 of 20 clozapine–treated patients as against 4 in the haloperidol control group (1). However, Bauer et al (4) found a comparable incidence of liver enzyme elevations for haloperidol, perazine and clozapine. Fisher–Cornelssen (2) found APh to be more frequently elevated in the clozapine group than in a chlorpromazine group. Kirkegaard et al (3) found moderate liver enzyme elevations in a number of cases and although these were not very significant compared with the control group there was a weak correlation with long duration and high doses.

Relatively little experience has been obtained with this agent since it was largely abandoned after reports of agranulocytosis in Finland.

(1) Gerlach et al (1974) *Acta Psychiatr. Scand., 50,* 410. (2) Fischer–Cornelssen et al (1974) *Arzneim.–Forsch., 24,* 1706. (3) Kirkegaard et al (1979) *Arzneim.–Forsch., 29,* 851. (4) Bauer et al (1983) *Pharmacopsychiatria, 16,* 23.

Loxapine

Causal relationship o

Five cases of hepatic injury were reported to the FDA in 1980 (1). Two were well–documented and demonstrated biochemically a hepatocellular pattern of injury. Onset was within 5–18 days of starting therapy. Recovery after discontinuation was reported in 4 patients.

(1) *ADR Highlights* (1980) *Aug. 14.*

Metiapine

Causal relationship o

Metiapine is a neuroleptic, resembling loxapine and clotiapine. Little experience has been obtained with this agent so far. Two studies comparing

268

metiapine with a control neuroleptic demonstrated occasional liver function abnormalities (1, 2). One patient developed ASAT/ALAT elevation at the end of the 6–week treatment period (1), while in the other study a patient had to be withdrawn because of a marked increase in aminotransferase levels after 12 days therapy (2). In both cases the causal relationship was uncertain.

(1) Steinbook et al (1975) *J. Clin. Pharmacol.*, *15*, 700. (2) Kramer et al (1975) *Curr. Ther. Res.*, *18*, 839.

B. HYPNOTICS/SEDATIVES/ANXIOLYTICS

B.1. BENZODIAZEPINES

Alprazolam

Causal relationship o/ +

Mild ALAT/ASAT elevation was observed 2 weeks after first intake. Rechallenge was positive (1). Jaundice has been rarely encountered as an adverse effect (2). No hepatic toxicity was seen in rats (200 mg/kg) (3).

(1) Roy–Byrne et al (1983) *Lancet*, *2*, 786. (2) Anonymous (1983) *Pharm. J.*, *230*, 47. (3) Watanabe (1981) *Preclin. Rep.*, *7*, 43.

Chlordiazepoxide

Causal relationship o

Hollister et al (6) observed ASAT elevation in 4 of 36 patients. Several case–histories of hepatic injury have been described (1–5), but none is completely convincing; mainly a cholestatic pattern was mentioned (1, 3–5), although hepatic necrosis has also been observed (2). Onset was within 6 weeks but mostly in 2 weeks (2–5). No immunoallergic signs were observed. Biopsy showed cholestasis (1, 4, 5), varying degrees of infiltration, with many eosinophils in 1 case (1), cellular unrest (1, 5) or more severe necrosis with collapse (2).

(1) Abbruzzese et al (1965) *N. Engl. J. Med.*, *273*, 321. (2) Pickering (1966) *N. Engl. J. Med.*, *274*, 1449. (3) Cacioppo et al (1961) *Am. J. Psychiatry*, *117*, 1040. (4) Lo

et al (1967) *Am. J. Dig. Dis.*, *12*, 845. (5) Kratsch et al (1972) *Z. Inn. Med.*, *27*, 408. (6) Hollister et al (1961) *Psychopharmacologia*, *2*, 63.

Clobazam

Causal relationship o

In a trial of 190 patients, mild liver enzyme changes occurred in 2 patients as against none in the placebo group (1).

(1) Donlon et al (1979) *J. Clin. Pharmacol.*, *19*, 297.

Clorazepate

Causal relationship o

A hepatocellular pattern of injury was observed in 1 case, appearing after 2 months of treatment; a chronic persistent hepatitis was still present 6 months after discontinuation (1). Biopsy showed mild centrilobular cholestasis, focal necrosis and portal–portal bridging fibrosis.

(1) Parker (1979) *Postgrad. Med. J.*, *55*, 908.

Diazepam

Causal relationship o/ +

Both a cholestatic (1, 3, 5) and hepatocellular (2, 4) pattern of injury have been described, starting within a few days (4), or one (1, 3) to several (1–3) months after initial intake. Rash, fever and eosinophilia were observed (1). The course was fatal in 1 case (2), ascribed to amitriptyline and diazepam. Biopsy showed marked centrilobular cholestasis (1, 3) with cellular unrest (3), acidophilic bodies (1), portal granulomas in a prolonged case (1), focal necrosis (4), and acute yellow atrophy (2).

Rechallenge was positive in 2 days (4). The surprisingly high percentage (100%) of signs of cholestasis in 11 patients with tetanus, treated with phenobarbital and diazepam (5), led some authors to assume that this combination might possibly enhance the production of hepatotoxic

270

metabolites of diazepam (6). This has not yet been confirmed.

(1) Klatskin (1975) In: Schiff (Ed), *Diseases of the Liver, 4th ed.* Lippincott, Phila-delphia. (2) Cunningham (1965) *Br. J. Psychiatry, 111,* 1107. (3) Fors et al (1968) *Läkartidningen, 65,* 4528. (4) Tedesco et al (1982) *Dig. Dis. Sci., 27,* 470. (5) Stacher (1973) *Wien. Klin. Wochenschr., 22,* 401. (6) Zimmerman (1978) *Hepatotoxicity,* p 395. Appleton–Century–Crofts, New York.

Flurazepam

Causal relationship o

Cholestatic hepatitis occurred 4 (1) to 6 (2) months after initial intake, with recovery in 6 weeks after discontinuation. Mild eosinophilia was observed (2). Biopsy showed canalicular and hepatocellular cholestasis, moderate hepatocellular unrest, and dense (1) or absent (2) portal inflammation.

(1) Fang et al (1978) *Ann. Intern. Med., 89,* 364. (2) Reynolds et al (1981) *Can Med. Assoc. J., 124,* 893.

Triazolam

Causal relationship o

Cholestatic hepatitis was reported, starting after 4 months of treatment and complicated by pancreatitis and renal failure, which ultimately proved fatal. Hydrochlorothiazide and amiloride were used concurrently. Biopsy showed intracanalicular bile plugs, portal tracts expanded by collagenous tissue and marked periportal pseudoductular proliferation (1).

(1) Cobden et al (1981) *Postgr. Med. J., 57,* 730.

B.2. BARBITURATES

Barbital

Causal relationship o/+

An occasional case of barbital–induced jaundice has been described (1).

It concerned a woman who developed a generalized rash and mucosal lesions and fever 2 hours after ingestion of a combination of aminopyrine and barbital. Cholestatic jaundice developed subsequently with moderate parenchymal damage, canalicular dilatation and casts. After a prolonged course of 7 months a rechallenge with phenobarbital was immediately followed by fever, rash and aggravating jaundice.

(1) Pagliaro et al (1969) *Gastroenterology, 56,* 938.

Methylphenobarbital

Causal relationship o/ +

Methylphenobarbital is metabolized to phenobarbital and may therefore be expected to induce an analogous pattern of injury. One case of jaundice, secondary to submassive necrosis, appeared $3^{1}/_{2}$ months after initial intake. No hypersensitivity symptoms were noted. Inadvertent rechallenge after partial recovery was held responsible for a relapse. Histology showed multiple areas of confluent necrosis and bridging with a 50/50 mononuclear/neutrophilic infiltrate (1).

(1) Shapiro et al (1980) *Am. J. Gastroenterol., 74,* 270.

Methyprylon

Causal relationship o/ +

Although methyprylon is not a barbiturate, it is included in this group because it resembles these compounds structurally. A case of hepatic dysfunction was reported after overdosage, with a mixed hepatocellular–cholestatic pattern. Biopsy showed periportal hydropic cell swelling and regeneration with moderate cholestasis (1). Mild ASAT elevation was seen in 3 of 10 intoxicated patients (2).

(1) Loiudice et al (1978) *Dig. Dis. Sci., 23, Suppl,* 33s. (2) Bailey et al (1973) *Clin. Toxicol., 6,* 563.

Phenobarbital

Causal relationship +

In spite of the widespread use of phenobarbital, symptomatic hepatic in-

272

jury is probably rare. Besides occasional liver enzyme elevations and the well–known ground–glass appearance due to hypertrophy of the endo-plasmic reticulum, rare cases of symptomatic hepatic injury have been reported. Both cholestatic (2, 5) and hepatocellular (3, 4, 6, 7, 11) injury have been reported. These reactions were frequently accompanied by rash (1–8, 11, 12) which may vary from a bullous eruption (1) to complete exfoliation (4). Moreover, fever (3–8, 11, 12), lymphadenopathy (3, 4, 6, 8)/ splenomegaly (5, 8), periorbital edema (4, 6, 11) and eosinophilia (3, 11) favor an immunoallergic mechanism. The reaction started within 5 weeks (1–7, 11, 12) and disappeared in several months, except in 3 fatal cases (4, 8). Rechallenge performed in 2 cases was positive (5, 7). Histolo-gy showed cholestatic hepatitis (5). In other cases, necrosis varied from mild and scattered (6, 7) to massive (4). In a case of chronic hepatitis, por-tal fibrosis was accompanied by intense inflammation with mononuclear cells (8).

By induction of the cytochrome P450 enzyme system phenobarbital may enhance the hepatotoxicity of co–administered drugs, e.g. paraceta-mol in overdosage (9, 10), probably due to the increased formation of tox-ic metabolites. Although it is a proven tumor–promoting agent in animal toxicity tests, there is no conclusive evidence for enhanced carcinogene-sis in man. Liver enzyme elevations secondary to acute porphyric attacks may be caused by the induction of δ–aminolevulinic acid synthetase (13).

(1) Weber (1925) *Br. J. Child. Dis., 22,* 280. (2) Birch (1936) *Lancet, 1,* 478. (3) Wel-ton (1950) *J. Am. Med. Assoc., 143,* 232. (4) McGeachy et al (1953) *Am. J. Med., 14,* 600. (5) Pagliaro et al (1969) *Gastroenterology, 56,* 938. (6) Weisburst et al (1976) *South. Med. J., 69,* 126. (7) Thirunavukkarasu et al (1979) *Gastroenterology, 76,* 1261. (8) Klatskin (1975) In: Schiff (Ed), *Diseases of the Liver, 4th ed,* p 604. Lippin-cott, Philadelphia. (9) Mitchell et al (1973) *J. Pharmacol. Exp. Ther., 187,* 211. (10) Wilson et al (1978) *Am. J. Dis. Child., 132,* 466. (11) Evans et al (1976) *Drug Intell. Clin. Pharmacol., 10,* 439. (12) Lane et al (1984) *South. Med. J., 77,* 94.

B.3. ALCOHOLS/ALDEHYDES

Ethchlorvynol

```
      CH=CHCl
       |
CH≡C-C-CH₂-CH₃
       |
      OH
```

Causal relationship o

In several textbooks, cholestatic jaundice has been reported after oral in-take, but unfortunately no references are given (1, 2). One report of acute intoxication following intravenous 'recreational' administration of 3 g was followed by dehydration, pulmonary edema and progressive liver en-zyme elevations (ALAT 2200 IU), peaking on the 16th hospital day. Hypo-tension and other drug use complicated this case–history. Biopsy was 'con-sistent with drug–induced hepatitis' (3). The outcome was not reported.

(1) *The Extra Pharmacopoeia, 28th ed*, p 792. Pharmaceutical Press, London, 1982.
(2) Harvey (1975) In: *The Pharmacological Basis of Therapeutics, 5th ed*, p 102.
Macmillan, New York. (3) Hurwitz et al (1980) *Vet. Hum. Toxicol., 22, Suppl 2*,
66.

Methylpentynol

$$HC\equiv C-\overset{\overset{\displaystyle CH_3}{|}}{\underset{\underset{\displaystyle OH}{|}}{C}}-CH_2-CH_3$$

Causal relationship o

Methylpentynol has been mentioned as cause of a pattern resembling
that of obstructive jaundice (1) but no details were given.

(1) Klinge (1979) *Klinische Hepatologie*, p 6.158. Thieme, Stuttgart.

B.4. CARBAMATES/MISCELLANEOUS

Chlormezanone

Causal relationship o

Cholestatic hepatitis has been reported but no details were given (1).

(1) Klatskin (1975) In: Schiff (Ed), *Diseases of the Liver, 4th ed*, p 604. Lippincott,
Philadelphia.

Ectylurea

$$NH_2-CO-NH-CO-\overset{\overset{\displaystyle C_2H_5}{|}}{C}-CH-CH_3$$

Causal relationship +

A mild icteric, cholestatic hepatitis was observed, starting 2.5 weeks
after initial intake with rapid recovery after discontinuation. Biopsy
showed portal infiltration and bile plugging of canaliculi (1). Rechallenge was positive in 2 days.

(1) Hochman et al (1958) *N. Engl. J. Med., 259*, 583.

Mebutamate

Causal relationship o

Mebutamate has been mentioned as a possible cause of cholestatic jaundice, but no details were given (1). The drug has been used as a hypotensive agent and as an anxiolytic.

274

(1) Klinge (1979) *Klinische Hepatologie,* p 6.158. Thieme, Stuttgart.

Meprobamate

$$H_2N-OC-O-H_2C-\overset{\overset{\displaystyle CH_3}{|}}{\underset{\underset{\displaystyle C_3H_7}{|}}{C}}-CH_2-O-CO-NH_2$$

Causal relationship o

Cholestatic hepatitis was reported in 3 patients, starting with fever and urticaria (1 pt) and followed by jaundice (3 pts) after 1–6 months of intermittent treatment. Recovery took place after withdrawal of the drug (1). See also 'Carisoprodol' (Chapter 24).

(1) Klatskin (1975) In: Schiff (Ed), *Diseases of the Liver, 4th ed,* p 681. Lippincott, Philadelphia.

C. ANTIDEPRESSANTS

C.1. MONOAMINE OXIDASE (MAO) INHIBITORS

Iproclozide

$$Cl-\langle\rangle-O-CH_2-\overset{\overset{\displaystyle O}{\|}}{C}-NH-NH-CH\overset{\displaystyle CH_3}{\underset{\displaystyle CH_3}{<}}$$

Causal relationship o/ +

Four cases of fatal hepatic necrosis were attributed to the use of this agent. Jaundice appeared after more than 1 month of therapy and within 10 days of starting treatment with an enzyme–inducing drug. Immunoallergic signs were absent (1, 2). Enhanced formation of toxic metabolites due to enzyme induction was suggested to be analogous to the interactive effect of rifampicin and isoniazid, of which the latter is a hydrazine compound like iproclozide.

(1) Pessayre et al (1978) *Gastroenterology, 75,* 492. (2) Opolon et al (1969) *Rev. Méd. Chir. Mal. Foie, 44,* 251.

Iproniazid

$$CO-NH-NH-CH\overset{\displaystyle CH_3}{\underset{\displaystyle CH_3}{<}}$$

Causal relationship + +

Although abnormal serum aminotransferase levels have been reported in up to 20% of recipients, the incidence of jaundice has been estimated at only 1% (1). The symptomatic cases invariably demonstrate a pattern of hepatocellular necrosis, often extensive and confluent but sometimes mild. Cholestasis is secondary to necrosis. Immunoallergic signs are very rare. In approximately 70% of the cases, hepatic injury starts within 1–3 months after initiating therapy. The case–fatality rate has been estimated at 15–20%. Most patients recover after discontinuation, but fibrosis or cirrhosis may develop (2), especially after continuation or repeated use (1). Iproniazid is converted to toxic metabolites, probably by oxidation of isopropylhydrazine, an intermediate (3). Covalent binding of these reactive electrophilic metabolites to liver macromolecules paralleled liver cell necrosis (3).

Although iproniazid has been abandoned in several countries, it is still in use in some (e.g. France), as demonstrated by several recent cases of hepatic necrosis (1, 4). In 4 of these 6 published cases, prochlorperazine had been used concurrently and the authors suggested that this agent might have been responsible for an increased production of toxic metabolites of iproniazid due to enzyme induction (4). Four patients had antimitochondrial antibodies of the M_6 type which is not organ– or species–specific but, so far, it seems to be specific for iproniazid (1, 5).

(1) Danan et al (1983) *Gastroentérol. Clin. Biol., 7,* 529. (2) Zimmerman (1978) *Hepatotoxicity,* p 395. Appleton–Century–Crofts, New York. (3) Nelson et al (1976) *Science, 193,* 901. (4) Capron et al (1980) *Gastroentérol. Clin. Biol., 4,* 123. (5) Homberg et al (1982) *Clin. Exp. Immunol., 47,* 93.

Isocarboxazid

Causal relationship o

Some cases of jaundice have been described in the medical literature, appearing one (1) to $3^1/_2$ months (2) after starting therapy. In 1 case there was a concurrent rash, but this was not thought to be drug–related (2). Biochemically, there was a mixed cholestatic–hepatocellular pattern. Histology showed focal centrilobular and periportal necrosis, mild cholestasis and portal zones heavily infiltrated with mononuclear cells and eosinophils (2). One patient was treated with phenytoin concurrently (1) which should be noted because of the latter's enzyme–inducing properties.

(1) Benack et al (1961) *N. Engl. J. Med., 264,* 294. (2) Knight (1961) *Am. J. Psychiatry, 118,* 73.

Mebanazine

Causal relationship o/ +

Little experience has been obtained with this MAO inhibitor. One study mentioned ASAT elevation in 3 of 33 treated patients as against none in the placebo group (1).

(1) Barker et al (1965) *Br. J. Psychiatry, 111,* 1095.

Nialamide

CO-NH-NH-CH$_2$-CH$_2$-CO-NH-CH$_2$

Causal relationship o/ +

An occasional case of jaundice has been attributed to nialamide (1). Jaundice appeared after 3 weeks of use and subsided within 3 weeks after discontinuation. The patient had had the same reaction to pheniprazine 5 months previously. Histology showed patchy necrosis, steatosis and infiltration with neutrophils and lymphocytes.

(1) Holdsworth et al (1961) *Lancet, 2,* 621.

Phenelzine

CH$_2$-CH$_2$-NH-NH$_2$

Causal relationship o

Some cases of hepatic injury have been reported, varying from a mild mixed pattern of hepatitis (1) to acute yellow liver atrophy (2). One report mentioned 6 fatal cases and 13 non–fatal ones in 750,000 patients (2), but these figures are probably too low.

One case concerns a 64–year–old woman who developed angiosarcoma (3). She had been treated with phenelzine for 6 years (15–45 mg/d). She had not been exposed to well–known iatrogenic causes of angiosarcoma such as thorium dioxide. Although a causal relationship is speculative, it should be noted that this agent has induced angiosarcomas of the liver in mice on a continuous daily dose of 1.3–2.4 mg (4, 5).

(1) Holdsworth et al (1961) *Lancet, 2,* 621. (2) Anonymous (1963) *Med. News, 41,* 4. (3) Daneshmend et al (1979) *Br. Med. J., 1,* 1679. (4) Toth (1976) *Cancer Res., 36,* 917. (5) Toth (1975) *Cancer Res., 35,* 3693.

Pheniprazine

CH$_2$-CH-CH$_3$
|
NH-NH$_2$

Causal relationship o/ +

Like iproniazid, pheniprazine has been associated with significant hepatocellular damage (1–5), often fatal (1–4). The appearance of signs of hepatic injury varied from 3 weeks to 7 months after starting treatment. As with other MAO inhibitors, immunoallergic signs were absent or not considered to be associated with the agent (4). One patient later had the same reaction to nialamide (2), whereas another had previously had the same reaction to iproniazid (2). Histology showed mostly extensive necrosis with collapse of the reticulin framework and neutrophilic and mononuclear infiltration.

(1) Holdsworth et al (1961) *Lancet, 2,* 621. (2) Beer et al (1959) *J. Am. Med. Assoc., 171,* 887. (3) Dominguez et al (1962) *Gastroenterology, 42,* 69. (4) Berkowitz et al (1961) *Am. J. Dig. Dis., 6,* 160. (5) Fentem et al (1961) *Br. Med. J., 2,* 1616.

Phenoxyproperazine

O–CH$_2$–CH–NH–NH$_2$
|
CH$_3$

Causal relationship o

Two cases of severe hepatic necrosis were seen after 1–2 months of therapy (20 mg/d). The outcome after discontinuation and treatment with corticosteroids was favorable (1).

(1) Cook et al (1965) *Lancet, 1,* 175.

Tranylcypromine

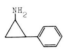

Causal relationship +

Tranylcypromine differs from other MAO inhibitors in the absence of a hydrazine moiety (HN–NH$_2$). Hence, hepatic injury is probably very rare but has been recorded. In 1 well–documented case, jaundice appeared approximately 6 weeks after starting treatment and normalized within 3 weeks after discontinuation. There was a mixed pattern of injury accompanied by mild eosinophilia. Rechallenge was immediately followed by marked liver enzyme elevation (1).

(1) Bandt et al (1964) *J. Am. Med. Assoc., 188,* 752.

C.2. TRICYCLICS

Amineptine

NH–(CH$_2$)$_6$–COOH

Causal relationship +

Amineptine has caused several well–documented cases of hepatic injury, mostly of a cholestatic pattern with jaundice (1–8). Many of these cases have been accompanied by fever (1–3, 7), eosinophilia of 5–15% (1–4, 6, 7), and less frequently by arthralgia (3). The onset is usually within the first 6 weeks of treatment but has varied from 1 day (after an overdose) to 90 days after starting intake. Histology mostly showed centrilobular cholestasis (1, 3, 8) and portal mononuclear infiltration. A rechallenge was positive in several cases (1, 3, 4, 6, 8). Although an immunoallergic mechanism seems possible, amineptine apparently has intrinsic toxic potential since several reports of overdosage mentioned signs of hepatic injury (1, 4, 5).

Although introduced relatively recently, many cases of hepatic injury have been attributed to this drug. Both the incidence and the pattern seem to differ from that of other tricyclics.

(1) Andrieu et al (1982) *Gastroentérol. Clin. Biol., 6*, 915. (2) Bel et al (1980) *Nouv. Presse Méd., 9*, 2356. (3) Bories et al (1980) *Nouv. Presse Méd., 9*, 3689. (4) Ramain et al (1981) *Gastroentérol. Clin. Biol., 5*, 469. (5) Bentata–Pessayre et al (1981) *Rev. Méd. Interne, 2*, 177. (6) Cleau (1981) *Gastroentérol. Clin. Biol., 5*, 1067. (7) Martin et al (1981) *Gastroentérol. Clin. Biol., 5*, 1071. (8) Bertrand et al (1982) *Gastroentérol. Clin. Biol., 6*, 946.

Amitriptyline

Causal relationship +

Cases have been reported of a mixed pattern with mild hepatocellular damage (1–3) but also of a predominantly hepatocellular pattern of injury (1, 4, 5). Concurrent rash and/or eosinophilia was reported in some cases (1, 2). A positive reaction to rechallenge was obtained in some reports (1, 4). A lymphocyte stimulation test with metabolite–containing serum from the patient was positive (6).

(1) Morgan (1969) *Br. J. Psychiatry, 115*, 105. (2) Anderson et al (1978) *J. Clin. Psychiatry, 39*, 37. (3) Biagi et al (1967) *Br. J. Psychiatry, 113*, 1113. (4) Yon et al (1975) *J. Am. Med. Assoc., 232*, 833. (5) Cunningham (1965) *Br. J. Psychiatry, 111*, 1107. (6) Namihisa et al (1975) *Leber Magen Darm, 5*, 73.

Desipramine

Causal relationship o

Jaundice was recorded during the first clinical trials but has remained poorly documented (1). In 1 report of fatal hepatic necrosis, desipramine and imipramine were used concurrently (2). In 2 more recent cases liver enzyme elevations were discovered 1–3 weeks after starting treatment. In one of them peripheral eosinophilia was present. Discontinuation resulted in rapid normalization (3). In a study of 46 patients on desipramine (2.5 mg/kg/d; mean 17.7 d), 4 developed mild ASAT elevation and 4 eosinophilia (4). This was not considered significant since high pre–treatment ASAT levels in 5 patients returned to normal.

(1) Council on Drugs (1965) *J. Am. Med. Assoc., 194*, 194. (2) Powell et al (1968) *J. Am. Med. Assoc., 206*, 642. (3) Price et al (1983) *J. Clin. Psychopharmacol., 3*, 243. (4) Price et al (1984) *Am. J. Psychiatry, 141*, 798.

Dimetacrine

Causal relationship o

Dimetacrine is an acridine derivative with a different structure from that of other tricyclics. Clinical experience with this agent is limited. One double–blind trial in hospitalized depressive patients comparing imipramine with dimetacrine demonstrated that the latter was less effective and caused a higher incidence of hepatic function abnormalities (1).

(1) Abuzzahab (1973) *Int. J. Clin. Pharmacol., 8,* 244.

Dosulepin (dothiepin)

Causal relationship o/ +

An occasional case of hepatic injury ascribed to dosulepin has been reported in the medical literature (1). A mixed cholestatic–hepatocellular biochemical pattern of injury with jaundice appeared 40 days after starting treatment with 75 mg/d dosulepin and benzodiazepines. Recovery was rapid after discontinuation. Some cases of acute intoxication in children have been noted, with cerebral edema and hemorrhage besides liver, renal and myocardial damage (2). Liver histology showed steatosis and focal necrosis in the centrilobular area.

(1) Porot et al (1980) *Psychol. Méd. (Paris), 12,* 2351. (2) Neoral et al (1981) *Kriminol. Forens. Wissenschaft, 44,* 31.

Imipramine

Causal relationship +

Cases of hepatic injury have been described with a predominantly cholestatic (1–5) but also with a, usually mild, mixed to hepatocellular (6–9) pattern. In some cases rash (10), fever (4, 5) or eosinophilia (10) was present concurrently. In 1 case there was also neuropathy and agranulocytosis (7). Readministration after normalization in 1 case was immediately followed by a relapse (9). A macrophage inhibition test was positive in the presence of the drug (6). Horst et al (11) described a patient with biliary–

280

cirrhosis–like abnormalities either caused, but more likely precipitated, by the use of imipramine (11). Antimitochondrial antibodies in this patient were absent (11). It should be noted that imipramine and chlorpromazine have the same side–chain and have a similar ring structure. The latter has also been associated with cases of biliary cirrhosis.

The incidence of hepatic injury due to imipramine and other tricyclics is unknown but has been estimated at approximately 1% (12). Andersen (5), however, found ALAT elevations, albeit mild, in 19 of 85 treated patients, whereas jaundice developed in 2 patients (5). The mechanism of injury is unknown. It might be interesting to know whether imipramine has the same cholestatic potency as chlorpromazine in animal toxicity tests since well–performed comparative studies have not yet been done, as far as we know.

(1) Short et al (1968) *J. Am. Med. Assoc.*, *206*, 1791. (2) Kuhn (1957) *Schweiz. Med. Wochenschr.*, *87*, 1135. (3) Lehmann (1958) *Can. Med. Assoc. J.*, *3*, 155. (4) Hoaken (1964) *Can. Med. Assoc. J.*, *90*, 1367. (5) Andersen et al (1959) *Acta Psychiatr. Neurol. Scand.*, *34*, 387. (6) Anonymous (1981) *Jpn. Med. Gaz.*, *18(8)*, 9. (7) Miller (1963) *Am. J. Psychiatry*, *120*, 185. (8) Moskovitz et al (1982) *J. Clin. Psychiatry*, *43*, 165. (9) Weaver et al (1977) *Dig. Dis. Sci.*, *22*, 551. (10) Mann et al (1981) *J. Clin. Psychopharmacol.*, *1*, 75. (11) Horst et al (1980) *Gastroenterology*, *79*, 550.

Opipramol

Causal relationship o

One case has been described of fatal hepatic necrosis 11 days after starting treatment. Since the drug was prescribed for general malaise, pre–existing disease in this patient may have been responsible, although pre–treatment APh values were normal. Autopsy showed a complete absence of hepatocytes (1).

(1) Van Vliet et al (1977) *Ned. Tijdschr. Geneeskd.*, *121*, 1325.

C.3. TETRACYCLICS/MISCELLANEOUS ANTIDEPRESSANTS

Amfebutamone (bupropion)

Causal relationship o

Amfebutamone is an antidepressant with a structure differing from that of other antidepressants. Little is yet known about its clinical usefulness, but according to clinical trials its side–effect profile is comparable to that of amitriptyline, except for a less sedative effect. In animal toxicity tests, chronic administration produced mild reversible hepatic injury (1), but so far no significant hepatotoxic effect has been reported in man.

(1) Tucker (1983) *J. Clin. Psychiatry, 44, Sect. 2,* 60.

Iprindole

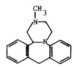

Causal relationship +

Some cases have been described of a cholestatic pattern of injury with jaundice (1–5), starting within 3 weeks after initiating treatment and mostly disappearing within 1 month after discontinuation. Some cases showed influenza–like prodromal symptoms (2–4), rash (1, 2) and eosinophilia (2, 5). A rechallenge was positive in 1 report (5). Histology, performed in 1 case showed centrilobular cholestasis without necrosis or inflammation (2).

(1) Young (1970) *Br. Med. J., 1,* 367. (2) Ajdukiewicz et al (1971) *Gut, 12,* 705. (3) Price et al (1970) *Br. Med. J., 1,* 238. (4) Harrison et al (1970) *Br. Med. J., 4,* 368. (5) Aylett (1971) *Br. Med. J., 1,* 112.

Mianserin

Causal relationship o/ +

Cases have been reported of a cholestatic or mixed pattern of injury with jaundice (1–3). Fever (1, 3) and neutropenia (1) accompanied hepatic involvement. The onset was within the first 3 weeks of therapy (2, 3) but in 1 case following 3 months (1). In another case concurrent use of baclofen may have been responsible (2).

In one of the cases cholestatic jaundice, accompanied by fever, appeared 11 days after starting treatment. After normalization of all values following discontinuation of mianserin, treatment was instituted with nomifensine. Four weeks later cholestatic jaundice reappeared, accompanied by marked ASAT/ALAT elevation and eosinophilia without fever. Histology showed centrilobular cholestasis, cellular degeneration and ballooning (3).

(1) Adverse Drug Reaction Advisory Committee (1980) *Med. J. Aust., 2,* 673. (2) Goldstraw et al (1983) *NZ Med. J., 96,* 985. (3) Zarski et al (1983) *Gastroentérol. Clin. Biol., 7,* 220.

Nomifensine

Causal relationship +

Several cases have been described of mild (1–6) to moderate/marked (3, 7, 8) hepatocellular injury. Fever is a prominent feature (1–8), often above 39°C, and may occur without signs of hepatic injury, analogous to methyldopa. Concurrent eosinophilia (1, 4), rash and conjunctivitis (4), and elevated IgE levels (3) have been noted. The onset is mostly within 2–3 weeks (1, 3–5, 7), but symptoms may appear later, although usually within 2 months (2, 8). A rechallenge performed in 4 cases was immediately followed by a relapse (1, 3, 4, 8). Histology showed a granulomatous pattern (2, 5, 7), although 1 case resembled chronic active hepatitis (3).

(1) Dankbaar et al (1980) *Ned. Tijdschr. Geneeskd., 124,* 2184. (2) Hunziker et al (1980) *Schweiz. Med. Wochenschr., 110,* 1295. (3) Nielsen et al (1981) *Ugeskr. Laeg., 143,* 1328. (4) Thomsen et al (1981) *Ugeskr. Laeg., 143,* 1331. (5) Weihe et al (1981) *Ugeskr. Laeg., 143,* 1330. (6) Enanth et al (1978) *Curr. Ther. Res., 23,* 213. (7) Haughton et al (1982) *Pharma Bull., 64,* 66. (8) Brandes et al (1980) *Med. Welt, 31,* 1607.

Trazodone

Causal relationship o/ +

Two cases of a mixed hepatocellular–cholestatic reaction have been reported (1, 2). The onset was 2–3 weeks after starting therapy (1, 2) and in 1 patient was accompanied by a mildly exfoliative rash (1). Histology showed canalicular cholestasis, acidophilic bodies, Kupffer cell hyperplasia and portal inflammation with eosinophils, neutrophils and mononuclear cells.

(1) Chu et al (1983) *Ann. Intern. Med., 99,* 128. (2) Sheikh et al (1983) *Ann. Intern. Med., 99,* 572.

Viloxazine

Causal relationship o

Jaundice and elevated aminotransferase levels have been reported (1).

Only a limited amount of experience has been gained with this drug so far.

(1) *The Extra Pharmacopoeia, 28th ed*, p 134. Pharmaceutical Press, London, 1982.

Zimelidine

Causal relationship +

Zimelidine is a new antidepressant which is claimed to inhibit the neuronal reuptake of serotonin more selectively than other drugs. In the medical literature, mild to moderately elevated aminotransferase levels, fever and jaundice have been reported (1–3, 5–7), usually appearing in 3 weeks after starting therapy. A clinical trial also showed a high incidence of liver enzyme elevations (8). In 1 case hepatocellular jaundice and fever recurred within 1 week after rechallenge (5). The Swedish Adverse Drug Reactions Advisory Committee in 1982 received 96 reports of of which 35 mentioned a generalized hypersensitivity reaction with fever and/or arthralgia/myalgia, rash and liver damage (see Table 1) within 3 weeks after initial treatment (4). Most patients used 100–200 mg/d. With the exception of mild jaundice in 1 patient, liver damage appeared to be restricted to ASAT/ALAT elevation up to 2–5 times the upper normal limit. Biochemically, the pattern was of a mixed cholestatic–hepatocellular type. Biopsy was performed in a few patients and showed biliary stasis and granulomatous hepatitis.

TABLE 1 *Hypersensitivity symptoms in 80 patients, possibly or probably related to the use of zimelidine (adapted from Ref. 4)*

Fever	43
Exanthema	23
Urticaria+Quincke's edema	5
Liver damage	26
Arthralgia/Myalgia	32

In at least 8 patients the hypersensitivity reaction has been followed by Guillain–Barré syndrome and, based on epidemiological evidence of an association with the intake of zimelidine, this drug has been withdrawn worldwide.

(1) Sommerville et al (1982) *Br. Med. J., 285*, 1009. (2) Coppen et al (1979) *Psychopharmacology, 63*, 199. (3) Aberg et al (1979) *Acta Med. Scand., 59*, 45. (4) *SAD-RAC Bull.*, 1983, *39/40*. (5) Simpson et al (1983) *Br. Med. J., 287*, 1181. (6) Ursing et al (1983) *Läkartidningen, 80*, 32. (7) Sawyer et al (1983) *Br. Med. J., 287*, 1555. (8) Wålinder et al (1983) *Acta Psychiatr. Scand., Suppl. 308, 68*, 147.

D. PSYCHOSTIMULANTS

Methylphenidate

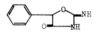

Causal relationship +

A hepatocellular pattern of injury was observed in 1 case, starting in the first week of intake (30 mg/d). Normalization occurred in 10 days after discontinuation. Rechallenge was positive within 2 days (2.5 mg/d) (1). Mehta et al (2) documented liver enzyme and bilirubin elevations during intravenous abuse of methylphenidate. Histology showed hepatocellular disarray and portal infiltration. A rechallenge caused re–elevation of laboratory values.

(1) Goodman (1972) *NY State J. Med., 72,* 2339. (2) Mehta et al (1984) *J. Clin. Gastroenterol., 6,* 149.

Pemoline

Causal relationship +

Pemoline is a central nervous system stimulant which has been used for a variety of conditions including fatigue, memory impairment and depression. It is still in use for the treatment of hyperkinesis in children. Approximately 2% of children show transient ASAT and/or ALAT elevations (1). In a study of 9 hyperactive children treated for 8 months these elevations reappeared after rechallenge with the drug (2). Tolman et al (3) in a study of 600 patients reported 2 patients with ASAT elevation, discovered 8 weeks after starting therapy and increasing the dose up to 150 mg/d. There was recovery after discontinuation and a prompt reaction to rechallenge with 75 mg/d. Lymphocyte stimulation tests were negative. In both patients BSP storage capacity was significantly decreased and transport maximum increased, the latter of which is unusual. Histology showed mild steatosis, focal necrosis and portal inflammation. Recovery after rechallenge was slow (2–4 months) (3).

(1) Sampson (1975) *J. Am. Med. Assoc., 232,* 1204. (2) Lopatin et al (1980) In: Dukes (Ed), *Side Effects of Drugs, Annual 4,* p 1. Excerpta Medica, Amsterdam. (3) Tolman et al (1973) *Digestion, 9,* 532.

23. Vasodilators

Introduction

The vasodilating agents show a large overlap with other cardiovascular agents. Several antihypertensives, for instance, have powerful vasodilating effects but are nevertheless discussed in a different section. Inclusion of an agent in one of these groups may be arbitrary. Vasodilators are often used in patients with complicated medical histories and on several other drugs. Therefore it may be difficult to assess the causal relationship between the intake of one of these agents and hepatic injury.

With some exceptions, most vasodilators are without significant hepatotoxic effects, but most of them, including new drugs such as ketanserin (4), have been associated occasionally with mild liver enzyme elevations. The most important examples discussed below are perhexiline, papaverine and the nicotinic acid derivatives. Very interesting is the pattern resembling phospholipidosis which has been described mainly in the French literature in patients on perhexiline. Analogous cases have been observed in Japan where 4,4′–diethylaminoethoxyhexestrol (Coralgil), also a vasodilator, has led to over 100, sometimes fatal, cases of hepatosplenomegaly, phospholipidosis and cirrhosis (1).

Besides nicotinic acid, nicotinyl alcohol (β–pyridylcarbinol), aluminium nicotinate and inositol nicotinate have been associated with hepatic injury (see 'Nicotinic acid'). Some other agents have been only occasionally associated with liver injury, e.g. azapetine (2), which is structurally related to the tricyclic antidepressants.

Sulmazole, a new vasodilator recently under trial, may possibly cause liver dysfunction (3). Diltiazem, a new calcium–blocking agent, has been associated with jaundice (5), but no details were given and we are not yet aware of a published case–history.

(1) Zimmerman (1978) *Hepatotoxicity,* p 510. Appleton–Century–Crofts, New York. (2) Klinge (1979) *Klinische Hepatologie,* p 6.158. Thieme, Stuttgart. (3) Hagemeijer et al (1984) *Eur. Heart J., 5,* 158. (4) Verstraete (1984) In: Dukes (Ed), *Side Effects of Drugs, Annual 8,* p 199. Elsevier, Amsterdam. (5) Tartaglione (1982) *Drug Intell. Clin. Pharm., 16,* 371.

Benziodarone

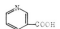

Causal relationship o

Benziodarone resembles amiodarone but lacks the diethylamino group. The agent is infrequently used, as far as we know. In 1964 it was withdrawn in the United Kingdom because of 11 cases of jaundice, appearing 8–16 weeks after starting treatment, which were reported to the Committee on Safety of Drugs (1). Few details were given and a causal relationship with the drug was debated.

(1) Cahal (1964) *Lancet, 2,* 754.

Nicotinic acid

Causal relationship +

Nicotinic acid and its derivatives have been used as both vasodilating and lipid–lowering agents, usually in a daily dose of over 3 g. In the treatment of pellagra a dose of 500 mg/d is sufficient and is not associated with significant side–effects. Several cases of jaundice have been reported (1–4, 6, 7, 10, 11), mostly with signs of hepatocellular degeneration or necrosis, sometimes massive (6), in patients treated with the high–dose regimen. The onset is often insidious with jaundice appearing after treatment for several months (1, 3, 5) to a year or more (2, 4, 6, 8, 10). In 1 case the onset of hepatic injury followed a dose increase on 2 successive occasions (11). Immunoallergic signs were absent in all cases. Histology showed, besides cholestasis and/or necrosis in most cases, portal and periportal fibrosis with signs of cirrhosis (10) and fibrosing pericholangitis (8).

Although most case–reports concerned nicotinic acid, nicotinyl alcohol (β–pyridylcarbinol) (8, 9) and aluminium nicotinate (3, 12) have also been incriminated of causing hepatic injury.

The incidence of hepatic injury appears to differ. In a group of 36 patients on nicotinic acid, 28% showed liver function abnormalities during treatment for more than 1 year with 3 g/d (4). Baggenstoss et al (7) noted 3 cases of jaundice in a group of 67 patients on 1.5–6 g/d; 2 of them had a pattern of cholestatic hepatitis on biopsy. Mishima et al (12) noted ASAT and/or ALAT elevation in 14% on 1.2 g/d inositol nicotinate. On the other hand, Zöllner et al (9) saw abnormal liver function tests in only 4% on nicotinyl alcohol.

The mechanism is probably toxic with an important role for individual susceptibility. The slow onset suggests chronic toxicity. There appears to be a dose–related effect; immunoallergic signs are absent. Baggenstoss et al (7) found evidence of focal cytoplasmic degradation of endoplasmic

287

reticulum and mitochondria in most of 8 patients on long–term therapy.

(1) Sugerman et al (1974) *J. Am. Med. Assoc., 228*, 202. (2) Rivin (1959) *J. Am. Med. Assoc., 170*, 2083. (3) Christensen et al (1961) *J. Am. Med. Assoc., 177*, 546. (4) Parsons (1961) *Arch. Intern. Med., 107*, 643. (5) Pardue (1961) *J. Am. Med. Assoc., 175*, 137. (6) Einstein et al (1975) *Dig. Dis. Sci., 20*, 282. (7) Baggenstoss et al (1967) *Gastroenterology, 52*, 314. (8) Pirovino et al (1980) *Dtsch. Med. Wochenschr., 105*, 1292. (9) Zöllner et al (1966) *Med. Klin., 61*, 2036. (10) Kohn et al (1969) *Am. J. Med. Sci., 258*, 94. (11) Patterson et al (1983) *South. Med. J., 76*, 239. (12) Mishima et al (1977) *Angiology, 28*, 84.

Nifedipine

Causal relationship +

Biochemically, a cholestatic hepatitis has been observed with jaundice and mildly elevated aminotransferase levels, starting within 14 days of treatment (1, 3). There was concurrent fever.

Rechallenge was positive within 1 day. A macrophage inhibition test was positive. Mast cell degranulation has been observed; a lymphocyte stimulation test was negative; no autoantibodies were present (2). A biopsy in 1 case showed subacute hepatitis against a background of alcoholic liver disease, but no further details were given (3).

(1) Rotmensch et al (1980) *Br. Med. J., 281*, 977. (2) Rotmensch et al (1981) *Z. Gastroenterol., 19*, 691. (3) Davidson (1980) *Br. Med. J., 281*, 1354.

Papaverine

Causal relationship +

Elevated APh and ASAT/ALAT levels were found in 27% (1) to 43% (2, 3) of patients (300–600 mg/d). Especially older people seem to be at risk (2, 3). Cases of a hepatocellular (1, 4) and mixed (1, 3) type of hepatic injury have been observed; chronic active hepatitis was reported in 1 case (5). Except for fever (1), no concurrent immunoallergic signs were observed. Onset was mostly within 5 weeks (1, 3, 4). Biopsy showed non–specific inflammatory changes (3, 4), focal necrosis with considerable eosinophilic periportal infiltration (1) or piecemeal necrosis and bridging fibrosis (5). An occasional granuloma was reported (3).

Rechallenge was positive in 2 days (1, 4) to 1 week (5). Accelerated and more serious reaction to rechallenge (1) suggests immunoallergy. Nevertheless, additional intrinsic toxicity is strongly supported by the high incidence of liver enzyme elevations.

(1) Rønnov–Jessen et al (1969) *N. Engl. J. Med., 281*, 1333. (2) Driemen (1973) *J. Am. Geriatr. Soc., 21*, 202. (3) Pathy et al (1980) *Postgr. Med. J., 56*, 488. (4) Chousterman et al (1980) *Nouv. Presse Méd., 9*, 1899. (5) Poupon et al (1978) *Gastroentérol. Clin. Biol., 2*, 305.

Perhexiline

Causal relationship + +

Perhexiline is usually started at 100–200 mg/d and lowered during the following weeks to months. It has a half–life of up to 12 days. Serum ASAT/ALAT/bilirubin elevations or abnormal BSP retention is encountered in a high percentage, varying from BSP retention in up to 75% (3, 4) to ALAT elevation in 30% (3) on 100–400 mg/d. In addition, several metabolic disturbances such as hypertriglyceridemia (5, 7, 8), elevation of free fatty acids (5) and hypoglycemia (6, 9, 10, 25) suggest a far–reaching influence on cellular function. In this context, weight loss (2, 11, 13, 15, 18, 19, 21, 22, 26) is interesting but remains unexplained. Many cases of symptomatic liver injury have been described (2, 12–28). The latent period to appearance varied from 3 months to several years, mostly insidiously with mild enzyme changes progressing to cirrhosis (1, 2, 12, 14, 16–19, 21–28). The case–fatality rate is high. No immunoallergic signs have been reported, except for a positive lymphocyte stimulation test in some cases (25, 28). Histology showed non–specific changes with diffuse steatosis and cellular hyperplasia (3) or, more frequently, a pattern resembling alcoholic hepatitis with necrosis and neutrophilic infiltration, Mallory's hyaline and beginning micronodular cirrhosis. Cholestasis is mostly absent. Several reports mentioned accumulation of triglycerides, gangliosides and phospholipids in the liver in the presence of numerous lysosomal pigmentary inclusions, of which several had a lamellar appearance. Ganglioside storage in nerve cells has also been noted (31). Indeed, neuropathy is often seen concurrently (2, 15, 16, 18, 20–22, 25, 26) and like the liver injury is probably secondary to impairment of lipid metabolism (32). Schwann, liver and endothelial cells appear to be sensitive (32). In an in–vitro assay, accumulation of gangliosides, phospholipids and cholesterol was noted in human skin fibroblasts with concentric lamellar inclusion bodies (32). Concurrent use of alcohol may have been responsible in some of the patients (14, 15), but others were teetotallers or used only minimal amounts. Discontinuation has led to recovery in some cases but others nevertheless developed progressive cirrhosis.

The drug or one of its metabolites is obviously an interesting but important hepatotoxin. Hepatotoxicity is probably indirect: with its long half–life and its apolar and polar ring structure, this drug has the ability to induce phospholipidosis like amiodarone and 4,4′–diethylaminoethoxyhexestrol. The high incidence of liver function abnormalities and the insidious course cast doubt on the drug's usefulness. If used, it has been

289

advised to start with 100 mg/d (18) or even less and to increase the dose only very slowly. Serum levels should not exceed 600 ng/ml (29). Concurrent use of alcohol should be discouraged. Regular assessment of liver enzyme levels is necessary.

(1) Hamchi et al (1982) *Acta Gastroenterol. Belg., 45*, 210. (2) Beaugrand et al (1978) *Gastroentérol. Clin. Biol., 2*, 579. (3) Poupon et al (1980) *Digestion, 20*, 145. (4) Howard et al (1976) *Br. Med. J., 1*, 133. (5) Dudognon et al (1979) *Coeur Méd. Interne, 18*, 129. (6) Schlienger et al (1978) *Coeur Méd. Interne, 17*, 631. (7) Bourrat et al (1975) *Nouv. Presse Méd., 4*, 2528. (8) Crevelier et al (1974) *Nouv. Presse Méd., 3*, 2182. (9) Roger et al (1975) *Nouv. Presse Méd., 4*, 2663. (10) Feldman (1974) *Nouv. Presse Méd., 3*, 2580. (11) Masoni et al (1975) *Am. Heart J., 90*, 145. (12) Forbes et al (1979) *J. Clin. Pathol., 32*, 1282. (13) Lewis et al (1979) *Gut, 20*, 186. (14) Roberts et al (1981) *Med. J. Aust., 2*, 553. (15) Paliard et al (1981) *Gastroentérol. Clin. Biol., 5*, 564. (16) Dawes et al (1982) *Lancet, 2*, 109. (17) Heathfield et al (1982) *Lancet, 1*, 507. (18) Hay et al (1983) *NZ Med. J., 96*, 202. (19) Pieterse et al (1983) *Pathology, 15*, 201. (20) Caruzzo et al (1980) *Am. Heart J., 108*, 270. (21) Beaugrand et al (1977) *Gastroentérol. Clin. Biol., 1*, 745. (22) Bonnet et al (1978) *Nouv. Presse Méd., 7*, 208. (23) Labram et al (1977) *Concours Méd., 99*, 5149. (24) Meullenet et al (1977) *Gastroentérol. Clin. Biol., 1*, 118. (25) Paliard et al (1978) *Digestion, 17*, 419. (26) Pessayre et al (1979) *Gastroenterology, 76*, 170. (27) Roche et al (1978) *Nouv. Presse Méd., 7*, 521. (28) Bertrand et al (1978) *Ann. Méd. Interne, 129*, 565. (29) Horowitz et al (1982) *Med. J. Aust., 2*, 9. (30) Lageron et al (1977) *Lancet, 1*, 483. (31) Pollet et al (1977) *Lancet, 1*, 1258. (32) Hauw et al (1980) *Virchows Arch. Abt. B. Cell. Pathol., 34*, 239.

Pyridinol carbamate

$H_3C-HN-CO-O-H_2C$ ⬡ $CH_2-O-OC-NH-CH_3$

Causal relationship +

Pyridinol carbamate is claimed to be a bradykinin antagonist and to have beneficial effects in the treatment of atherosclerosis. It has been used mostly in Japan. ASAT and/or ALAT elevations have been reported in up to 10% of cases in some studies (1).

Of 30 cases of hepatic injury reported to the Japanese Ministry of Health, 23 occurred between 1 and 3 months after starting treatment (2). Rechallenge in 11 patients resulted in relapse within 21 days in all of them, in 9 patients within 10 days. About half the cases recovered within 1 month after discontinuation. Some patients had fever and eosinophilia. Histology showed mild reactive or focal hepatitis (2) or a viral–hepatitis-like pattern with mononuclear infiltration and slight hepatocyte swelling (3). In some there was bridging necrosis (2). Although the mechanism is unknown, dose independence, a positive lymphocyte stimulation test (2, 4), a prompt reaction to rechallenge (2, 3) and irreproducibility in animals strongly suggest immunoallergy. The Japanese authorities estimated the incidence at 0.73% (2), but this may be higher due to possible underreporting. Aminotransferase elevations are probably more frequent and assessment every 2 weeks for the first 6 months has been advised (2).

(1) Mishima et al (1977) *Angiology, 28,* 84. (2) Anonymous (1976) *Jpn. Med. Gaz., 13,* 8. (3) Litvin et al (1977) *Lancet, 1,* 1257. (4) Namihisa et al (1975) *Leber Magen Darm, 5,* 73.

Suloctidil

```
     OH
     |
     CH-CH-CH3
        |
        NH-(CH2)7-CH3


  S-CH(CH3)2
```

Causal relationship o/ +

Markedly elevated aminotransferase levels to a level consistent with mild hepatitis were reported in 3 of 20 patients. Biochemically, a hepatocellular pattern was seen (1). A case of hepatocellular injury was noted by Perrin et al (2, 3). After 5 weeks of treatment, jaundice appeared. Immunoallergic signs were absent. Histology showed diffuse hepatocellular degeneration with ballooning and necrotic cells, centrilobular cholestasis and a neutrophilic portal infiltrate. Readministration was followed by a relapse on several occasions and finally the patient developed cirrhosis and died. An additional case in an alcoholic patient was doubtful (3).

(1) Schouten et al (1982) *Eur. J. Clin. Pharmacol., 22,* 559. (2) Perrin et al (1983) *Gastroentérol. Clin. Biol., 7,* 1042. (3) Beaujard et al (1984) *Presse Méd., 13,* 1218.

24. Muscle relaxants

A. Central relaxants
B. Spinal/skeletal relaxants

Introduction

Muscle relaxants comprise two important groups: those affecting neuromuscular transmission used primarily in operative procedures and those used for reducing muscle spasm.

The depolarizing and non–depolarizing muscle relaxants used to facilitate muscle relaxation during operation have not been held responsible for hepatic injury and are probably not hepatotoxic. Hepatic injury sometimes observed after their use in certain cases may be ascribed mostly to concurrently used anesthetic agents, transfusion, operation or complications. Some of these agents, especially suxamethonium, have been associated with malignant hyperthermia. In these cases a significant rise in ASAT and LDH concentrations may accompany a rise in creatinine phosphokinase; ALAT remains normal because the enzymes are of muscular origin.

Drugs used in the treatment of muscle spasm diminish skeletal muscle tone and involuntary movement. Some of these drugs act selectively on the central nervous system (e.g. carisoprodol and chlorzoxazone), whereas others have a direct action on muscle fibers (e.g. dantrolene) or have a predominantly spinal action (e.g. baclofen).

Most cases of hepatic injury have been associated with agents used to reduce muscle spasm and have generally involved a hepatocellular type of injury. With the exception of zoxazolamine, which was withdrawn following several cases of fatal massive necrosis, and dantrolene, hepatic injury by these agents has been reported only rarely. Chlorzoxazone (see below) and metaxalone (1), both structurally related to zoxazolamine, have only rarely been reported as a cause of jaundice.

(1) *The Extra Pharmacopoeia, 28th ed,* p 986. Pharmaceutical Press, London, 1982.

A. CENTRAL RELAXANTS

Carisoprodol

$$H_2N-OC-O-H_2C-\underset{\underset{C_3H_7}{|}}{\overset{\overset{CH_3}{|}}{C}}-CH_2-O-CO-NH-CH\overset{CH_3}{\underset{CH_3}{<}}$$

Causal relationship o

Mild jaundice and erythema multiforme developed approximately 2 weeks after a 3–day course of carisoprodol in 1 patient (1). There was rapid recovery. Biopsy showed scattered foci of acidophilic degeneration and cellular unrest. See also 'Meprobamate' which resembles carisoprodol structurally.

(1) Klatskin (1975) In: Schiff (Ed), *Diseases of the Liver, 4th ed,* p 604. Lippincott, Philadelphia.

Chlorzoxazone

Causal relationship o

A hepatocellular type of injury with jaundice has been reported, with normalization in 6 weeks after which biopsy showed only slight fibrosis (1). No further details were given. The Swedish Adverse Drug Reaction Advisory Committee received several reports of hepatic injury, probably caused by a combination of dextropropoxyphen, acetylsalicylic acid and chlorzoxazone (2). Although the last may also have been responsible, the first agent was considered to be the more likely cause. It should be noted that this drug bears a strong structural resemblance to zoxazolamine which has been abandoned because of severe hepatic necrosis (see below).

(1) Bjørneboe et al (1967) *Acta Med. Scand., 182, Fasc. 4,* 491. (2) *SADRAC Bull.,* 1983, *38,* 1.

Zoxazolamine

Causal relationship o/ +

Acute hepatocellular necrosis (1, 3–5) and cholestatic hepatitis (2) have been reported. Jaundice appeared within 5 weeks (1–3) or after several months (1, 4, 5). Most patients died (1, 3, 5); the others recovered in 2–3 months. No immunoallergic signs were observed. Biopsy showed diffuse (4), centrilobular, hemorrhagic (1) and massive (3, 5) necrosis, early fibrosis (4), and mononuclear (3–5) and eosinophilic (3) infiltration.

Other drugs had been given intravenously in the preceding period (3,

5), suggesting that needle–transmitted viral hepatitis may have played a role in these older cases.

(1) Hoffbauer et al (1958) *Gastroenterology, 34,* 1048. (2) Jasper (1960) *Am. J. Gastroenterol., 34,* 419. (3) Carr et al (1961) *N. Engl. J. Med., 264,* 977. (4) Eisenstadt et al (1961) *J. Am. Med. Assoc., 176,* 874. (5) Lubell (1962) *NY State J. Med., 62,* 3807.

B. SPINAL/SKELETAL RELAXANTS

Baclofen

$H_2N-CH_2-CH-CH_2-COOH$

Cl

Causal relationship o

Five patients were reported with mildly elevated aminotransferase levels, 1–2 months after starting treatment; there were no symptoms. A lymphocyte stimulation test was positive in 1 case (1). In a patient with cholestatic jaundice, appearing 3 weeks after starting therapy with baclofen and mianserin, both drugs could have been responsible (2). In another case ASAT/ALAT levels started to rise in the first 6 weeks of therapy, gradually increasing to a highest ALAT value of 414 IU/l over the next few months. Discontinuation was followed by a rapid decline with normalization in approximately 1 month (3).

(1) Anonymous (1981) *Jpn. Med. Gaz., 20 May,* 12. (2) Goldstraw et al (1983) *NZ Med. J., 96,* 985. (3) Chui et al (1984) *Clin. Pharm., 3,* 196.

Dantrolene

N-CH   NO$_2$

N   O

O   NH

Causal relationship +

A mainly hepatocellular (1, 3, 4, 6, 9) or mixed (2, 4, 7) pattern of injury has been observed. Fatality (3, 5–7) is estimated at 28% of cases with overt hepatic injury (6). Immunoallergic signs were absent. Injury mostly developed after several months of treatment (2–7, 9) and resolved in 1–5 months after discontinuation in non–fatal cases. Biopsy varied from mild spotty necrosis (2, 4, 6) to confluent necrosis with lobular disarray and bridging (1, 4, 7, 9) and massive necrosis (3, 6). Chronic active hepatitis and cirrhosis were demonstrated in several patients (6). A picture resembling that of ascending cholangitis was seen in 2 patients (4).

Rechallenge, performed in some cases, was positive in 2–4 weeks (1, 6). A trial for 60 days in 1044 patients showed hepatic injury in 1.8% of cases of which 0.6% were icteric and 0.3% had a fatal course (6). All fatalities occurred after more than 2 months of treatment (57% within 6 months). All patients were more than 30 years old (6). Doses of >300 mg/d seemed to be associated with more frequent and severe hepatic injury. Dose–dependence, however, was not confirmed by others (4, 8) and several other reports mentioned injury at lower doses (1, 4, 5, 8, 9). Roy et al (10) showed that dantrolene caused a significant decrease in hepatic mixed–function oxidase system activity and in cytochrome P450 content. They suggested that dantrolene or one of its metabolites acts as an electrophilic agent, forming stable complexes with hepatic protein. The observation that phenobarbital pretreatment decreases binding to hepatic protein suggests that dantrolene rather than its metabolites was responsible (10).

(1) Ogburn et al (1976) *Ann. Intern. Med., 84,* 53. (2) Schneider et al (1976) *J. Am. Med. Assoc., 235,* 1590. (3) Donegan et al (1978) *Dig. Dis. Sci., 23, Suppl,* 48. (4) Wilkinson et al (1979) *Gut, 20,* 33. (5) Goodman et al (1977) *NY State J. Med., 77,* 1759. (6) Utili et al (1977) *Gastroenterology, 72,* 610. (7) Cornette et al (1980) *Acta Neurol. Belg., 80,* 336. (8) Molnar et al (1978) *NY State J. Med., 78,* 1233. (9) Lundin et al (1977) *Drug Intell. Clin. Pharm., 11,* 279. (10) Roy et al (1980) *Res. Commun. Chem. Pathol. Pharmacol., 27,* 507.

25. Vitamins

Introduction

The main indication for vitamin therapy is a latent or manifest deficiency state. Unfortunately, several vitamins are abused in excessive amounts on irrational grounds, thereby producing acute and chronic intoxications. This may present a diagnostic problem since abuse is either not considered as such or is completely denied, in which case the assessment of blood levels may confirm the diagnosis.

High doses of vitamin A are therapeutically employed for the treatment of psoriasis, ichthyosis or acne, but as an 'over the counter' preparation it is often abused as a remedy against the common cold. Recent assertions that it has antineoplastic activity will probably enhance its abuse as soon as the lay public becomes fully aware of this still unproven claim.

The most important potentially hepatotoxic vitamins are vitamin A and nicotinamide/nicotinic acid (the latter is discussed with the vasodilators in Chapter 23). High doses of pyridoxine have been associated with ASAT elevations (1). Menadione and its water–soluble derivatives have been reported to compete with bilirubin; excessive jaundice in neonates has been ascribed to this effect and to its hemolytic properties (2).

(1) Westerholm (1980) In: Dukes (Ed), *Side Effects of Drugs, 9th ed,* p 632. Excerpta Medica, Amsterdam. (2) *The Extra Pharmacopoeia, 28th ed,* p 1635. Pharmaceutical Press, London, 1982.

Nicotinamide

Causal relationship +

Nicotinamide does not have a vasodilating effect, unlike most other nicotinic acid derivatives (1). It is however highly likely that its hepatotoxic potential in high doses is the same (see Chapter 23). Winter et al (2) noted very high ASAT/ALAT concentrations and hyperbilirubinemia in a patient on 3 successive occasions which proved to be preceded by a dose increase to 9 g/d. These values returned to normal after a decrease to 3 g/d. A subsequent challenge with 9 g/d was followed by a relapse. Histology showed swollen parenchymal cells in the centrilobular area and bridging fibrosis with only a few inflammatory cells.

(1) *The Extra Pharmacopoeia, 28th ed*, p 1635. Pharmaceutical Press, London, 1982. (2) Winter et al (1973) *N. Engl. J. Med., 289*, 1180.

Vitamin A

Causal relationship +

Acute hypervitaminosis A with clinical signs of toxicity has been reported to occur after the intake of 1–2 million IU (1, 2) in adults, whereas children may become intoxicated at much lower doses. It is mainly associated with central nervous system (CNS) symptoms such as drowsiness, irritability, delirium and convulsions (1).

Chronic hypervitaminosis A may occur after long–term administration of doses as low as 10,000 IU/d (1). Higher doses for prolonged periods cause malaise, CNS symptoms, skin and musculoskeletal changes; signs of hepatic involvement in the form of hepatomegaly are frequent. In a review of 80 cases in the literature, hepatomegaly was reported in 11 cases (2). Usually liver enzyme concentrations are normal or mildly to moderately elevated, whereas jaundice is absent. However, the skin may be discolored orange–yellow.

More worrying are reports of perisinusoidal fibrosis and cirrhosis after the intake of high doses for 1 to several years (4, 5, 7, 8, 12, 19, 20); in one report cirrhosis was discovered $3^1/_2$ years after a course of 70 million IU for 7 weeks (6). Usually these cases also show extrahepatic signs of chronic vitamin A intoxication but these may be absent (20). Others have noted portal hypertension and ascites without histological signs of cirrhosis (3, 9, 11, 14, 17), in 1 case accompanied by pleural effusion (14). In most of these cases the clinical features disappeared or improved after discontinuation, but in 1 case ascites remained despite this (9). Several authors point to an increase in perisinusoidal lipocytes (Ito cells) with varying degrees of perisinusoidal fibrosis with collagen in the space of Disse. In some cases this accumulation of lipocytes is the main feature (11, 15, 17), whereas in other cases fibrosis extends to the portal area (9). Sinusoidal dilatation may be present (4). Some reports mentioned fibrous thickening of central vein walls (4, 9, 14).

Blood levels are often elevated but were below normal in a patient with a decrease in retinol–binding protein (16). Vitamin A fluorescence of biopsies is diagnostic. Quantification of vitamin A in liver tissue may show massive amounts of up to 19,000 IU/g (16).

The portal hypertension is supposed to be secondary to obstruction of sinusoids due to an increase in the number and size of lipocytes (9). Possibly these cells are precursors of fibroblasts (10) and thereby responsible for the perisinusoidal fibrosis.

An interesting suggestion is the possible unmasking effect of acute intercurrent liver disease on hypervitaminosis A. By a decrease in the production of retinol–binding protein, lipoprotein–bound retinyl esters increase accompanied by signs of enhanced toxicity (13).

In a study of rats on vitamin A supplements in amounts considered harmless, chronic alcohol administration induced lesions in the liver which are uncommon on alcohol alone. Necrosis, inflammation and numerous myofibroblasts appeared in association with abundant collagen fibers. Retinol–binding globulin was decreased. The authors conclude that alcohol and vitamin A may have a mutually potentiating adverse effect on the liver (18).

(1) Westerholm (1980) In: Dukes (Ed), *Meyler's Side Effects of Drugs, 9th ed*, p 632. Excerpta Medica, Amsterdam. (2) Goeckenjan et al (1972) *Dtsch. Med. Wochenschr., 97*, 1424. (3) Baadsgaard et al (1983) *Dan. Med. Bull., 30*, 51. (4) Babb et al (1978) *West. J. Med., 3*, 244. (5) Frøkjaer (1981) *Ugeskr. Laeg., 143*, 2038. (6) Fleischmann et al (1977) *Dtsch. Med. Wochenschr., 102*, 1637. (7) Jacques et al (1979) *Gastroenterology, 76*, 599. (8) Eaton (1978) *Am. J. Hosp. Pharm., 35*, 1099. (9) Russell et al (1974) *N. Engl. J. Med., 291*, 435. (10) Popper et al (1970) *Am. J. Med., 49*, 707. (11) Kistler et al (1977) *Schweiz. Med. Wochenschr., 107*, 825. (12) Tholen et al (1980) *Leber Magen Darm, 10*, 193. (13) Hatoff et al (1982) *Gastroenterology, 82*, 124. (14) Rosenberg et al (1982) *Clin. Pediatr. (Philadelphia), 21*, 435. (15) Farrell et al (1977) *Dig. Dis., 22*, 724. (16) Weber et al (1982) *Gastroenterology, 82*, 118. (17) Guarascio et al (1983) *J. Clin. Pathol., 36*, 769. (18) Leo et al (1983) *Hepatology, 3*, 1. (19) Le Marchand et al (1984) *Gastroentérol. Clin. Biol., 8*, 116. (20) Verneau et al (1984) *Gastroentérol. Clin. Biol., 8*, 121.

26. Miscellaneous and non–orthodox agents

A. Miscellaneous agents
B. Non–orthodox agents

Introduction

This Chapter comprises a variety of agents which are used for diverse purposes. Several miscellaneous drugs have been associated with hepatic injury, the most important being isaxonine and agents used in alcohol–aversion therapy, i.e. disulfiram and calcium carbimide. Especially the progressive fibrosis which has been associated by Vazquez and co–workers with continuous carbimide treatment in alcoholics is a matter of concern. Nitrefazole, a recently marketed alcohol–aversion agent, was withdrawn in the Federal Republic of Germany following reports of severe liver and bone marrow damage (15).

The term 'non–orthodox agents' is chosen from a Western point of view since many of these agents are considered as orthodox in developing countries. Although most of them have not been tested in adequate clinical trials, the doubt is not so much about their pharmacological effects as about the irrational and unproven claims that are made by the producers and the uncritical lay public.

Since the use of non–orthodox medicine is becoming increasingly popular, the adverse effects of these agents will also become important in the differential diagnosis made by the hepatologist.

Besides non–drug remedies such as acupuncture, which may be responsible for the transmission of viral hepatitis (1), some non–orthodox medicines are injurious to the liver. Most of these are pyrrolizidine alkaloids which have a direct hepatotoxic effect. Only occasionally has an immunological reaction to non–orthodox agents been suggested, e.g. by a positive lymphocyte stimulation test in cases of Shohakuhi–associated jaundice (13) and Kinshigan–associated liver enzyme elevation (16). Although the relatively few reports, e.g. about comfrey (2–4) or herbal tea (5), which reach the large medical journals of the developed countries suggest an infrequent problem, there are in fact more than 350 plant species containing pyrrolizidine alkaloids. Plants containing these alkaloids have a worldwide distribution and their widespread use in the de-

299

veloping countries has even led some authors to believe that the high incidence of chronic liver disease in some areas may be related to their regular intake (6). This is however speculative and difficult to prove or disprove since most people in these areas are exposed to several sources of hepatic injury. Nevertheless, such suggestions deserve serious consideration.

Besides the agents discussed below, others have been associated with signs of hepatic injury, e.g. gossypol, a male contraceptive developed in China which has caused ALAT elevation in a number of patients (7). Pennyroyal or squawmint, which is the source of pulegium oil, has been associated with a case of fatal hepatic and renal failure in a woman who ingested 30 ml (8). Its hepatotoxicity is known from animal toxicity tests (14). Vulto et al (9) pointed to the high concentration of arsenic, lead and other heavy metals in several non–orthodox medicines (9). Indeed, cases of idiopathic portal hypertension have been reported after ingestion of bhasams, an Ayurvedic agent, in which there was a high liver concentration of arsenic (10). It is well known that chronic ingestion of arsenic (e.g. Fowler's solution) (12) may cause hepatoportal sclerosis with non–cirrhotic portal hypertension and also cirrhosis and it is obvious that the modern hepatologist should be aware of these exotic causes. It should be re–emphasized that we are discussing 'medicines'. Many other environmental toxins ingested for non–medical reasons or accidentally (e.g. cycads, safrols, *Amanita phalloides* and other mushrooms etc.) are not discussed here.

Finally, it should be realized that many non–orthodox drugs are not pure pharmacological agents but merely mixtures often containing small amounts of well–known drugs. For example, Chuifong Toukuwan, propagated as a herbal antirheumatic, was found to consist of phenylbutazone, phenacetin, aminopyrine, dexamethasone, indometacin, diazepam and hydrochlorothiazide (11). Although no data have yet been published, one should reckon with the possibility of liver damage in patients who have previously experienced an immunoallergic type of hepatitis to one of these agents.

(1) Kobler et al (1979) *Schweiz. Med. Wochenschr., 109,* 1828. (2) Mattocks (1980) *Lancet, 2,* 1136. (3) Roitman (1981) *Lancet, 1,* 944. (4) Anderson (1981) *Lancet, 1,* 1424. (5) Kumana et al (1983) *Lancet, 2,* 1360. (6) Arseculeratne et al (1981) *J. Ethnopharmacol., 4,* 177. (7) Qian et al (1980) In: Turner (Ed), *Clinical Pharmacology and Therapeutics,* p 489. Macmillan, London. (8) Gunby (1979) *J. Am. Med. Assoc., 241,* 2246. (9) Vulto et al (1982) In: Dukes (Ed), *Side Effects of Drugs, Annual 6,* p 416. Excerpta Medica, Amsterdam. (10) Datta et al (1979) *Gut, 20,* 378. (11) Dukes (1980) In: Dukes (Ed), *Side Effects of Drugs, Annual 4,* 341. Excerpta Medica, Amsterdam. (12) Franklin et al (1950) *Am. J. Med. Sci., 219,* 589. (13) Tozuka et al (1983) *Acta Hepatol. Jpn., 24,* 1035. (14) Gordon et al (1982) *Toxicol. Appl. Pharmacol., 65,* 413. (15) Anonymous (1984) *Dtsch. Apoth.–Ztg, 124,* 1178. (16) Sato et al (1984) *Acta Hepatol. Jpn., 25,* 574.

A. MISCELLANEOUS AGENTS

Alrestatin

CH$_2$COONa

Causal relationship o

Alrestatin is an aldose reductase inhibitor. It is used experimentally in the treatment of cataract and polyneuropathy in diabetes mellitus. It lowers intracellular levels of sorbitol and galactitol. In a study of 9 patients 1 developed a photosensitivity reaction and biochemical evidence of hepatic injury which resolved within 6 months after discontinuation (1).

(1) Handelsman et al (1981) *Diabetes, 30,* 459.

Calcium carbimide (cyanamide)

Ca=N-C≡N

Causal relationship o/ +

Besides a report of acute cholestatic jaundice in 2 patients (5), most reports of calcium–carbimide–associated hepatic injury concern chronic reactions. In 1979, Vazquez et al (1) reported cytoplasmic inclusions in patients treated with calcium carbimide and disulfiram for alcohol–aversion therapy (1). At first, these observations were mainly ascribed to disulfiram (1) but later to calcium carbimide (2). Subsequent studies (3, 4), reports (6) and animal toxicity tests (5) have confirmed these findings.

The inclusion bodies stain positive with PAS and methenamine silver (1). These consist of round or kidney–shaped, well–demarcated areas which have a similar ground–glass appearance to that of hepatocytes seen in other conditions (3). These bodies resemble those seen in Lafora's disease (3). On electron microscopy the bodies are not membrane–bound; they contain much glycogen located in beta–granules, secondary lysosomes, lipid vesicles and residues of degenerating organelles (3). In addition, Koyama et al (6) reported hyperplastic endoplasmic reticulum with irregular figures and cisterna dilatation.

In a study of 42 liver biopsies from 39 alcoholics on calcium carbimide, these cytoplasmic inclusions were noted in all biopsies (4). Unfortunately, this study did not include a control group of biopsies from alcoholics not on calcium carbimide treatment. Fibrosis was observed in all cases, with a degree of severity varying from active periportal fibrosis with cholangiolar proliferation and inflammation (Stage I), via portal–to–portal bridging (Stage II), to a pattern of nodular regeneration (Stage III). The incidence of these stages was clearly related to the duration of therapy with an average of 6 months for Stage I, 19 months for Stage II and 52 months for Stage III. According to the authors, alcoholic liver disease was absent (4). This seems likely since alcoholic fibrosis starts mainly around the central vein. Moreover, steatosis and Mallory's hyaline were mostly absent, whereas γ–GT levels were normal. Vazquez et al (2) suggested that breakdown of the smooth endoplasmic reticulum and mitochondria could account for the inclusion bodies. See also 'Disulfiram'.

(1) Vazquez et al (1979) *Histopathology, 3,* 377. (2) Vazquez et al (1980) *Lancet, 1,* 361. (3) Vazquez et al (1983) *Liver, 3,* 225. (4) Moreno et al (1984) *Liver, 4,* 15. (5) Iglesias et al (1983) *Gastroenterol. Hepatol., 6,* 417. (6) Koyama et al (1984) *Acta Hepatol. Jpn., 25,* 252.

Disulfiram

Causal relationship +

Several cases of liver injury (1–7) have been described, mostly of a clear hepatocellular pattern. In cases where rechallenge proved a causal relationship (1–5, 7) the onset of the first episode occurred within 8 weeks. Rechallenge was positive mostly in 4 days (2–5). Eosinophilia (3, 4), transient urticaria (1) and fever (3) were relatively infrequent. Biopsy showed hepatocellular degeneration (1), focal (3, 4) or extensive (2, 3, 6) necrosis with bridging (2), and a periportal distribution of inclusion bodies with a ground–glass appearance (PAS–positive, orceine–negative) was seen in 19 patients with disulfiram or calcium carbimide therapy (8). Vazquez et al (10) previously ascribed this pattern also to disulfiram but later to calcium carbimide (see above). One may speculate that the inclusion bodies are related to the consequences of alcohol–aversion therapy rather than to a particular agent *per se*. Ethanol intake does not seem to be a prerequisite since the lesions could be reproduced in rats – with and without ethanol intake – receiving high doses (8–16 mg/kg) of calcium carbimide (12).

Although the difficulty of proving drug–induced hepatic injury in alcoholics is obvious, disulfiram has been demonstrated as a cause on the basis of rechallenge, its pattern and its occurrence during abstention. Moreover, in a study of 24 patients, not with alcohol abuse but with nickel dermatitis, hepatic dysfunction developed in 2 (8%), 1 of whom had biopsy–proven hepatitis (11).

According to Moussavian et al (9), disulfiram may aggravate steatosis, especially in zinc–deficient alcoholics (9).

(1) Keeffe et al (1974) *J. Am. Med. Assoc., 230,* 435. (2) Eisen et al (1975) *Ann. Intern. Med., 83,* 673. (3) Ranek et al (1977) *Br. Med. J., 2,* 94. (4) Morris et al (1978) *Gastroenterology, 75,* 100. (5) Kristensen (1981) *Acta Med. Scand., 209,* 335. (6) Schade et al (1983) *Arch. Intern. Med., 143,* 1271. (7) Knutsen (1949) *Tidsskr. Nor. Laegeforen, 69,* 436. (8) Bruguera et al (1982) *Hepatology, 2,* 682. (9) Moussavian et al (1982) *Hepatology, 2,* 727. (10) Vazquez et al (1979) *Histopathology, 3,* 377. (11) Kaaber et al (1983) *Contact Dermatitis, 9,* 297. (12) Guillen et al (1984) *Lab. Invest., 50,* 385.

Isaxonine phosphate

Structure: pyrimidine ring —NH—CH(CH₃)—CH₃·H₃PO₄

Causal relationship + +

Isaxonine has been used in France since 1981 for the treatment of several forms of peripheral neuropathy, mostly in a daily dose of 1–1.5 g. It has been claimed to stimulate regeneration of peripheral nerves. Several cases of a hepatocellular pattern of injury, sometimes mild (9) but often severe, have been ascribed to isaxonine since its introduction (1–8). In most cases, jaundice appeared within 2 months after starting treatment (1–8) but occasionally after several months (6, 7). The reaction was fatal in approximately 30% of these reported cases (2, 4, 6), but of course a definite case–fatality rate cannot be based on the literature alone. Fever (2–6), mostly up to 39°C or more, and eosinophilia (2, 3, 5, 6) were frequently reported. Rash was mentioned in 1 case (6). A rechallenge, performed in some cases, was positive (2, 4, 6) often promptly after readministration. Lymphocyte stimulation tests and basophil degranulation tests were negative (3).

Histology invariably showed hepatic necrosis, often extensive, but with a predominance in the centrilobular area. Only 1 report mentioned diffuse necrosis (8). Infiltration was mostly mononuclear. Sharp zonal margins were not mentioned. Cholestasis may be present (8). Steatosis as seen in 1 report (5) may have been partly caused by concurrent treatment with corticosteroids (5). Granulomas were noted in 1 case (5).

Activation of isaxonine by cytochrome P450 yields a reactive metabolite which binds covalently to liver microsomal protein (10). This reaction was enhanced by both phenobarbital and 3–methylcholanthrene pretreatment (10). Addition of glutathione decreased the amount of protein–bound metabolite (11). The metabolite, however, had only limited hepatotoxic potential in mice (11). In man, either another metabolite is a cause of liver injury or the above–mentioned metabolite–protein complex acts as an antigenic stimulus, generating an immunoallergic reaction in vulnerable individuals. According to the clinical and histological pattern, including the prompt reaction to rechallenge and signs of hypersensitivity, an immunoallergic mechanism seems likely. Fabre et al (3) suggested that isaxonine might possibly have an effect on the excretory function of the hepatocytes because their patient had a pure cholestatic reaction which preceded the necrotic period (3), but their experience has not yet been confirmed.

(1) Papazian et al (1983) *Presse Méd., 12,* 770. (2) Ben Mami et al (1983) *Gastroentérol. Clin. Biol., 7,* 193. (3) Fabre et al (1982) *Thérapie, 37,* 671. (4) Alcabes et al (1983) *Presse Méd., 12,* 2696. (5) Zarski et al (1983) *Gastroentérol. Clin. Biol., 7,* 430. (6) Baud et al (1983) *Gastroentérol. Clin. Biol., 7,* 352. (7) Mallet et al (1983) *Gastroentérol. Clin. Biol., 7,* 429. (8) Hirtz et al (1983) *Rev. Méd. Limousin, 14,* 109. (9) De Lumley et al (1983) *Rev. Méd. Limousin, 14,* 11. (10) Lettéron et al (1984) *J. Pharmacol. Exp. Ther., 229,* 845. (11) Fouin–Fortunet et al (1984) *J. Pharmacol. Exp. Ther., 229,* 851.

Ritodrine

HO—⟨ ⟩—CH(OH)-CH-CH₃
        |
        NH-CH₂-CH₂-⟨ ⟩—OH

Causal relationship o

Ritodrine, as a sympathicomimetic agent, is not a likely candidate for causing hepatic injury. Nevertheless, a case of hepatic injury has been ascribed to the use of this drug in a primigravid woman treated with 160 mg p.o. over a 36–hour period for pre–term labor. Despite this she delivered her baby. Two days later she developed scleral jaundice, hemolytic anemia, hypokalemia, leukocytosis and elevated liver enzyme levels. Spontaneous recovery followed after 1 week. Other possible causes were not found by the author (1).

(1) Alcena (1982) *Am. J. Obstet. Gynecol., 144,* 852.

Theophylline

Causal relationship o

Theophylline is not a known hepatotoxin and even in overdosage liver damage is absent or trivial compared to effects on the central nervous system. In a recent report of 9 children on therapeutic and well–tolerated doses of theophylline, all developed signs of toxicity when becoming ill during an influenza epidemic. Blood levels were in the toxic range and there were ASAT elevations in 7 of them. The author concluded that the ASAT level may serve as a predictive tool in the detection of theophylline toxicity (1), but this conclusion seems premature. The role of the underlying viral illness is far from clear in these cases. Moreover, it is unclear whether hepatic injury is the consequence or, due to impairment of metabolism, the cause of theophylline toxicity.

(1) Schuller et al (1981) *Immunol. Allergy Pract., 111,* 27.

B. NON–ORTHODOX AGENTS

Mistletoe
Causal relationship o/ +

Parenchymatous hepatitis was observed after several weeks ingestion of a herbal medicine containing mistletoe. Biopsy showed a pattern resembling chronic active hepatitis with 'piece–meal' necrosis, dense infiltration with lymphocytes/plasma cells, and distortion of liver architecture (1). Readministration resulted in recurrence after about 10 days.

(1) Harvey et al (1981) *Br. Med. J., 282,* 186.

304

Pyrrolizidine alkaloids

RCOO   (9)
      CH₂OCOR

Causal relationship + +

Pyrrolizidine alkaloids (PA) are discussed in this book since they are found in many herbal remedies used in non–orthodox medicine. PA are very common constituents of plants in every part of the world, especially those belonging to the Crotalaria, Heliotropum and Senecio genera (1).

Their ability to induce hepatic injury in man is unequivocal and has been reported after drinking a tea for 'childhood disease' (2) or for psoriasis (3) as well as after ingestion of contaminated cereals (4, 5). The hepatic injury is reproducible in animals and has led to the loss of grazing cattle (6). In an extensive compilation Smith and Culvenor (7) listed over 350 plant species containing PA. This was up to 1980 and one may expect many more to be added to this list since several thousands of plant species are known in the botanical families in which PA have been detected (8). Many of these plants, with exotic names like *t'u–san–ch'i*, are used in herbal products which are becoming increasingly popular in Western countries. This may present the hepatologist with a problem since their composition is often unknown and their PA content will therefore have to be analyzed. In a study of 50 medicinal plants purchased from herbal drug stores, 3 proved to contain PA (9). Feeding trials in rats demonstrated disruption of centrilobular veins with surrounding hemorrhage and congestion. The authors suggested that the high consumption of PA–containing products could contribute to the high incidence of chronic liver disease in Asian and African countries.

Not all PA are equally hepatotoxic. There is a structural basis for this. According to McLean et al (6), there are 3 important criteria: (a) the presence of a C_1–C_2 double bond (see structural formula), (b) esterification of at least one hydroxyl group (C_7/C_9) and (c) a branched carbon chain in the acid moiety of the ester may be associated with enhanced toxicity. Their relative toxicity is: cyclic esters (2 bonded esters) > diesters > monoesters > no esters.

PA may cause veno–occlusive disease. Patients suffer from vomiting and severe abdominal pain. There is abdominal distension, hepatomegaly and often rapidly developing ascites. Venous collaterals directly visible on the abdomen are often very prominent. Jaundice and fever are infrequent (2, 4–6, 10). Stuart and Bras (10) followed up a group of 64 patients with acute veno–occlusive disease due to bush–tea intoxication: 27% died in the acute phase of liver failure, usually within 4 weeks; approximately 50% recovered completely; of the remaining group, approximately one–third progressed to cirrhosis (10). This progression may be facilitated if intake is continued. In a follow–up of the outbreak of veno–occlusive disease in India in 1975–1977, Tandon et al (5, 13) reported a 5–year survival of only 51%.

Histology shows hemorrhagic necrosis in the centrilobular zone with congestion and sinusoidal distension and dilatation. The central veins are disrupted and occluded. In the chronic form, collateral vessels develop in the surrounding parenchyma; fibrosis starts from the central area instead of the portal zone and may end in a characteristic pattern of cirrhosis ('reversed lobulation') (2–6, 10). In animals, besides the above–mentioned changes, megalocytosis may be seen secondary to an abnormality of cell division (6). This has not been demonstrated in man. A carcinogenic action of PA has been demonstrated in rats (8), which may develop liver tumors.

The injury is probably secondary to dehydrogenation of the pyrrolizidine nucleus to highly reactive pyrrolic derivatives, rather than N–oxidation or epoxidation (6). There is a species difference in susceptibility to pyrrolizidine toxicity which correlates with the production rate of pyrrolic metabolites, as measured in liver samples (11). These metabolites are preferentially formed in the centrilobular area and – at least of some PA in some animals – their toxicity is enhanced by the enzyme inducer, phenobarbital (11). This centrilobular localization is confirmed by the fact that pyrroles administered via the mesenteric vein cause portal rather than centrilobular necrosis (6), unlike the parent compound. The precise mechanism of action is unknown, but there is little doubt about the strong alkylating capacity of the pyrrolic metabolites. The appearance of hemorrhagic necrosis within 12 hours (6) after an overdose (with the parent compound) suggests a direct toxic effect of metabolites on cell organelles or disruption of the membrane. Downstream damage to the central veins confirms the overwhelming of protective mechanisms by excessive amounts of toxic metabolites. It has been demonstrated that several reactive pyrrolic derivatives may cross–link DNA strands in vitro (12). Their antimitotic and carcinogenic actions, however, according to McLean et al (6), are more likely to result from specific interactions with vital cell components (6).

(1) Robins (1982) *Prog. Chem. Org. Nat. Prod.*, *41*, 115. (2) Bras et al (1954) *Arch. Pathol.*, *57*, 285. (3) Kumana et al (1983) *Lancet*, *2*, 1360. (4) Mohabbat et al (1976) *Lancet*, *2*, 269. (5) Tandon et al (1976) *Lancet*, *2*, 271. (6) McLean et al (1980) In: Farber et al (Ed), *Toxic Injury of the Liver, Part A*, p 517. Marcel Dekker, New York. (7) Smith et al (1981) *J. Nat. Prod.*, *44*, 129. (8) Schoental (1982) *Toxicol. Lett.*, *10*, 323. (9) Arseculeratne et al (1981) *J. Ethnopharmacol.*, *4*, 159. (10) Stuart et al (1957) *Q. J. Med.*, *26*, 291. (11) White et al (1973) *Chem. Biol. Interact.*, *6*, 207. (12) White et al (1972) *Biochem. J.*, *128*, 291. (13) Tandon et al (1984) *Lancet*, *1*, 730.

Seatone

Causal relationship o

Jaundice appeared 3 weeks after starting treatment with this product, derived from the green–lipped mussel, which is used for arthritis in Australia (1). Biopsy showed epithelioid granulomas with giant cells and focal necrosis. Granulomas were found in both the lobuli and portal tracts; portal fibrosis was observed. Indometacin had been discontinued 3 weeks previously.

(1) Ahern et al (1980) *Med. J. Aust., 2,* 151.

INDEX

Age/Sex:
Suspected drug (trade name):
Route:
Daily dose:
Underlying illness/Reason for drug use:

Latent period (if possible, give dates)
First intake – First sign/symptom
Discontinuation drug – Normalization
Readministration drug – Relapse

Signs/Symptoms (including extrahepatic ones: if possible, date of appearance of each sign/symptom in brackets)

Clinical investigation (imaging procedures etc.)

Biopsy

Laboratory values (please include normal values in brackets)

Dates								
Values								
ASAT/ALAT (normal:)								
APh (normal:)								
Bilirubin total/conjugated								
γ-GT/5-NT								
Albumin/ gamma-globulin								

Other values (e.g. leukocytes/eosinophils)

Other possible causes excluded or unlikely

Viral causes (hepatitis A,B, infectious mononucleosis, cytomegalovirus or others)

Hypotension, cardiac failure, malignancies, operation, underlying liver disease, transfusions, alcohol abuse

Bacterial/other microbial causes (sepsis, parasites etc.)

Other drugs used (include dates of administration)

Comment or other relevant remarks

Send this report to: The Authors of *Drug-Induced Hepatic Injury, c/o B.H.Ch. Stricker, Medical Officer,*
PO Box 439, 2260 AK Leidschendam, The Netherlands

(Please fill in your name and address for reply)

NAME: ....

ADDRESS: ....

COUNTRY: .... DATE: ....

REPORT of SUSPECTED DRUG-INDUCED HEPATIC INJURY
(please report only associations not included in the book; even suspicions may be important)
N.B. *May be typewritten in English, French, German or Dutch*

Age/Sex:
Suspected drug (trade name):
Route:
Daily dose:
Underlying illness/Reason for drug use:

Signs/Symptoms (including extrahepatic ones: if possible, date of appearance of each sign/symptom in brackets)

Clinical investigation (imaging procedures etc.)

Biopsy

Latent period (if possible, give dates)

First intake – First sign/symptom
Discontinuation drug – Normalization
Readministration drug – Relapse

Laboratory values (please include normal values in brackets)

Dates								
Values								
ASAT/ALAT (normal:)								
APh (normal:)								
Bilirubin total/conjugated								
γ-GT/5-NT								
Albumin/ gamma-globulin								

Other values (e.g. leukocytes/eosinophils)

Other possible causes excluded or unlikely

Viral causes (hepatitis A,B, infectious mononucleosis, cytomegalovirus or others)

Hypotension, cardiac failure, malignancies, operation, underlying liver disease, transfusions, alcohol abuse

Bacterial/other microbial causes (sepsis, parasites etc.)

Other drugs used (include dates of administration)

Comment or other relevant remarks

Send this report to: The Authors of *Drug-Induced Hepatic Injury*, c/o *B.H.Ch. Stricker, Medical Officer*,
PO Box 439, 2260 AK Leidschendam, The Netherlands

(Please fill in your name and address for reply)

NAME: ....

ADDRESS: ....

COUNTRY: .... DATE: ....

REPORT of SUSPECTED DRUG-INDUCED HEPATIC INJURY
(please report only associations not included in the book; even suspicions may be important)
N.B. *May be typewritten in English, French, German or Dutch*